DRINK URINE AND LIVE HEALTHY

D1882441

DRINK URINE AND LIVE HEALTHY

Dr C.S. Rayudu (Yogasree)

GenNext Publication

© **Author**

All rights reserved. No part of this book may be reproduced, stored, adapted, or transmitted in any form or by any means, electronic, mechanical, photocopying, micro-filming, recording or otherwise, or translated in any language, without the prior written permission of the copyright owner and the publisher. The book is sold subject to the condition that it shall not, by way of trade or otherwise, be lent, resold, hired out, or otherwise circulated without the prior publisher's written consent in any form of binding or cover other than that in which it is published.

The views and opinions expressed in this book are author's own and the facts reported by him have been verified to the extent possible, and the publishers are not in any way liable for the same.

ISBN : 978-93-8022-273-8

Price : ₹ 350

First Published, 2016

Published by

GenNext Publication
5, Ansari Road,
Darya Ganj, New Delhi-110002.
Ph. : 9811692060
E-mail: gennext@hotmail.com

Printed at : G. Print Process, Delhi

Cataloging in Publication Data—DK

Courtesy: D.K. Agencies (P) Ltd. <docinfo@dkagencies.com>

Rayudu, C. S., 1946- **author.**

Drink urine and live healthy / Yoga Shree Dr C.S. Rayudu.

pages cm

ISBN 9789380222738

1. Urine—Therapeutic use. 2. Urine—Therapeutic use—India. 3. Self medication. I. Title.

DDC 615.36 23

CONTENTS

Pedagogical Features of the book 7

1. Just a Minute 11
2. Frequently Asked Questions (FAQ) 17
3. Know Your Body and Make It Healthy 19
4. Ancient and Historical Overview 25
5. We All Have Drunk Our Urine and Born 35
6. What is Piss 39
7. What is Urinopathy 41
8. Physical Characteristics of Human Urine 45
9. What are All Contained in Human Urine 47
10. Principles and Philosophy of Urinopathy 53
11. Top Ten Reasons to Urinopathy 57
12. Methods of Using Urine 59
13. Medicinal Secrets of Urine and How It Works 63
14. Quality and Taste 71
15. Is Human Urine Poisonous–No 73
16. Is Urine a Waste Product–No 75
17. Safety and Efficacy of Urinopathy 79
18. How Urine is Formed and Produced 83
19. Role of Kidneys–Nephrons and Urine Bladder 85
20. Urine Testing – Urinalysis 89
21. Why Should You Drink Urine 91
22. Choosing Your Own Therapy 93
23. Urinopaths 99
24. Model of Care 101
25. Checklist Towards Auto-Urine 103
26. People are Shy 105
27. How Can You Overcome the Barriers to Drinking Your Own Urine 107
28. Science Validates Urinotherapy 109

29. Rise and Fall of Urinopathy Movement 117
30. A Note About Doubts on Urinopathy 121
31. Benefits Conferred by Shivambu 125
32. Urine is a Life Force 127
33. Urine–the Unknown Medicine 129
34. Urine Urea–A Natural Drug 135
35. A Traditional and a Nature Cure 137
36. Drink Mid-stream Urine 139
37. Drink Morning Urine 141
38. Preserved Urine 143
39. Urine the Mysterious Liquid 145
40. Mystic Power 147
41. Animals' Urine 149
42. What Conditions can Urinopathic Medicine Treat 151
43. When Can You Expect Result 157
44. Success Stories 159
45. Urine–A Doctor of Divinity 161
46. Urine-Your Personal Doctor 163
47. Curable Diseases 171
48. Cancer 185
49. AIDS/HIV Positive 201
50. Self-Therapy 215
51. Leading Personalities 219
52. The Urine and Immunity Connection 225
53. Describing About Urinopathic Medicine 229
54. Is Urine Therapy Really Essential Today 233
55. What The Future Holds For Urinopathy 237
56. Why The Therapy Not Popular 241
57. Exceptions 245
58. Urine–The Medicine For Physical Immortality 247
59. Body Mind Spirit Medicine 251
60. Mental Illness and Physical Disorders 263
61. Pranic Healing 281
62. Dangers of Drugs 299
63. Epilogue 321
Index 325

Pedagogical Features of the book

As the world spins into the first decade of twenty first century, dramatic changes are occurring in the human health arena. The pace of deteriorating human body is so rapid that the ability to change has now became a necessity.

In this book, I examine the major trends in health care industry and forces that are changing the health service landscape and challenges in this new millennium.

Welcome to the exciting world of health of mankind. In this book to start you off, I will introduce you to the basic concepts of priceless, and drugless self-natural therapy.

Thank you for giving up your time to read what I have to say about urinopathy. You are our beneficiary, the target of our service efforts, it is you I aim to delight.

I believe that exciting new changes are coming in the healthcare industry and that I can help teach, present and future human race to maintain and promote well-being better.

You are about to begin an exciting useful and necessary understanding, the exploration of health. Health is an exciting because it combines the science, art of chosing therapy with many other disciplines.

To set the stage, let us first look at historical overview in the book of our traditional household medicinal practice depicted in the text.

Welcome to the Self-therapy

Urinopathy, a healthcare system provides an authoritative, comprehensive, practical introduction to health enhancement, longevity and deageing. It is designed to help the readers learn about and apply the basic concept and practice to prevent the deteriorating health condition as it is used in a wide variety of complaints.

Powerful Theme in Health Philosophy

Fast changing life styles, dietary styles, occupational styles, technological advancement, migration, immigration, urbanisation, industrialisation, cultural and environmental shifts are causing profound changes in health. As the health conditions change, so must the physicians who serve it. These new developments signify a brand new world of health opportunity and health service providers for forward thinking.

In the light of these developments, urinopathy a hidden ancient remedy builds on powerful new health theme that go to the heart of modern medical theory and practice.

The principles and philosophy of urinopathic medicine unearths the medicinal secrets and tells the stories that reveal the drama of modern healthcare field. I think it is important to show how alternate health strategies are the best practices and upcoming natural drug change and continuously evolve.

Audience of the Book

This modest handbook of self-therapy is designed for use in Naturopathy, Ayurveda, Oriental Medicine, Drugless Therapy, Alternative, Complementary, Traditional, Nature Cure Therapy courses. It will also be useful for allopathic physicians practising Urinopathy who want to update their knowledge, about the alternate therapy in their practice, diversify, adopt multi-therapy and who wish to improve their ability in treating their clients.

To cater to the needs of both general readers, practitioners, physicians, drinkers, propagators, crusaders, sympathisers, activists in the advancement of urinotherapy movement, the subject matter has been discussed in conceptual-cum-analytical and practical manner. It is the aim of the book to help any drinker, new entrants and readers develop skills to understand and self-practice to live with good health and normal living.

Focus of the Book

To create a book that differentiate itself from other books in terms of coverage, presentation, utility, and with an equal focus on theory and practice with real life examples, I write this book with the following objectives:

1. To explain the nature of Urinopathy and its interaction with other pathies and therapies.
2. To review the changing role of the physicians and their position in the healthcare hierarchy.
3. To focus on the health enhancement, maintenance, promotion, self-responsibility and principles as an operationally desirable health strategy.
4. To demonstrate to the readers that the practice of therapy is simple to understand relevant in practice and interesting to learn.
5. To help physicians appreciate the logic for making better health service to the public.
6. To develop concepts and theories of self-therapy in a lucid way so the readers could grasp them very easily and able to put into practice.
7. To provide a book that has a comprehensive coverage for urine therapy subject.

Learning Aids

I have taken great care to offer the readers new features on this new subject to every topic of theory and practice package. The following is the list of specific features of the book.

1. Looking Ahead : Previewing the concepts. The beginning of each chapter briefly previews topic concepts, links them to concepts in previous chapters, describes chapter learning objectives and introduces the chapter opening health related story.

2. Looking Back : Reviewing the concepts. A summary at the end of each chapter reviews modern medical concepts with urinopathic application.

3. Opening Stories : Each chapter starts with a dramatic health story that introduces the topic material and sparks the reader interest.

4. Real Health Highlights : Go behind the scenes for an indepth scientific look at real healthcare practices at individual and household level.

5. Discussion and Application : Each chapter contains a body of discussion relevant and urine application exercises, relating to modern medical science equivalent, covering major chapter concepts.

6. Health Connection : Each chapter in detail covers the philosophy of urinopathic medicine and ends with an interactive allopathic exercise that relates to cover concepts of each topic specific.

7. Key Terms : Key terms of Amaroli equivalent in medical terminology are highlighted within the text, clearly defined under each topic or theme in which they appear to avoid duplication and overlapping.

8. Case Studies : Patient cases, recovery stories, success studies for specific diseases as available are provided wherever necessary such as cancer, AIDS, etc. These case histories create confidence and motivate the entrants of urine-therapy movement in real terms.

9. Medical Efficacy : The medicinal properties of urine according to scientific proof and curative efficacy qualities of urinopathic medicine are systematically explained in every topic. This new feature is designed to help the readers to get confidence in the therapy.

10. Literature Background : The major problems for non-popularity of urine therapy is scanty literature, availability, lack of awareness and information and other factors. List of books, written by experts on the subject, research findings, reports, opinions, so far available appear in a separate chapter which provide strong support to the therapy. It is an extensive bibliography provides quick reference to the new subject to the readers, researchers, policy makers, practitioners, propagators, crusaders, leaders leading the movement as well as sympathisers.

11. Examples : They are an important components of the books' learning system, clearly set off from the text. Examples provide an immediate and concrete demonstration of how to use urine, methods and how it works.

12. Review Option : The book gives scope to review, which appears at the end of each core topic as a part of presentation, challenge readers to stop reading and test their understanding by practice before they move on to the next topic.

13. Value Feature : Each section ends with a focus on value feature, which means explaining how the topic's content relates to the individual's goal of health enhancement. This feature helps reinforce understanding of the link between readers's action and use value.

No self-therapy book can consistently meet users needs without continual feedback from drinkers, physicians etc. I write users to relate their experiences using to this and its package to me. Your constructive criticism will help me to improve the quality of the book.

No book is the work only of its author. I owe the pioneers of urinetherapy, scientists, researchers, yogis, who identified the major issues of medicinal properties of urine and developed it, its concepts, practice, procedure by actually using.

Dr C.S. Rayudu

Address :
D. No. 28-3-393
Sarada Nagar
Anantapur (PO) 515001
Andhra Pradesh (India)
Phone : Land : 08554-272182
Cell : 9848618095
E-mail ID : rayudu.choudem@gmail.com

1
Just a Minute

This small book in your hands is about medicinal secrets of urine, how it is wasted and how it is useful for good health and normal living of human beings. Truly speaking, most of us have probably never thought of urine as a valuable drug.

You have never thought that there was anything medicinal drug in a glass of urine? Right here is an interesting topic for you.

So, now you know there is some medical secrets to than that meets the eye.

Urine is a good alternative in a place where water is scarce or shortage.

Urine therapy is proved to prevent and cure a variety of common, acute, chronic, degenerative, as well as opportunistic infections associated with HIV/AIDS, VDS, etc. Accordingly, urine drug cures a wide range of human ailments ranging from Arthritis, Cancer, AIDS, Hepatitis, Multiple-scleroses, Eczema, Psoriasis, Diabetes, Herpes, Adrenal failure, Colitis, Lupus, Pancreatic insufficiency, Fills Immunity Deficiency, Inflammatory Troubles, Respiratory Congestion, B locked Nasal Passages, Nose, Eye, Ear disorders, Asthama, Ache, Throatache, Ache, Sores, Sinus, Bronchitis, Candid, Pelvic inflammatory ills, etc. The list of curable diseases with urine is exhaustive.

This book is written as a brief introduction to urinopathic medicine for people to be more informed about the health treasure, long hidden, and now unearthed and what it offers and how best to use to serve mankind.

Continuing with our life-long involvement in healing process, today we are going to shift focus on inward healing system. This book on self-healing is about how to use and understand what it is really trying to tell you.

It is not the subject just to read and put in mind, it actually alters the biological and physiological response.

Our predecessors have enjoyed its benefits, without even knowing it. How is that? What is that? You ask. Many misunderstood about it. How to manage your health yourself?

Urinotherapy is an old Indian form of medicine. It deals with drinking one's own urine for therapeutic purposes. According to ancient Indian medical therapy, it is the earliest form of household practice.

Drinking urine is an inexpensive way to gain vitality, health. A drugless drug, priceless, natural, self-therapy. It is unfortunate in India that the most medicinally valued drug has remained hidden long as such the entire ailing human race has been deprived of this divine panacea.

Truly speaking, it is a boon, God's gift to our poor country while millions of people lack an effective medicine. Today common man is at the crossroads, under healing crisis with innumerable, incurable diseases, many poor families are ruined because they cannot afford the modern costly medicines.

In my search for natural therapy which is difficult to find, I am impressed very much by urotherapy which is very appealing. In my yogic life experience, I have found that this is the appropriate therapy. In the days to come of new diseases, non-availability and non-working of modern medicine, the only therapy that can rescue the coming generation is this therapy only.

In recent years due to failure of modern medicine in treating emerging innumerable and incurable diseases, a bit of an oddball, urine is gaining popularity, which has now wide recognition from different cross sections of the society in combating the menaces of human race and maintaning good health.

To your surprise, in advanced countries, some multinational pharmaceutical companies are manufacturing several types of drugs and injections from urine. To illustrate, Urokinase, an injection, is meant to treat cardiovascular diseases by dissolving blood clots, preventing heart attacks. Antineoplaston, a substance of urine, is wonderfully working for treatment of cancer. Another substance found in urine is named as Dehydroepi and Roster-one, it is relating to testosterone. Profasi meant for infertility patients, likewise pergonal. There are many such anti-AID/HIV, anti-obesity, anti-bodies, anti-ageing property drugs made from urine.

The biochemical analysis of urine revealed that there are many compounds well proved by scientific research that have tremendous therapeutic value. If that urine is taken into the body it has the efficacy to boost the immunity system prevent and protect the body from diseases, stimulate treatment in a very special and unusual way, and keep the drinker in a unique position.

In the vast globe, millions of people who are under healing crisis, poor at crossroads cannot afford modern costly medicine. Laymen, poor, illiterates are interested just in quick recovery without any cost and they would not mind using harmless urine therapy.

We should follow the footsteps of our predecessors. We are grateful to all our *yogis*, the unknown *yogis* who discovered the hidden secrets of therapeutic value of urine and made us aware of it. It is a right opportunity to acknowledge them who have preserved this health science strove through the centuries and those a few who are practicing even today standing tall amidst crisis.

In this book, I have made a humble effort to explain the secrets of body's science and its medicine, in a simple way, with a hope that it will greatly benefit the people at large since our body has a fabulous unknown capability to heal itself.

This is the only 'Future Medicine' in time to come which may be used as an alternative to costly medicine. What cannot be cured by the own urine of the body cannot be cured by any other medicine.

As long as mankind survives, this therapy will exist, co-exist, co-terminus. It is really a book to the mankind of this *yuga*. Human body is a supreme creature of this nature having capability of detoxifying agent and creating anti-bodies to fight against its own antigens.

If these natural substances of urine are used properly, good health, longevity can be enjoyed. However, those who are already suffering from incurable, degenerative and opportunistic diseases may use urine drug. Similarly, wasting of excess of these urine substances leads to a national loss.

Nature designed to excrete urine from the body. But any attempt to reinject it into the body would lead to disease-free body.

The modern medicine has many drawbacks, such as dangerous side effects, after-effects and ill-effects, as a result in the long run it destroys the natural immunity system thereby leading to breed degenerative new diseases like cancer, AIDS, arthritis, sinus, etc.

It is interesting to know that even many allopathic, ayurvedic doctors are treating their clients, and recommending auto-urine therapy. Several such instances are referred to in this book in appropriate contexts.

The drinkers of urine have formed associations locally, regionally, nationally and at international level. The members periodically gather to organise seminars, workshops, conferences to promote awareness as well as to bring out latest developments in this area of therapy. The first world Conference on Urine Therapy in India was organised in February 1996. The Second World Conference on Urine Therapy was organised in Germany in 1998. Today, it has become a common feature to have such meetings locally and regionally, and at national level. People gather, share and exchange views, knowledge and experiences.

Many diseases which could be cured under allopathy, ayurveda, homeopathy or by any other therapy until now have been treated, prevented, alleviated or completely cured by urotherapists. For some incurable diseases there is no other alternative except urine therapy.

Urine has superior quality of harmless treatment and works for preventive maintenance. It has sustainability quality. The use of urine means using natural products and energy in way that it does not harm the body. It continues to work for a long time and cures the root cause of the disease. The cause of the malady is removed from the body rather than simply suppressing the symptoms, as the modern medicine does.

People have a feeling of aversion to drink urine because of smell. How does it taste? What does it taste? Regular urine drinkers know well how does it taste? They never say bad about it. They like it as sweet odour.

Really, it always smells good only. Meet people who have drunk enough urine, and good practitioners, they really know what does it taste like. Because of its colour, smell, temperature, piss and orthodox beliefs and barbarous superstitions, we consider that it is not good, not drinkable. It is not at all bad.

Because it is of salty taste, you feel that urine is dirty to taste.

The growth and evolution of this therapy as a science is an interesting story since time immemorial. Urinopathy is the science which deals with the study of urine and its therapeutic properties. When this study relates to the auto-urine consumption, we call it urinopathy, which is the subject matter of this book.

When we think of auto-urine therapy, we must also think, that to learn it, practise it, we must have an idea how could urine be a therapy? The subject of this self-therapy is very simple, self-explanatory and it is possible for any one to practise. Therefore, no one should nauseate, disgust, hate, feel shy to read and use it. But every one should try to learn and it is the only medicine and cure to face innumerable incurable diseases in the days to come.

My close association with many *yogis* for years, and my personal experience of using my own urine for ailments has enabled me to understand why this therapy has not been popular, and why the general public are not aware of it.

I have spared no pains to minimise technicalities and follow scientific way of writing, but at the same time, I have attempted to make the therapy easily understandable. The topic on historical review, ancient documentary evidences, texts has been made interesting to convince the readers that it is an ancient household medicinal practice.

The nature of urine, and how it is a therapy has been treated in one part, and in the other part the contents of urine, along with the description of methods of taking or using urine also have been explained. How urine works in prevention and curing of ailments, as required by every reader, has also been described in detail along with illustrations. Some of the topics in this book are novel, and useful to the readers. Many other topics also provide all the necessary information in support of the therapy. The efforts put in this volume would convince the people and they would be amply benefited by it.

The title of the book on Urinotherapy, popularly called as " Auto–urine therapy", outlined in this book is an entirely traditional, natural self-system of healing and prevention. This book includes nature, scope, uses, practice of this therapy supported by scientific evidence. It also deals with the diseases successfully treated with urine therapy.

It also provides the fabulous efficacy of urine therapy, as well as historical and ancient roots. This book is a valuable handout for growing number of new entrants in whom it instils confidence and motivates.

"The Yellow Fountain", the most fundamental book to date on urine therapy, user-friendly guide is most helpful to the beginners.

I owe a great deal to Dr T. Narayana Swamy, former Director of B.C. Study Circle, Anantapur, A.P., the reviewer, for having gone through the manuscript and offered useful suggestions for its improvement and presentation. He provided literary assistance immensely at all stages in the production of this book. The book is much better because constant of his constant efforts.

C.S. Rayudu

2

Frequently Asked Questions (FAQ)

- What do you need to know about urine?
- What is the true difference between allopathy and Urine therapy.
- What is the novelty?
- What led to this therapy?
- Why should we avoid it?
- What is its background?
- Does urine make you healthy?
- Are drinkers less succeptible to illness and others not so?
- Why the people do not drink it, what are rights and wrongs with them?
- What is the way to increase its longevity?
- Does the therapy maintain its validity?
- What is the mechanism behind its working?
- What are the measures of success?
- Why do people take risk with their health, when it works like panacea?
- How is the therapy described, defined and explained?
- How do drinkers do and cure themselves?
- Are there any clinical investigation results and empirical findings?
- How does the therapy explain its efficacy and effectiveness?
- What is the future agenda?

3

Know Your Body and Make It Healthy

The human body indicates the physical structure of the human being, male, female and child. The body has many parts with different weight, temperature, size, fat, colour and shape. The study of the body in medical science is called anatomy. It is the science that deals with the study of the form and the structure of human body, known as human anatomy.

The human body is made up of innumerable organs and each part or organ is subject to one or other ailment or disorder.

The body-made urine can help the body in the process of curing and also in maintaining all the organs, glands, tissues and endocrine system, that produces harmones in proper working order, so that the drinker of urine will have good health and long life.

As the detailed study of the human body with innumerable of parts, organs, glands is out of scope in this volume, a mere outline of the body will be discussed in the following paragraphs in order to have an overall idea about our own body.

1. Nucleus

It is the central part of an atom in which neutrons and protons are bound together that contain most of its mass, and carry a positive electric charge.

In biological sense, it is the central part of a cell, containing the genetic material, connected with genes. They are the units in the cells that control the physical characteristics of a living person. It is the executive centre of the cells. The shape, size and number of the nuclei vary from cell to cell.

2. Cell

It is the smallest unit in the body of a living person that can exist on its own. The human body is made up of cells. For instance, red blood cells and white blood cells. Each of the small sections together forms a larger structure. So, it is the smallest structural and functional unit of the human body, a unit of a multi-cellular organism. Cells play an important role both singly and collectively in the life cycle of the human being.

The shape and size of cells may vary. They may be globular, columnar, spindle-shaped, cuboidal or may be of any modified form, surrounding the nucleus as jelly like mass known as cytoplasm. The cytoplasm along with nucleus is called protoplasm and, put together is called structure of a cell.

Reproduction of cells takes place through division of cells into which one other cell divides into two-daughter cells each of which again divides into two and thus multiplication goes on until full growth is attained.

3. Tissues

A tissue is the mass of cells that forms different parts of human body. Many cells of similar structure and functions together form a tissue. It is an assemblage of cells, which are held together by inter cellular substances. It is made up of cells. A human body is an arrangement of group of tissues. A human body is made up by the following elementary tissues, namely:

1. Epithelial tissues
2. Connective tissues
3. Selerous tissues
4. Blood
5. Lymph
6. Muscular tissues, and
7. Nervous tissues.

4. Organs

An Organ is a part of the body that has a particular purpose. A number of tissues unite to form an organ; such as heart, brain, sense-organs like eyes, ears, nose, sexual organs etc.,

5. System

A group of organs put together form the human system. An organised set of organs, which are connected and interlinked work together to have a body. A human system is like a computer-system, solar system, expert system, eco-system and public address system. A system may have a number of sub-systems to form an integrated structure. For instance, the human system has a number of sub-systems which together form a full system. Such sub-systems are digestive system, skeletal system, muscular system, respiratory system, etc.

Sub-systems

6. Muscular System

The muscular system of the human body is connected with the muscle called musculature which is a system of muscles in the entire body or part of the body. A muscle is a piece of body-tissue that you tighten and relax in order to move a particular part of the body. The system forms the muscles of the body. The muscle or the flesh is an internal part of the body-mechanics which is mainly concerned with causing movements. It causes locomotion which puts greatest demand on muscles, besides production of body-heat. It consists of several muscle fibers, grouped into bundles.

The muscle fibres are classified variously as striated and non-striated, cardiac, voluntary, involuntary, somatic, and visceral. When muscles are damaged or disorganised, disordered, the muscle fibers lose their regenerative power. The urine prevents damages and cures common diseases. It also repairs, regenerates and rebuilds the tissues. As a result, the full return of functions takes place.

The science of muscular system is called mycology. There are 600 muscles present in the body and form 40 per cent to 50 per cent of the body weight.

7. Nervous System

It is the system of all the nerves in the body. A specialised tissue organisms in the body, made with nerve cells are known as nerve fibers. A nerve cell with its process is called neuron. The cell that carries information between the brain and other parts of the body is called neuron. It is also known as functional cell.

It is the function of this system to control and coordinate.

Neurosis is a mental illness, with which a person suffers from strong feeling of fear and worry.

On the basis of whole nervous system, it is broadly sub-divided into two types. There are:

1. Central Nervous System (CNS) – Brain, Spinal cord, Cranial nerves 12 pairs, signal nerves 31 pairs.
2. Peripheral Nervous System (PNS)–Sympathetic and parasympathetic system.

The PNS is concerned with receiving, correlating and integrating incoming nerve impulses, orientations and coordination of PNS which has 43 pairs of spinal nerves.

The sensory organs constitute group of informers. The entire nervous system has two main units as :

1. Sensory or information unit, and
2. Motor or executive unit. They are integrated within the CNS.

8. Skin System

The skin forms the generalised protective coverings over the body surface. It is the outer covering of the body and continuous mucous membrane at all the openings of the body. Around all natural holes and openings, the skin becomes continuous. In the adult male, the skin forms about 1.8 sq m in surface area, in adult female 1.6 sq m. The thickness of the skin varies considerably from place to place like lymphatic membrane, eyelids, nose, nail. The rest of the skin varies generally from one mm to two mm in thickness.

There are two layers as outer epidermis and inner endodermis. It is made up of multiple layers of epithelium. Dermis contains hair follicles, melanin pigments, capillaries, nerve endings, sweat glands and sebaceous glands.

Skin protects underlying structures, excretes salts, metabolites like urea, regulates body temperature, secretes sweat, sebum and acts as sensory organ of the body. The colour of the skin varies from race to race, from country to country, person to person and mainly depends on the pigment present in the body. Skin is rich in blood vessels. Hair are present everywhere except on some places like palm, sole of the foot, etc.

9. Respiratory System

Another smaller part of human system is respiratory system. One's own urine is the best drug for many ailments of human respiratory problems like sinus, bronchitis, asthma and other respiratory related ills. This system is connected with breathing and respiratory tract.

The main function of this system is to the supply of oxygen and removal of carbondioxide from the cells. The whole activity is concerned with the air passages and lungs. The oxygen of the air is absorbed by the blood. It consists of the organs of respiration, i.e., lungs. The human respiratory system is associated with a series of stages.

The parts which are involved in air passages are nose pharynx, larynx, trachea, bronchi and lungs. The respiratory stages are inhalation, exchange of gas and exhalation. The cycle of respiration takes place 15 times per minute in normal adults.

The total air capacity of lungs is about five litres. Only 400 ml of air is inhaled and exhaled every time. 150 ml of air remains in the respiratory passage in each turn of respiratory cycle.

10. Digestive System

One of the sub-systems of the human system is digestive system which is involved in the digestion of food. It is a process that changes the foodstuffs we eat into substances that your body can use to produce energy for the maintenance of life, growth, immunity and repair of the tissues. It deals with the organs involved in the act of swallowing, digestion, ingestion, absorption of food, assimilation of food, excretion, elimination of the non-absorbable food residue that is the stool. It consists of a long tubular structure with two openings. One serves for in take of food and the other for the excretion of non-absorbable food residue. The opening is the mouth, and exit is anus. The whole tract from mouth to the anus is called alimentary canal. The whole canal with its associated glands is included in the digestive system.

The mouth, vest tube, lips, cheek, teeth, tongue, hard palate, soft palate, salivary gland , parotid gland, sub-mandibular gland, sub-lingual gland, pharynx, oesophagus, abdomen, peritoneum, lesser sac, omentum, stomach, lever, gall-bladder, bile duct, intestines, duodenum, travsverse colon, rectum.

The longest portion of the digestive tube measures about 21 feet in length.

11. Excretory system

This system is connected with urine or the parts of the body through which urine passes. Urination is a natural activity of the body to get rid of urine from the body at urinals. This system consists of two kidneys, two ureters, one urinary bladder, and one urethra, and the nephrons which are deposited in kidneys. Each kidney is made up of about one million nephrons. The kidneys purify blood, maintain water balance and regulate concentration of salts.

Ureters are the ducts which drain urine from kidneys. Urine bladder is a reservoir of urine. Urethra is a canal out-passage. An adult can urinate about one to two litres of urine per day.

12. Circulatory System

A sub-system of a human body relates to the circulation of the blood, by the blood vessels in the body. The blood vessels are hollow tubes carrying blood. The arteries carry blood away from the heart to the body. All the arteries contain oxygenated pure blood. The veins carry blood from the periphery to the heart. They contain deoxygenated impure blood.

The heart is an automatic muscular pump which consists of four chambers. The heart distributes oxygenated blood to different tissues of the body. A heart attack occurs when a coronary artery is blocked as a result of which the supply of blood to the heart muscle is reduced or stopped.

It produces two types of sounds like "*lub lub*" and "*dup dup*" respectively indicating a dull but a lengthier and a sharp but short sound. The normal blood pressure of a healthy person is 120/80 mm of mercury. During every heart beat the heart pumps 70 ml of blood. The total volume of blood pumped in each minute is about five litres (70x70=490 ml).

13. Skeleton System

Auto-urine therapy helps in curing many ailments of the bones of the human being. The structure that supports the body of a person is called skeleton. A human skeleton consists of 206 bones, which are arranged in a distinctive pattern. These bones are grouped into trunks or vertebral bones, ribs, sternum, limb bones, skull bones. It is a locomotive system called osteology, osteoarthritis, a disease that causes painful swelling and permanent damage to the joints of the body. Especially the hips, knees, thumbs and other ailments can be cured and prevented by auto-urine.

14. Reproductive System

This is concerned with the process of producing babies. The system is different for male and female which called:

(1) Male Reproductive System.

(2) Female Reproductive System.

1. Male Reproductory System

It has sub-systems, (1) External genital organs and (2) Internal genital organs.

1. External: Penis, testes, epidermis and vasdeferens.
2. Internal: Ductus deferns, seminal vesicle, prostate gland.

2. **Female Reproductory System**

It has external organs : vulva, monspubis, labia majora, limbia minora, clitors. Internal : uterus, uterine tube, ovaries, mammary glands, menstrual cycle.

15. **Endocrine System**

A gland is an organ in a person's body that produces chemical substance for the body. The glands secrete hormones which are directly send into blood. These glands do not have ducts, which is a tube in the body through which liquid passes. Hence these glands are called endocrine glands. This system is made up of endocrine glands some secrete only one hormone, while the other glands secrete more than one hormone.

The human body has eight types of glands which secrete their own hormones. They are :

1. Pituitory gland in the brain.
2. Pineal gland in the brain.
3. Thyroid gland in the neck.
4. Parathyroid gland in the neck.
5. Thymus gland in the thorax.
6. Pancreas gland in the abdomen.
7. Suprarenal gland in the abdomen.
8. Sex gland in testes in males, in ovaries and in the pelvic region in females.

In the case of a person who is suffering from chronic ailment, poisonous substances are found in tissues, intestines. It means he has a high level of toxicity. The best method is administering urine enema that removes, sweeps out poisonous materials from the body, tissues, intestines, etc. The body easily absorbs a number of readily available vital substances deposited in the urine.

10. **Complementary to Each Other**

Method of using urine either for prevention or treatment can broadly be divided into two categories. Thus, based on the observation as how to use, they are called as:

Urine Therapy

Internal Application and External Application

Both the methods are complementary and different but together form a useful and holistic combination of qualities. Therefore, we can use one or two or more than two methods depending on the need and the nature of ailment. All are equally important for optimal result. These are only different ways to applying urine.

4

Ancient and Historical Overview

Indian Origin

The traditional medicine played an important role in Indian Hindu society, knowledge about the types and extent and characteristics of natural healing practices and practitioners were very limited and remained as secrets in those days. There are a number of natural medical practices that reflect the diversity of Indian cultures. Indian traditional medicine is concerned not only just with suppressing or masking the symptoms of disease but to eradicate the cause of malady, with the prevention, curing, promotion of human physical, spiritual, social, mental, emotional and material well-being. The many categories of traditional medicinal practice dealing with these different aspects of health include :

Varient branches of *yoga*, meditation, *rasa sadhana*, spiritual healing, *mudras*, *satkriya*, *suryanamaskar*, semen withdrawals, natural diet, auto-urine therapy, herbs, etc. both for preventive, curative and maintenance.

Among these health care practices auto-urine therapy is considered to be the most powerful medical system because one's own urine is a life force, vital power, serum. Unfortunately, little has been done in recent decades to utilise, enhance and develop the beneficial aspects of urine therapy, including relevant research to explore possibilities for its gradual integration into mainstream modern medicine to address emerging chronic, acute, degenerative, opportunistic infections, innumerable and incurable diseases like cancer, AIDS, arthritis, sinus, bronchitis, asthama, etc. So, urinopathy today is a traditional part of national heritage, as culturally acceptable household medicinal practice. The vast majority of Indian population live in rural areas, where healthcare coverage is low, many people follow urine therapy due to the cultural acceptability. Even today it exists and continued to use over many centuries. Nevertheless this modality as primary healthcare system, it has been neglected its therapeutic potential with no side effect.

India has a long history of urinopathic medicine to cure diseases. Indian traditional medicine is concerned for a holistic medicine for the protection, promotion of human physical, spiritual, social, behavioural and material well-being. The object of this topic is to review history of practice of traditional urinopathic medicine in India. The therapeutic properties of urinal and its beneficial references are found in several ancient Hindu Scriptures like *Vedas*, *Mahabharata*, *Purunas*, *Yoga* texts, etc.

Damara Tantra

Urotherapy is an ancient practice as it finds mention in many ancient texts of India. One of such books is *Shivambu Kalpa Vidhi, Damara Tantra.* The word *shivambu*, literally means, 'water of Lord Shiv'a, a Hindu God, pure water, one's own water.

Many urine therapists in India often speak of drinking *shivambu, swamootra panam*, means, 'drinking one's own urine, which is considered as water of auspiciousness. It is a nature's elixir, or divine nectar. Indian people consider urine as an auspicious object because it is something sure prevent and cure health problem. They believe God, Lord Shiva, because it is who designed and advocated. Besides, it is later mentioned about it in many other old texts.

Damara Tantra is an age-old Sanskrit text which contains 107 stanzas, refers about the benefits of urine. '*Shivambu Kalpa*' as referred to in the text means urine therapy. It suggests, among other uses and prescriptions, massaging one's own skin with concentrated urine. Urotherapy is practically as old as man himself. So, it is a divine manifestation of cosmic intelligence. The spiritual advantage is to unleash the power of *kundalini*, sending it straight into the *sahasrara* to the third eye to bring instant enlightenment.

The spiritual practitioners drink the midstream of their morning urine. But urine is a divine nectar of a number of holy men in India where urine therapy has been practised for thousands of years. Though not in the name of urine-therapy, but as a natural diet ancient Indians have been practiced for thousands of years, but lack of publicity, it has merely fallen a bit into obscurity in recent past. The practice of urine drinking in India is not new, does not introduce anything new or original. It has been popular throughout the centuries in India. This is in no way completely a new therapy.

Urine therapy as a medicinal quality has been well-documented in many ancient Hindu texts, it has a long proven record of its incredible power to heal an amazing variety of human ailments. Urine has supernatural healing qualities, it is named as divine nectar. It means the miraculous curing powers of urine that cannot be explained by the laws, or medical science and that seems to involve God or miracle. It has supernatural force, strength, a vital force.

Shivambu

Shivambu, or urinecare is advocated by Lord Shiva considered to be the father of auto-urine medicine known in medical history. The text is a comprehensive philosophy and system of primary healthcare. His approach emphasised diet, herbs, seasons, naturopathy as ways to improve and maintain good, long health. Urinopathic medicine grew quickly, with wide acceptance and was practiced later by *yogis*.

Shivambu says :

Yada Yada hi Swasthyasya Hanirbhavati
Manava Abhyuthanamcha Roganam
Tadatmanam Srujamyaham.

It means -

"O helpless human being ! Whenever there is total loss of health and presence of monstrous of diseases [in this *kali yuga*], I manifest myself".

Another verse :

Sarva Chikistsaparityajya
Mameka Sharanam Mama.

It means :

Abandon all therapies and seek refuge in me alone.

Amaroli

Urinotherapy is also known as '*amaroli*', which is an integral part of the tradition of yoga. In Indian yogic tradition, urine therapy may be called as amaroli. The word 'amar' means 'the state of being immortal'. It implies the practitioner of urine is believed to live long. Longevity increases, it does not cause death or likely to cause it soon, our lives considerably long without disease, decay, figure change, and with strength and stamina. In tantric religious traditions, this practice is called 'amaroli'. Among Hindus, urine drinking is a common practice in ceremonies performed by a group of people, often for religious purposes, there is a scientific reason also for drinking their own urine.

The practitioners in ancient days believed and realised its efficacy by drinking urine. They enjoyed the fact of seeming to see or hear something, somebody, that is not really there. It is called hallucination. Urine acts as a harmless drug that affects people's minds and makes them see and hear things that are not really there.

In ancient times, or early days in rural areas, many people used to practice this therapy.

Therefore, in tantrik yoga culture, urine drinking is termed as amaroli. The word comes from the root word Amar which is immortality, undying, imperishability. Amaroli is, therefore, a practice designed by first users of urine to bring about immortality to life. But it does not mean that a person will never die, live forever, instead it means that one will enjoy healthy life. It implies drinkers would not die a premature death with illness, disorders, very common now a days.

Yoga Texts

Yoga, a Hindu philosophy, which has a number of branches, teaches how to control body and mind, good health, and normal living in the belief that one can become united with the spirit of the universe through this way. Yogic teachings, techniques practices include urine therapy as a natural medicine for prevention and curing of all ailments, which is a panacea for ailing human race.

It is an ancient spiritual practice, designed to promote meditation. The ancient Hindu and *yoga* texts that mention about the importance, using methods, curing several diseases. In *Shivambu Kalpa*, Lord Shiva discoursed that, the practitioner of *yoga* should take it before proceeding with his other rituals.

First users

First drinkers of urine are *yogis*, who have a long history of urinopathic medicine and have developed ways and procedures to cure diseases. They are concerned not only with curing of diseases but also with the protection, longevity, deageing and promotion of human physical, spiritual, social and mental well-being.

It is widely believed in India, that the knowledge of health and medicinal secrets of urine are given and designed by God, Lord Shiva which is not only well-documented but passed orally from *guru* to disciples, father to a child, and thus the healing knowledge has been guarded by certain families, households, communities or social groups. Health and urine are seen as a gift of God, or the will of God and many Indians believe generally that their ancient texts as holy books help to keep them healthy.

As we understood urine today scientifically as bio-chemistry, they believed that in addition it contains supernatural life forces in treatment. This scenario is even more applicable to many conditions as the last resort which are outside the scope of modern medicine like cancer, HIV, etc. The use of urine as a therapy in practice has a supernatural power, has been around us as even today, for a much longer time in the practice of Indian traditional medicine.

Life Style of Yogis

It is to be believed that drinking one's urine in the morning was an ancient yogic practice designed to promote meditation. It is a life style, the custom and behaviour that are considered typical of a yogic group. The pineal gland, produces a chemical substance, a hormone called melantonin. The gland secrets at about two am, but this production is being shut off when the eyes are exposed to bright sunlight.

If this hormone is taken orally or given intravenously, it provokes tranquility, quite and peace. *Yogis* in India lead a tranquil life by taking urine. So, this hormone of urine is a tranquiliser, a fast acting tranquilising natural drug. It is used to reduce anxiety, worry. It also heightens one's visualisation. Even scientific studies proved that there are high concentration of melantonin hormone in the first morning urine.

Pre-dawn Urine

This is the reason why *yogis* used to consume pre-dawn autogeneous melantonin. It slows down brain wave activity. This is the secret behind the alleged benefits ascribed to auto-urine drinking by ancient texts of the yogic religion.

Yogis follow the discourses of Lord Shivạ contained in *Shivambu*. Accordingly, after cleansing the mouth, and performing other essential morning functions, they used to drink one's own urine. The sagacious practitioners used to get up when three quarters of the night elasped and passed urine, drank facing the east.

Meditation

The effect of drinking one's own urine on meditation has been known in India for many centuries. It has been confirmed by experience of the various types of changes occur in the body and mind concentration during meditation or yogic practice.

In recent years, the interest in the Science of Yoga, drinking before practising, its effect on mind and result have shown much beneficial outcomes. In addition, the *yogis* are seen to experience powers that appear supernatural. It reduces strain and stress. In meditation, the mind becomes immobile and can be directed towards total calm and peace.

But the practice is very personal. They do not open up their secret to others except to other disciples, or co-practitioners of *yoga*, meditation. But today it has become a public interest, attracted strong media attention and social interest. There is a wide reaction from the public.

It has been practiced by *yogis* in India for thousands of years. There is good record of ancient literature in support of it. Curing with urine is india's traditional medicine popular. There is a lot of paper evidence, public experience about this, India's traditional households may not still need some were convincing. People are ignorant but people who are aware are enthusiastic about trying it themselves, but very personal. People of modern generation are re-discovering this traditional medicine.

In practice in India, it is popular to call as *amaroli*. The people in yogic life, from whom the practice actually came, found that one's own urine is a food, medicine, restorative and transformative agent, strengthens the aura-powers. They further experienced that the mind is less inclined to think as it behaves like a monkey; the spiritual energy is kept high, and the progress towards the *samadhi* is smoother. For this reason, spiritual aspirants more depend on natural elixir, urine.

The importance of urine and herbal mixture practices are indicated by the fact that people of traditional cultures depend on them for their primary healthcare. Besides its role in healing, the practice is helpful in preventing the evil eyes and omnel overcoming demons, maintaining clear eyesight, visualisation, good memory, long life as well as a large family and faithful members.

Urinopathy has evolved out of the ancient healing traditions of earlier *yugas*, with its roots firmly grounded in yogic life styles. Today, it is also with an expanded and scientific understanding from modern sources. It is now recognised by mainstream medicine as a valuable and effective treatment for a variety of disorders. Its principles and philosophy have been found since the time immemorial, even today. But in past recently it was overlooked in general healthcare. However, it is now once again gaining popularity as a primary healthcare, just as it was for many thousands of years back. Urine-use is based on historical medical practice. There are well-defined procedure, benefits, that are well-documented in ancient texts dating back nearly 5,000 years and other monographs. However, this is not always the case, and in a number of countries, the knowledge and practice still exist.

Ayurveda

Ayurveda is a branch of medical science, of traditional medicine, concerned with environment of all the plants, that exist in the universe not made and used by the people for health. It uses medicinal herbs, plants helpful in the process of healing illnesss or infection. Ayurveda also has recognised and has accorded its approval to the drinking of urine as a therapeutic measure. It regards urine therapy as an effective antidote that controls the effects of a poison or disease.

The consumption of one's own urine as medicine was a popular method and widely used in early days.

About 200 years ago, our medicinal practices were largely dominated by urine therapy and herbal medicine. However, the medicinal age of urine and herbs went into a rapid decline in India, when more predictable synthetic drug were made commonly available. In contrast, many known people continued to benefit from the rich knowledge of medicinal urine. Even today, it is still used by a large majority of traditional households.

Yogic practices play a large part in the healing process for Indians such as meditation and going to the temples. Along with them, urine is also used for a wide variety of diseases, prevention, good health and normal living. Indians believe that (mid stream) urine drinking cures when it is drunk in the early morning.

Bhavprakasha is one of the volumes of Ayurveda. In this, urine is termed as killer of all poisons, anti-poison. It also referred urine as a chemical element which can rejuvenate even an old person. In another words, it says that urine purifies blood and cures all skin diseases, infections, affections.

Reference of urine therapy is found in almost all the volumes of Ayurveda, namely, SUSHRUT, HARIT, BHAVPRAKASH, GAJNIGHANTU, YOGRATNAKAR, BHAISHAJRATNAUALI, RAJNIGHANTU, VAGBHATT, DHANVANTARI NIGHANTIU, and others. Dear readers, what a painful paradoxical surprise that it is though mentioned in all the volumes of Ayurveda and others, it still remained hidden for centuries. It was never lost, for the truth is indestructible, hence it always exists. Urine mixed with ayurvedic knowledge can prove to be tremendously beneficial.

Lord Shiva discoursed the secrets of the variant uses of herbal plants or power or liquid mixed with auto-urine for additional benefits. For example, it recommends ayurvedic plants like gaduchi, tinospora condifolia, harade, terminalia, chebula, sulphur, masha, koshtha, terminalia belavica, phylonthus embica, etc.

Botanical medicine or phylotherapy was a corner stone of traditional medicine along with urine long before the development of synthetic pharamaceuticals. The fact is that most of the drugs are also derived from medicinal plants. Modern scientific investigations have substantiated many of the early uses of medicinal plants as recommended in *Shivambu,* and have increasingly found ways to use them in treating modern diseases. *Shivambu* recognised long before the benefits of urine and herbs in medicine as a means of providing affordable primary healthcare to the people of ancient times. Herbs and urine are characterised by their low toxicity and lack of accumulation in the body. If used it offers powerful, safe and effective approach to healing with no side effects. Although, this medical system dates back to about 5000 years, it is scientifically being recognised now.

Medicinal plants, flowers, powders, extracts are used according to *Shivambu* principle in modern Ayurvedic medicine. Many plants, substances have powerful medicinal properties as urine, which address to a variety of problems simultaneously. The biological-organic nature of urine-herb substances are compatible with body's own chemistry. Hence, the mixture can gently be effective with no side effects, so urine-herbal medicine has been the primary medicine used by most of the human community as culturally accepted. Herbal auto-urine as a medical art remains as secret medical choice even today. The single chemically derived drugs may cure only in one condition, but herb-urine medicines are able to cure a variety of problems.

So, what we have to understand here is that *Shivambu* medicine is a healing philosophy that is complementary to Ayurvedic medicine. Tree bark, dried herbs, urine has the ability to keep your home cure.

Other References

The therapeutic value of urine has been mentioned not only in Hindu scripts, but references are also there in other religions and their texts.

The Holy Bible recommends urine therapy. The Bible is the holy scripture of the Christian religion consisting of the Old Testament and the New Testament. It contains some important information on the subject of urine, this we can refer to support.

A verse reads : Drink water from thy own cistern,
Flowing Water from thy own well.

The word 'cistern' means 'a container' in which water is stored in a building, specially one on the roof or connected to a toilet. In present context, cistern is urine bladder.

The Bible says : *The Life or Life force of Flesh*
is in blood, and
As urine comes from the blood
It contains that life force.

Jesus said : *It is not what goes into a man*
Which defiles him so much as
What comes out of him.

Rabshakeh said : *Hath my master sent me to thy master*
And to thee to speak these words?
Hath he not sent me to the men
That sit upon the wall,
That they may eat their own
Dung, and drink their own piss with you. **[Isaiah 36:12]**

Prophet Muhammad advocated drinking camel's urine as a medicine in several verses of Islamic Scriptures for medical purposes.

Abu Honifa referred as He said that it is disliked, but not forbidden, to drink the urine from camels. Abu Yusuf commented, He said that urine from camels can be consumed for medical purposes.

In Roman times, there was a tradition among the Gauls to use urine to whiten teeth [Your Teeth, Egnatius, Poem by Catullus].

Evidences are there in adavanced and civilised country like France, people practice urine therapy. Customarily, soaked stockings in urine are wrapped around the neck in order to cure strep throat, an infection of the throat. Urine cure effectively.

In Sierra Madre, Mexico, it is reported that the farmers prepare a soft substance spread on a cloth, sometimes heated, and put on the skin to reduce the pain or swelling for broken bones by having a child urinate into a bowl of powder burnt and black of any plant that is grown for its grain. The mixture thus made into a paste is applied to the skin.

A country, very popular in traditional and oriental medicine, in China, there is also a institute called Institute of chinese Traditional Medicine. In some parts of southern china, the faces of babies are washed with urine to protect the skin.

More than three million Chinese drink their own urine in the belief, it is good for their health, [*Xinhua*, official news agency]. It is according to the official news agency. There is a Chinese Association of Urine Therapy.

Yang Lian Sheng, a professor from the Liaoning Institute of Traditional Chinese Medicine, was quoted as saying that urine is more sanitary than blood.

Engineer Zhu Jinfu told at a seminar he had been drinking his own urine since he was 13, and had lived a healthy life for the last 58 years. Many of his forefathers had also lived to a ripe old age [Reuters].

Urine One of the Thousand Noble Things

It is advisable to refer to some evidences of the medicinal value of urine well-known in western countries. The modern source as to the value of urine as a preventive and curative agent can be found in a book titled "*One Thousand Noble Things*". It was published simultaneously in England, Scotland and Ireland, in the beginning of the nineteenth century.

In this book, there are several useful quaint citations of urine therapy as excellent remedy for many human ailments like distempers, dropsy, jaundice, deafness, numbness, chaps, sores, joints, itches, etc.

Advent of Industrial Medicine

Allopathic medicine is called by various names as industrial medicine, modern medicine, pharmaceutical drugs emerged to meet the diseases and disorders of industrial hazards, or occupational diseases. It has an history of not more than 200 years.

Long ago, there were no chemical drugs and people used herbs, and urine. In their own way of life, they depended on traditional medicine including urine therapy and they helped themselves. Today allopathic medicine and qualified doctors have taken over. They were highly conversant with a wide diversity of plant medicine, usages, and other elements of nature-based preventatives and therapeutics. It was the only major known source of medicine for the people of the days.

However, in the post-industrial world, there were a number of notable historical events that led to the decline of drinking urine. Colonialism, industrialisation, urbanisation, political transformation, migration, immigration, the arrival of industrial medicine, change of socio-economic and traditional ways of life styles undermined the long-standing healing household traditions.

The combined impact of these factors and many known and unknown forces, in addition to major deterioration in health status played havoc on cultural knowledge and practices and undermined the previous healthcare system, balance and harmony in cultures. Many of the older life practices also have been lost, and the indigenous knowledge of self-cure systems started disappearing.

Today in the scientific laboratories, experts are conducting analytical procedures to determine the medicinal constituents that are present in the urine solution. By experimenting its useful medicinal properties in hormones, enzymes are isolated and extracted and standardised injections in modern fashion are made and sold in the market in some countries today.

5

We All Have Drunk Our Urine and Born

No exception, every one of us have drunk our own urine when we were in the womb of the mother. As foetus babies survived by drinking of its own urine. We were ignorant of it, but it is a system created by God. Womb is an organ in woman where a baby grown before born. We drank our own urine which in medical literature is called in the form of amniotic fluid. The bulk share and volume of this liquid is urine only. The baby lives by taking this liquid from pregnant women's womb to survive. Amniocentesis is also a medical test conducted that involves taking some liquid from pregnant woman's womb in order to find out, if the baby has particular illness or health problem.

This fluid is nothing but the bulk of it is foetal urine. It is a vital substance for the development of a baby in the womb. So, drinking urine is a natural process, which is a very basic of human existence. But now at this age, we have forgetten our origin of baby growth, today we nauseate, disgust, hate and feel shy to listen urine therapy and even to drink. However, we all have drunk, breathed-in, grown, swimmed in urine pool, inside the womb. On the part of human being, drinking urine certainly is not unusual, especially in a way it is difficult to understand God's art of creation.

So, this is not something strange about drinking our own urine, because we are not familiar with it, because we have forgotten our foundation of existence, origin of growth. Today we have recognised it as a popular therapy, we have an unpleasant physical feeling, not feeling comfortable to situation. To say auto-urine drinking is connected with the earliest origin of life's existence in the womb of the mother itself. The primary medical treatment the baby receives is the first from urine. The liquid substance surrounding the baby in the woman womb is mainly urine. The bulk of amniotic fluid is fetal urine only.

It has a powerful healing effect on the body of the baby. A higher amount of amniotic fluid in the womb is correlated with better health, more energy and size, and growth of baby. The molecular structure of the liquid is more organised full of hormones and fetas urine is thus crystalline like substance containing a high level of cosmetic, medicinal nutrients and therapeutic properties.

Bag of Urine

In the body of a pregnant woman, there is what is called sack, is shaped like a bag, has thin skin around it, that contains this liquid. This bag grows slowly and begins to fill with the liquid two weeks after fertilisation. Two and half months later, the liquid contains the following substances :

Proteins, Carbohydrates, Lipids, Urea, Electrolytes, Phospholipids. All these substances contribute a lot to the growth of the baby.

The baby begins to swallow during eight-eleven weeks and begins to urinate. So, the foetus begins to get rid of her urine from the body in the womb of the mother only. In this pool of baby's own urine, the baby breaths-in, swims-in and swallows urine. The baby swallows majority of urine and the remaining fluid remain, inside the womb until the baby is born. The liquid in the womb in the form of urine is inhaled and exhaled and swallowed by the baby. The Urine fills the lungs of the baby and promotes the maturation of lungs for nespiration after birth.

Baby the Mysterious

The precious origin of the urine-filled fluid still remains unsolved mystery not even known to the medical science. It is probably of mixed maternal and foetal origin, God's creative secret. The most intelligent self-mechanism of baby creation is very difficult to understand or explain, a strange phenomenon is a urine system. The medicinal and metabolic functions of the baby urine in pregnant woman's womb is one of the great unsolved mysteries of the human evolution. It has become a secret knowledge even today, a spiritual belief that cannot be explained or proved in a scientific way. But public experience of its therapeutic properties is the only practical way of explaining its medicinal quality.

A person understands, believes the fabulous medical qualities that are beyond normal human understanding. This is the reason why urine therapy is a speculative therapy having spiritual powers or qualities that are difficult to explain, but only the results are the explanations in its favour as a natural therapy.

The composition of the liquid in the womb includes :

Water	:	98-99 per cent,
Solid	:	1-2 per cent.

The solid constituents of the urine associated with baby are as follows :

1. Organic Constituents

Protein	:	0.30 gm percentage
Glucose	:	20 mg percentage
Urea	:	30 mg percentage
NPN	:	30 mg percentage

Uric acid : 4 mg percentage

Creatinine : 2 mg percentage

Total lipids : 50 mg percentage

Hormones : Protactine, insulin, renin.

2. **Inorganic Constituents**

Sodium, Chloride, Potassium.

3. **Suspended Particles**

Lanugo, exfoliated squamous epithelial cells, vernix caseosa, cast off amniotic cells, cells from respiratory tract, urinary bladder and vagina of the foetus.

By the end of the period of three months when a woman is pregnant, the nephrons are active to secret urine.

Near term of pregnancy, the urine production rises to 650 ml per day. The volume of this liquid increases as the baby grows. The volume of fluid is highest nearly 34 weeks after conception. At 34 weeks, the volume of fluid is nearly 800 ml. The volume of fluid declines to roughly 600 ml at 40 weeks which is normally the amount when the baby is born.

Very early in human development, a clear fluid collects in amniotic cavity surrounding embryo. The volume increases rapidly with the growth of product of conception increasing about five ml at 12 weeks of pregnancy. At 20 weeks, its volume is about 400 ml and at 34 weeks, it reaches a peak of near a litre. During the last few weeks of pregnancy, its volume decreases and at 43 weeks the range varies from 100 to 600 ml.

During the early phase of foetal development, the amniotic fluid is probably an extension of total extracellular fluid space, the baby skin acting as a semipermeable membrane. After the mid-pregnancy, increased cornification and stratification of the skin prevents diffusion, the foetal urine then becomes the major contribution to the amniotic fluid and baby's swallowing is probably the major route of the fluid removal.

Towards the term, saliva and lung fluid may also make contribution towards composition of fluid.

Importance of the Urine to the Babies

- Urine fully surrounds the human baby in the womb. Urine is a primary medical treatment that naturally baby receives. The baby never faces any illness or health problem, because the urine prevents. Baby breaths-in always in urine. The lungs of the baby develop only with the help of urine.
- The medicinal qualities of amniotic fluid protects the body, prevents and cures all health problems. It is a natural therapy to the baby, cures quickly.

- The skin of the baby is smooth, pleasant and soft because of cosmetic properties of the urine. Foetus urine is a natural drug, considered very helpful likely to cause good health to the baby. The skin is very beautiful. The urine-based fluid contributes to the softness of the skin,
- Any pre-birth surgery effects are cured, healed quickly, and any mark or scar that is left on the skin after an operation would disappear quickly, due to therapeutic quality of the urine-based liquid.
- Baby swims-in, in the urine pool for months together.
- Baby in the womb is protected in several ways by this vital substance of foetus urine.
- The baby comes in contact with urea in the urine at an early age. Urine-filled liquid is the nourishing and protecting substance. The fluid around the baby protects the developing baby and acts as shock absorber. It acts as a cushion/against blows to the mother's abdomen, protects the foetus from extraneous injury. The surrounding substance allows the baby for easier movement in different directions.
- Liquid helps the baby to develop normally, promotes muscular, skeletal development. It also assists the foetus from heat loss. The fluid contains also foetus cells which can be examined for genetic defects. The liquid can be taken for amniocentesis, a test procedure, that can reveal many aspects of baby's genetic health, illness, general health.
- Recent research studies reveal that the fluid contains considerable quantity of stem cells which are useful for future human application. These stem cells can be preserved in cell banks. An adequate and balanced quantity of the liquid is good both for the mother and the baby. Too little, or too much can be a cause or an indicator of problems for mother and baby. If the liquid is too little the babies can develop problems of the limbs, clubbing of the feets and hands under developed lungs, life-threatening conditions, fatal and the baby can die shortly after birth, infection, kidney dysfunction, kidney malformation and other baby problems may be caused.
- Urine liquid maintains a balanced temperature. It prevents adhesion between the foetal parts and bag called sack. Though negligible, urine has a nutritive value because it contains proteins, and salt contents. It ensures adequate water supply to the baby. The fluid flushes the birth canal at the end. It has a septic and bacterial action, protects the baby and prevents ascending infection to the uterine cavity. The examination of fluid gives useful information about the well-being and also maturity of the baby.
- Facilitates dilation of the cervix during labour. It has got enzymatic activities for steroid hormonal metabolism.

6
What Is Piss?

Piss – A Heavenly Nectar and Elixir

Urine is an unused liquid that stores in the urine bladder. Every one urinate, to get rid of it from the body, called urination.Urinary track is connected with the parts of the body through which it passes.

The word 'piss' is used to mean 'to urinate'. More polite way of expressing this is to go to the toilet or go to the bathroom. I need to pee means to pass liquid from the body.

Urine is a mixture solution of many constituents like water, urea and multiple quantities of several hundreds of substances like minerals, proteins, nutrients, hormones, vitamins, enzymes, metabolites, including cortico-steroids. There is not only a scientific evidence, but also long prevailed public experience of therapeutic use of urine.

It contains 95 per cent water, 2.5 per cent urea and the rest 2.5 per cent mixture of hundreds of substances. A body fluid, by-product of blood.

All these chemical substances put together to form urine fluid. The molecular structure of urine is the composition of these valuable medicinal substances which have been excreted by the body not because they are waste products but they could not be used by the body at a particular point of time, or because they were present in excess of requirement to the body. It is not only a tonic, but also antiseptic, and a cure for a number of human ailments of modern days.

In Shivambu Kalpa, Lord Shiva, discoursed that auto-urine is a heavenly nectar.

Heavenly means, something that is connected with heaven. In Hindu religion, it is a place believed to be the abode of Gods where pious people go when they die. The secret of urine pious making and excretion is the process designed by the creator which is a medicinal secret.

Heavenly nectar is a mixture of chemical substances, liquid that is produced by the body. It is a thick juice of many constituents of the body. So, human urine is a natural elixir, a magic liquid that has fabulous medicinal qualities to prevent and cure illness or to make people live long, physical immortality, it is an elixir of life.

Urine is a serum, the thin liquid in the body tissues, taken from the blood when the rest has clotted in body tissue and is used to protect from diseases.

Human body has the most advanced and scientific mechanism. It takes care of its health, has auto mechanism to make its own medicine. Bodily disorders are cured by bodily medicine. It is an interesting story, to know about autogenous drug. What is this urine you have to discover? What is this therapy that helps ailments? What is it that you actually have to know?

This is what I thought to do in this book. But you must also absolutely need to know more hidden truth! What I discovered is that urine is not a waste water, we think it is. In this book, I explain that it is a medicinal substance we are wasting, as we are completely unaware what it is please be aware about your own urine which has enormous theraperutic and medicinal properties.

Everyone of us must have a common knowledge, or scientific study of urine and its use as medicine. Urine with such wondrous preventive and curative properties, it is unfortunate that we are not bothering, even the science also. It is amazing even after knowing well its medicinal value. Human body is a multi-million dollar high-tech pharmaceutical company which turns the foodstuffs and water we take into drugless natural drug in the form of urine. It has medicinal value, urine is tonic, a penacea for modern and future ailing human race. But drinkers knew well about urine secrets. A golden fluid.

It is a free, or priceless, much cheaper than the water, whisky, buttermilk, a life saver, a healer of last resort. It is always available, it is always with you, at all places, supplies at all times. A wonder drug is deposited in our bladder only. It is a multi-billion dollar medicine bag, the urine bladder. It is a panacea, something that will solve all the problems of a particular situation. Urine is like a sweet liquid that is produced by flowers and collected by bees for making honey. It is the elixir of life or youth. A fabulous magic liquid which has potential to cure illness.

7
What is Urinopathy?

Urine therapy is called by variant names as Auto-Urine Therapy, Urotherapy, Urinotherapy, Auto-immune Therapy, Uropathy, Intrinsic Medicine, Naturopathic Urine Therapy, Urine Therapy Lifeforce, also known in India as *Amaroli* and *Shivambu*. Urine is the water of Hindu God Lord Shiva , hence it is called *Shivambu.*

Therapy means the treatment of physical problems, disorders, an illness or ailments. In all these cases patients usually undergo some sort of natural drug therapy, means treatment by using drugs, may be alternative and complementary medicines. But in case of auto-urine therapy, the patients do not use factory made or other medicine. Urine therapy is a curing method, wherein treatments that do not use drugs, but uses one's own urine which is a drugless drug. In this system of medicine the urine therapist, a specialist who treats a particular type of illness or disorder or problem by recommending to risk patient's own urine.

Uro-therapeutics is a newly emerging branch of medicine concerned with the treatment of diseases. Human urine has therapeutic characters, and urine therapy has been designed to help to treat human ailments–the therapeutic medicinal properties of urine helps in preventing, curing wide range of human disorders and rebuilds immunity system. Hence, it is popularly called auto-urine therapy.

There is a lot of confusion in the minds of many people as to the difference between this therapy and urology. Urology is a branch of modern medical science, which is a scientific study of urinal system only. An ancient therapy, refers to various applications of human urine for medicinal or cosmetic purposes, it includes various methods of using it like internal and external application.

A person who is drinking urine as a therapy is a practitioner. Therefore, urinotherapy, refers to multifarious uses of urine like prevention, curing and cosmetic purposes. Many advocates, the urine therapy as panacea for all human ailments and there is practically no disease that urine would not cure.

Therapy

Under this healthcare practice, the patient drinks his own urine. Urinopathic medicine is use as diet massaging, life-style change and cutting edge natural therapies to enhance his body's ability toward off and combat disease. It acts on the patient as a complex, interrelated system as a whole person, not an organ. It blends the best traditional, natural, alternative medicine approaches not only to treat disease but also restores health.

It is based on basic principles, such as healing power of the body, treating causes of diseases instead of suppressing symptoms, customisation, educating patient, treating whole body, prevention and cure. Therapy is a proactive drug that saves money, pain, misery, lives with no side-effects. It focusses on holistic, proactive, prevention and comprehensive treatment. It removes inherent barriers to good health by helping to create a healing internal and external environment.

Its main emphasis is on naturopathic medicine and use of traditional alternative healing agents in its basket. So, the therapy has become customised health management strategy. A practice of healing by natural methods combines traditional therapies used for centuries to heal not only physically, but also mentally, emotionally and spiritually to keep a person's body to balance and optimal health.

The body reuses the constituents of urine after reintroducing into it, such as vitamins, minerals , nutrients, hormones, amino-acids, enzymes, proteins, etc. It ensures as many aspects of a person as possible or treating the whole person, but not just relieving a set of isolated ailments. The premise behind urine therapy is to find out the root cause of human ailment and address rather than treating on symptomatic cure. It would cure most, if not all known sicknesses and diseases. It has been called as natural tonic, vitamin rich solution, because of its recognised ability to build immunity.

Urine is a vital force, has innate ability, promotes self-healing, cleansing, self-repair. The immune, hormonal nervous, detoxification, elimination, pathways, excretion are the basic systems of the body, must always be in balance to be in healthy state. The urine therapy focusses mainly to restore, repair them. The biological balance is the main feature of any health system. It prevents, treats the drinkers holistically taking into account his bio-chemistry, biomechanics and emotional predisposition.

The urine of each individual has his or her own unique substances with innate ability of self-healing power. It is an individualised treatment protocol. The philosophy of this therapy is to develop optimal wellness of an individual. Prevention is the ultimate goal. The principle of urinopathic medicine is of wellness enhancement but not disease curing.

There is a lot to be learnt about urine, which is under active research in other countries. Approximately 25 years ago, medical profession was under the impression that urine is waste product. They also believed that urine containsed no therapeutic properties. Now urinopathic medicine is used even for curing cancer. Today it is recognised that it has many health benefits. There are many different yoga schools, institutions, both traditional as well as modern that teach about urine as one discipline.

New research findings show that urine is better than modern medicine in respect of many human ailments. New trials support the effectiveness of this therapy for cancer, cardio, etc. There are many published clinical trials and scientific research papers about the effectiveness of urinopathy. They give new scientific evidence to the old therapy that urine is bad.

The list is exhaustive of several diseases. Urine therapy prevents or cures ailments, enhances, improves longevity, deteraging, cleans bowels, intestines, alimentary canal, improves quality of skin.

Urine bathing, enema, throat disorder, effective against the flu, common cold, broken bones, whitening teeth, tooth-ache and other mouth problems, dry skin, psoriasis, sinus, skin diseases, cancer, aids, cardiovascular complaints, allergies, animal and snake bites, asthama , bronchitis, hypertension, burns, wounds, injuries, chemical intoxication, chickenpox, enteritis, constipation, pneumonia, dysentery, edema, Eczema, eye irritation, conjunctivitis, sight disorders, fatigue, gonorrhea, gout, blood urine, smallpox, immunological disorders, infections, infertility, baldness, insomia, jaundice, hepatitis, kapori's, sarcoma leprosy, lymphatic disorder, urticaria, morning sickness, hangover, nosal disorders, congestions, obesity, papilloma virus, opportunistic infections associated with VDS, HIV, parasitoses, respiratory disorders, gastric ulcer, rheumatism, birthmarks, strokes, lumbago, typhus, gastritis, cold sore , tuberculosis, tetanus, foot fungus endocrine related diseases, ulcerative colitis, pelvic inflammatory diseases, adrenal, digestive problems, exhaustion, excessive weakness, menstruation disorders, miscarriage, prostate trouble, arthritis, glaucoma, cataract, malaria, diptheria, scarlet fever, scurvy, bed wetting, mucus colitis, pyorrhea, gangrene, etc. about 175 known diseases are effectively cured with urine therapy.

8

Physical Characteristics of Human Urine

Normal urine of a person has some features like appearance connected with urine that actually exist or present and can be seen, felt, touched etc., rather than things that only exist in a person's mind. It is a tangible substance having some physical properties such as colour, weight, shape etc. The study of natural ingredients of the body reveals some medicinal qualities. It has typical features of all biological characteristics.

However, the following are the glaring physical characteristics of normal urine:

1. Volume

The quantity of urine that is collected and pissed out is the volume of urine. The amount of it is one of the physical characteristics of urine. The actual quantity of urine of a person per day is affected by factors such as:

- Recent quantity of fluid intake into the body like water and other drinks and food.
- Diet
- The intensity of temperature.
- Blood pressure
- General health
- Mental state
- External temperature

The typical normal volume of urine is 1-2 liters per normal adult.

2. Colour

The appearance of urine is the way it reflects. Some times colour of the urine also indicates the health condition of a person. It reveals an interesting and exciting medicinal quality of urine; typically it shows yellow amber. But generally it varies considerably according to recent and concentration of urine. Taking more quantity of water usually tends to reduce the concentration and therefore makes it to have a light colour. On the other hand, drinking less water generally tends to increase the concentration of urine thereby making it to have a dark colour.

The colour of urine in a way is affected by many factors like type of food, fatty, colours also. But normal human urine has a colour of lemon or butter. An infectious tropical diseases, and other diseases that make the urine turn in variant forms of yellow, fairly yellow, thick yellow, dark yellow, hard clear yellowish brown, yellowish brown colour.

Urine is a good indicator of hydration. Generally urine should be colourless. When there is too little water in the body it indicates bright yellow to orange urine. The water soluble like vitamins including B and C complex, temporarily the urine may turn into bright yellow colour.

3. Smell

The urine is the liquid that people can smell with their noses. It has the ability to produce smell. Human urine is chemical-mixed substance mixed with nutrients, with a very strong smell. As said earlier the smell of the urine of person on a day depends on the quality of diet one takes. Based on it, it may have an unpleasant odour a fishy, musty pungent, nasty house odour stench of rotten meat, stink of stole sweat, a neck of beer and tobacco or pleasant like a herb with a delicate fragrance. Generally, many people dislike mainly because of its odour, having unpleasant smell. The smell of urine may provide useful health-information.

For example, urine of a diabetic person may have the smell of fruity odour because of the presence of ketones, which are organic molecules of a particular structure. Similarly fresh urine has a strong odour, like the urine of a child. Urine containing ammonia has strong smell.

4. Acidity

The feature of urine having acidity is common. Acid is a chemical compound that contains hydrogen, which has a bitter sharp taste. It has the nature of having a sour taste because of containing acid which is generally unpleasant. Acid and Alkali are the two substance solutions in urine. A diet containing high proteins may result in more acidic urine. A vegetarian diet generally produces more alkaline. Urine PH is the measure of the acidity or alkalinity of a liquid. Pure water is natural. It means that it contains neither acid nor alkali called PH7. Urine may have strong alkali and strong acid.

5. Density

It is the degree to which urine is dense. It is dense like dense smoke, dense fume, dense population, indicating heaviness in relation to its size. It indicates the thickness of urine liquidity. It is also called specific gravity. Urine density is the ratio between the weight of a quantity of a urine substance and the weight of the same volume of distilled water.

Though urine is water, it contains some other substances. Nutrients in urine are dissolved in the water, so its density or thickness is dense or heavy. The density of normal urine is in the range of 0.001 to 0.035.

9

What are All Contained in Human Urine?

Is urine a waste product ? Does it contain anything? Urine contains something and many things. It has that thing, many things inside, inherent and part of it. What are they, very interesting to know. The urine bladder in which it is stored, a collection of valuable medical secrets of good health is extremely valuable to human beings. It has invaluable drugs, that are found hidden and extremely useful which is being extracted as waste product.

You may wonder to know, such things as follows:

1. Minerals

Natural human urine possesses mineral substances which are naturally present in the solution not formed from and matter outside. For example salt. Some minerals are also present in the food and water we take and in the human body collected in urine which are essential for good health, that otherwise go waste. The scientific study of urine analysis of minerals revealed these facts.

2. Hormones

A hormone is a chemical substance produced in the body which ends up as an integrated part of urine that actually encourages growth and influences the cells and tissues to function. A hormonal imbalance in the body may lead to many dangerous consequences. For instance, oestrogen is a female sex hormone. While hormonal changes are occurring during the pregnancy, urine therapy works as a hormone replacement therapy. During pregnancy, the urine is full of oestrogen and projestrogen hormones which are being extracted for preparing injections which is useful for infertile women. Other hormones contained in urine are catechol amines, hydroxy-steroids, 17-catasteroids, erythropoietine, adenylate cyclase, prostag landin's sex hormones, etc. Urine possesses other hormones called: Urokinase, erythropoietine, adenylate cyclase, prostaglandin, sex hormones, growth hormones, insulin, etc.

Professor Jean Rostande repeatedly stressed the biological singnificance of these substances known as hormones. The activity of hormones in urine which are filtered through the kidneys to pass out in urine has totally revolutionised the subject of urine-therapy.

The discovery of hormones has far-reaching benefit in curing many emerging incurable diseases. Multiples of hypophysical hormones, the hormones of the adrenal and hormones of sexual glands, urokinase, antineoplastons have been found in normal urine. Human urine possesses unlimited quality of substances having medicinal properties. From treatment point of view urine substances have fabulous power over the human organism.

Ellis Barher remarks, "Our body distils the most wonderful medicines and provides the most perfect serum and antibodies." Thus, today its use is identified in all forms of diseases: particularly it is sure-cure medicine for cancer, AIDS, etc.

There are over 100 other substances that are usually present. They have considerable medicinal value. The many other components of normal urine are the solubles that are dissolved in the water component of the urine. These can be divided into two categories according to their structure, size and electrical charge.

Production of hormones in the body requires lot of energy and time. Reusing means that readily available hormones can be reabsorbed which conserve energy, save time and improve immunity system. The energy required to produce new hormones can be conserved. Reintroducing into the body will have a favourable effect on the level of health and the level of resistance. Hormonal balance can naturally be maintained.

Yet another valuable hormone substance usually present in human urine is erythro-poietine. Its medicinal property is that it stimulates the bone marrow to increase the rate of production of erythrocytes, that is, red blood corpuscles. So, auto-urine therapy is beneficial to the patients of anaemia. A hormone present in urine is useful, because its substantial function is to coordinate the actions of all the hormones in the body through the production of a substance known as cyclic AMP. Prostaglandin is a hormone which in female is useful for the contraction of the muscles of the uterus, in which babies develop before they are born. According to some scientific studies, this hormone acts as a contraceptive also. Besides, urine contains sex hormones, insulin, and growth hormones.

It is believed that there is strong possibility of existence of several other hormones which are not yet discovered, and which are useful for treatment of many modern incurable ailments. Multiples of extremely small quantities of hormones and medical substances which are present in the urine have been found to be of great benefit to the body, if it is used properly.

3. Nutrients

Usual regular food along with self auto-urine therapy provides one a nutritionally balanced health. It is very good for you, as it contains many of the substances which help the body to grow. It is a tasty and nutrious solution.

Many people suffer from a serious nutrient deficiency which results in concerned disorders. Infact urine supplements nutrients. Urine contains a substance that is needed to keep a person alive and help to grow. Fully nutrients contained urine, when reintroduced into the body, it grows with ready made available nutrients from the urine. The practitioner will be well-nourished in good physical condition with regular drinking.

It is the food that is needed to stay alive, to develop and grow stronger, stay healthy. Many children starve due to lack of nourishment which results in ill-health because of lack of food or lack of right and balanced food. A poor condition of health is caused by lack of food or lack of right type of food.

For instance, we can find in urine calcium, creatinine, glucose, iodine, iron, nitrogen, inositol produced in certain quantities per day.

Dr A.H. Free published a book in the year 1975, titled "*Urinalysis in Clinical Laboratory Practice*" in which he presents a few nutrients found in urine. They are in milligrams per day, as follows:

Alanine, total	38	Argomome, total	32
Ascorbic acid	30	Allantion	12
Amino acids total	21	Bicarbonate	140
Biotin	35	Calcium	23
Creative	1.4	Cystine	120
Dopamine	0.40	Epinephrine	0.01
Folic acid	4	Glucose	100
Glutamic acid	308	Glycine	455
Inositol	14	Iodine	0.25
Iron	0.5	Isine, total	56
Magnesium	100	Manganese	0.5
Methionine, total	10	Nitrogen, total	15
Ornithin	10	Pantothenic acid	3
Phenylalanine	21	Phosphonus, total	9
Potasium	2.5	Proteins, total	5
Riboflavin	0.9	Tryptophan, total	28
Tyrosine, total	50	Urea	24.5
Vitamin B6	100	Vitamin B12	0.03
Zinc	1.4		

4. Vitamins

Vitamins are natural substances found in human urine that are very essential part of health which help us to grow and stay healthy. There are many different vitamins. Urine is rich in multiples of ample quantity of vitamins. Vitamin deficiency may lead to many health hazards. The vitamins that are available in urine are vital for health as they give full of energy, enthusiasm and freshness, which are legitimate, essential for staying alive. Urine contains proteins, vitamin B-6, B-12.

5. **Proteins**

Sufficient quantity of proteins are also essential for every one to eat which help them to grow and stay healthy. Urine naturally contains proteins. Protein is a natural substance usually found in meat, eggs, fish, some vegetables and also freely produced in the body through urine. There are many different proteins and they are essential. Essential protein deficiency is the main cause for health disorders or problems.

6. **Vitality**

Drinking one's own urine considerably enhances the vitality of a person. The vital components of urine are necessary for the physical body to be orderly and balanced and to keep healthy. It is vital that it keeps you in normal biological functioning state. The medicinal qualities are necessary not only for staying alive, but also for keeping wonderful freshness, vigour and exthusiasm.

7. **Enzyme**

Urine contains a biological substance usually produced by the body deposited in urine, which helps in happening a chemical change and happen more quickly, without changing itself.

8. **Metabolites**

Every body has its own metabolism which is strengthened up by the substances of urine. The metabolic process is a chemical series of steps in living things that converts or changes food into energy or life-force for growth. It turns food into new cells, energy and other produce, by means of chemical process.

9. **Carbohydrates**

Other substance that may be found in small amounts in normal urine are carbohydrates. It is a substance such as sugar or starch that consists of carbon, hydrogen and oxygen. Carbohydrates provide as bread, potatoes and rice that contain a lot of carbohydrates.

10. **Pigments**

A chemical substance which exists in natural urine gives skin a particular colour. The presence of pigments in skin that cause a person to be of particular colour. Every person appears in natural colour according to the character of pigments present in the body: for instance, pigments in skin, hair, leaves, etc.

11. **Mucins**

They are a group of large, heavily glycosylated proteins found in the urine.

12. Urine Constituent Substances

The liquid has multiples of rich drug qualities having therapentic value. A medicinal thing consisting of many sepatate things combined, intrinsic together. The urine is formed by a chemical reaction of many elements in fixed proportion relative to one another. For instance, common salt is a compound of sodium and chlorine. It is a water solution combination of different things, formed into a substance made by mixing other substances together.

The following are the average quantities of various substances in 100 milliliters of urine as reported in Introduction to Biochemistry by Dr Phron.

Urea nitrogen	682.00	Urea	1459.00
Creatinin nitrogen	36.00	Creatining	97.20
Uric acid nitrogen	12.30	uric acid	36.90
Amino nitrogen	9.70	Ammonia nitrogen	57.00
Sodium	212.00	Potasium	137.00
Calcium	19.50	Managanesium	11.30
Vhlotifr	314.00	Total sulphate	91.00
Inorganic sulphate	127.00	N/10 Acid	27.80

13. Colloids

In addition to the above multiple quantities of substances are found in plenty in urine which are useful for building immune function with therapeutic value. There are many invisible other constituents in urine. They are called "colloids" in blood. They are protits and somatids. They are very small particles. Much research attention had not been made in this area of study. As a matter of fact, these particles are very small, unfilterable by something like the most complex and intricate kidney process.

So, they naturally just got passed through the kidneys out of blood. With the help of these colloids incurable, degenerative diseases can be cured. When the urine is reingested into the body under urinetherapy, the body receives additional doses of these constituents of urine, and is able to prevent and cure numerous incurable ailments of human beings. The curing potentiality of these colloids has been proved by using modern scientific procedures. In this way experts say that urine is the body's own perfect medicine.

Urine contains 95 per cent of water.

14. Solubles

The other five per cent are solubles. Solutes are chemicals that are dissolved in the water. Some of these chemicals of the urine are the result of normal bio-chemical activity that takes place in the cells of the body. Other solubles are found due to chemicals originated outside the body such as modern medicinal drugs.

The Solubles found in human urine may be classified as follows:

(1) Ions, (2) Organic Molecules, (3) Inorganic molecules.

The nature of these solubles is briefly explained below to understand the structure of the urine.

1. Ion

It is an atom or a molecule with a positive or negative electric charge caused by its losing or gaining one or more electrons. Electorn is a very small piece of matter with a negative electric charge found in all atoms. Ion is a single element that is positively or negatively charged due to loss on acquisition of one or more electrons from or to the outer-levels of the atoms. Ions are atoms or groups of atoms that have either lost some outer electron, hence have a positive electric charge or have gained some outer electrons and hence have a negative electric charge. They have formed groups from only a small number of particles. They are:

I. Individual Elements

1. Sodium (Na),
2. Potassium (K),
3. Chloride (CI),
4. Magnesium (Mg),
5. Calcium (Ca)

II. Small Groups

1. Ammonium (NH4),
2. Sulphates (So),
3. Phosphates (H_2Po_4, HPO_4, PO_4).

2. Organic Molecules

A molecule is the smallest unit, usually consisting of a group of atoms, into which a substance can be divided without a change in its chemical nature. A molecule of water consists of two atoms of hydrogen and one atom of oxygen (H_2O). Organic chemicals mean natural chemicals produced by the body which the urine contains. It means not artificial chemical produced out side the body by using pharmaceutical drugs.

Natural human urine has several organic chemicals. Many atoms that have joined together form a group of atoms called "molecule". Organic molecules are formed from groups, rings, or chains of carbon atoms that are the 'building blocks' of the living things.

1. Urea (CON_2H_4 OR (NH_2)2 CO),
2. Creatinine,
3. Uric acid ($C_5H_4N_4O_3$),
4. Other substances and molecules.

By analysis of the urine, we can identify many substances found in normal urine. The biochemicals found in human urine are predominatly the end-products of nitrogens of metabolism process. These include urea, uric acid, and creatinine. Other components of urine include sodium chloride, i.e., common salt, etc.

10

Principles and Philosophy of Urinopathy

The practice, philosophy and principles of urinopathic medicine are based on the principles listed below. These principles are built up, based on the result of practice of urinopathic medicine.

1. Healing Power of the Body

The practice of urinopathy identifies and recognises the inherent ability of the individual's body to heal itself. It is based on the premises and the self-healing power of the body. It is in this way that serves the public and enriches the practice. It is the centuries-old knowledge of the body and understanding the health and human system and scientific knowledge of substances of human urine.

It is the role of urinopathic physician to know the medicinal and healing properties of the urine and enhance the self-healing process. It establishes, maintains and restores health. It is the patent's right as well as inherent responsibility for his own health. It is the inherent healing process in the person that is ordered by nature. So, the body is capable of healing itself. The urinopathic medicine removes obstacles to healing, recovers, facilitates and augments this inherent natural tendency of the body.

2. Treat a Cause

The allopathic approach is mainly concerned with to suppress, or masking symptoms of ailment than to eradicate the cause of malady. The urinopathic medicine seeks to treat the root cause, and remove the underlying cause of the disease rather than eliminating temporarily or surpressing symptoms.

For every illness, there will be root cause. Urinopathic medicine seeks to cure the causes of diseases. There are many causes for an illness like physical, mental, emotional, genetic, environmental, social and other factors like heredity, susceptibility, spiritual, personal, sensitiveness and risk factors. The multifactoral nature of human body demands a holistic medicine like urine. Urine medicine considers the whole person taking all these factors into consideration. It studies both the health as well as the disease. It removes the cause of illness.

Germs are not only the reason for any disease. They are present in every human healthy body. Disease may be produced by the weakened body's inability, accumulated toxins, incorrect life style, poor diet, improper care of the body, drugs and narcotics consumption, etc.

3. Do Not Harm

There is no harm in drinking one's own urine. It does no harm to the individual. So far no drinker of urine has reported any side-effects, after effects or ill-effects of auto-urine therapy.

But these effects are very much present in modern medicine, leading to destruction of one's own immune system, further resulting in degenerative, opportunistic infections like AIDS/HIV positive. It adopts no force or intervention to diagnose and treat, and repeat each individual's self-healing process. The urine substances minimises the risk of harmful effect of, and needs no human intervention. It stimulates the patient's vital force to promote healing, supplementing and replacing the function of the vital force.

No risk of side effects, least human intervention in treatment.

4. No Risk of Side Effects

The duty of a doctor is to educate the patients about the damages of a drug and drugless drug, which is of priority. They have to show something how to do for, keep health good, so that they will be able to do it themselves, and persuade natural, self-healing, priceless way, have a good health and normal living, to take responsibility for their own health. But not to prescribe a drug repetitively. The physicians also encourage our traditional, body made medicine and the therapeutic potential of human urine. He educates the patient the self-responsibility for one's own health. It has powerful therapeutic potential.

5. Treating the Whole Person

The basic principle of urine therapy is that it has a holistic approach to life. The urine as a medicine treats the whole body of an individual but not a part or organ or sub-system of the body. It treats the complete body of a person rather than just the symptoms, effects of a disease. Urine as a medicine is considered healthy, because it is in a simple form, has not been refined or made in a factory with materials, and does not contain artificial substances.

It is like whole food, whole grain and considers every thing in general. It is a medicine that is complete in itself. In fact, it treats for the total health including physical, mental, emotional, genetic, environmental, social, spiritual and other relevant factors. Urine takes care of harmonious and amicable functioning of all aspects of the individual. It considers all factors of the body and make ups a person's whole life and safeguards his health and well-being.

6. Prevention

The underlying philosophy of urine therapy lies in its act of prevention of illness happening to the body. It will not recognise to deal with the problem primarily after it has affected the body. Urine is preventive medicine and avoids possible affection, compared to curative medicines.

The principle is based on a proverbial saying that "Prevention is better than cure". The urine ingested into body, acts to create a healthy environment for an individual and prevents illness to the body. Human body is susceptible easily to ailment and urine intervenes always and releases antibodies to prevent diseases.

11

Top Ten Reasons To Urinopathy

1. Do you want a natural health management package for you?
2. Are you concerned about reactions, danger of drugs, side effects, after effects, ill effects of modern medicine?
3. Do you want optimal health, wellness, bodys' performance, protection of your immunity system resistance power?
4. Do you want fact sheet of natural healing power of your body ?
5. Do you want to get back to balance of your derailed hormonal, nervous, detoxification, elimination, bio-mechanism, bio-dynamism and mental predisposition?
6. Do you know, today more people than ever before are seeking Indian alternative medical health care approaches than pharmaceutical medicine?
7. Are you informed choices about what type of remedies will be most functional and beneficial to your health?
8. Do you know that your body has such a powerful, innate, instinct, self-healing ability? And how to remove the barriers to your self-healing ?
9. Do you know how to eat, what to eat, exercise, relax, stressless living and nurture yourself physically and emotionally?
10. How does urinopathic medicine act as panacea for modern ailing human race?

12

Methods of Using Urine

1. Oral

Ingestion means taking through mouth. Urine is clear, safe and drinkable. There are many urine drinkers who consume regularly like coffee, tea or beer. It can be drinkable in repugnancy cases mixed with milk, water or juice, with some fragrance. Oral consumption is a very common practice for many people like soft drink. Many have a drinking problem because of its colour, taste and smell. Hence, they hesitate. I wish something good luck to drink, health or misery as you lift your glass and then drink it. Drink up and let us live healthily.

Come on, drink up your nectar juice, Which is like manna from heaven.

2. Massaging

Fresh urine or stored urine can be used for massaging, rubbing and pressing a person's body with the hands, to reduce or relieve the pain in the muscles and joints. Urine massage helps the pain-aching muscles, and make them feel better than before. Pour urine or sprinkle on troubled part of the body and move hands on it backward and forward over a surface, pressing firmly. By doing so, it relieves pain in joints, shoulders, elbows, nose etc. At the same time it enters into the body through skin hair holes and works like medicine.

It can be used for treating skin disorders, with short-period massaging. Later it should be washed off immediately after 20-30 minutes with warm water.

Boiled urine is best for massaging. Boiled urine gets reduced to 1/4th of original volume.

This is light and fine extraction, concentrated and excellent for massaging.

3. Sniffing

Yet another way of using urine for medicinal purpose is urine sniffing. It means to breath the urine in, through the nose either by making a sound or without making sound. while breathing urine in through the nose, you enjoy its smell and find difference in your sense of smell.

Sniffing the fresh morning urine is the best medicine. The habit of breathing in the urine prevents and cures nose problems, disorders like sinus, nose congestions etc. Cold is a common illness that affects the nose and or throat making you cough, sneezing etc.

The air that comes suddenly and noisily out through your nose and mouth in a way that you cannot control is a common complaint of a ill person, because he has a cold. You will be sneezing all through the day. For cough and violent sneezing problems urine is good enough to be accepted and to be practised seriously.

Any hollow space in the bones of the head that is connected to the inside of the nose is a symptom of disease known as sinus disease. It gives a painful swelling of the sinuses, called sinusitis, blocked sinuses.

One's own urine is an effective medicine which relieves nasal congestion, track blocked with blood muscles or other material, Nasal is an organ connected with the nose gives nasal passage the blocked passage will be cleared by urine. An illness or cough, when you have cold, makes you cough often is a common seasonal disorder.

Its other forms are coughing nervously, hooping cough, bronchiatic cough, forcing out air suddenly and noisily through your throat can effectively be curved by sniffing urine.

When urine is inhaled through the nose, it cleans the upper part of the bronchial tube.

4. Bathing

One can do bathe with urine by mixing it with water. You put the water in and then wash your whole body by using bath tub or container. Fill the bath tub with water. It is an act of washing your whole body by sitting or lying in water mixed with urine, water mixed with urine becomes a liquid solution that smells pleasant and will not make lot of bubbles like soap bath. It is a bath which is better than bubble bath in the water as it is more hygienic and antiseptic. All skin disorders disappear and the skin becomes soft and shining.

You can wash your hands, legs or any part. A long container or bath-tub with urine liquid mixed with water, whole of the body can be washed. Remain in it for a short period of time.

When you wash your body with it you can say that you have bathed with urine which is called urine bath. You can also bathe another person for example a baby, clean a wound or swim in the urine pool. Bathe everyday to be healthy and beautiful.

In Japan many modern Japanese women are said to engage in urine bathing. In the seventeenth century Aristocratic French women reportedly bathed in urine to beautify their skin.

5. Urine Pack

For treatment of wounds and other skin disorders urine pack method can be used for external application. A strip of fabric or surgical cotton soaked in urine can be used for dressing a part of the body that has been hurt in order to protect or support or cure it. A urine pack can be used to wrap a bandage around the affected area, because it is injured wound, burnt, infection etc. Do not tie the bandage around the wound too tightly but gently tie for safety. A piece of soft material that absorbs liquid can be used for treating.

Also dip piece of cotton in urine for some time, so that it becomes completely wet, after absorbing urine and wrap the soaked cloth around the wounded part.

The wet cotton pack absorbed with urine is used to cure parts of the body that are injured, wounded or infected. Please pour urine drops frequently to keep it wet, and to prevent drying put the urine pack on the wounded body part and take off after a prescribed period of time. You can certainly find the improvement.

6. Gargle

It is a gargling process, putting small quantity of urine and to gargle in order to wash inside your mouth and throat. It is to move the urine around the mouth and at the back of your throat for some time and spitting it out. So urine can be used for gargling as it has antiseptic character. Gargle urine mixed with salt also. Please hold urine firmly and use force in order to move the urine to all sides. All kinds of throat inflammation can be solved by gargling with urine.

Urine should be kept in the mouth as long as possible as per convenience but not less than 15-30 minutes. To fight gum problem, tongues and other mouth disorders, gargling with fresh urine is an effective and priceless easy self therapy. Gum disease of either of the firm areas of flesh in the mouth to which teeth are attached is the common problem.

7. Washing

Every one has to keep body clean, no smell, swat smooth, fresh and protect from skin disorders and infections. For this we are spending much for soaps, creams, lotions, medicine etc. We can use drugless free drug to make body clean using urine and usually without shampoo or soap. You can wash your hands, legs, face, dirty hair, wounds, injuries and make yourself clean and hygienic. It can be washed without losing colour or being damaged. This swat washes the skin removes marks by washing.

8. Injecting

It is the process where urine is injected into a person's body by using a syringe. It is like:

Injecting oneself with insulin

Injecting adrenalin into muscle

Treating with penicillin injection

Administering anesthesia by injection.

When urine is injected into the body, it is like injecting fuel, energy, force nutrients, hormones etc., into the body.

Dr Salaria, a popular surgeon , Ahmedabad, Gujarat, India practised this method and gave injection of the patient's own urine before undertaking surgery.

The object is to forestall any risk of overburdening or harming the heart during or after the surgery.

9. Enema

In this method urine is put by a separate tube, like saline solution, into a person's rectum . Rectum is the opening through which solid waste leaves the body. Enema is given in order to clean out the bowels. The objectives are:

- Giving especially before medical operation.
- Cleaning out the bowels.
- Administering in a condition of being unable to get rid of waste material from bowels easily, a case of constipation.

In the case of a person who is suffering from chronic ailment, poisonous substances are found in tissues, intestines. It means he has a high level of toxicity. The best method is administering urine enema that removes, sweeps out poisonous materials from the body, tissues, intestines etc. The body easily absorbs a number of readily available vital substances deposited in the urine.

10. Complementary to Each Other

Method of using urine either for prevention or treatment can broadly be divided into two categories. Thus based on the observation as to how to use, they are :

Urine Therapy

Internal application External application

Both the methods are complementary to each other methods that are complementary and different but together form a useful and holistic combination of qualities. Therefore, we can use one or two or more than two methods depending on the need and the nature of ailment. All are equally important for optimal result. These are only different ways to applying urine.

13

Medicinal Secrets of Urine and How it Works

1. Prevention

A saying goes "An ounce of prevention is better than a pound of cure", or "Prevention is better than cure".

To protect and prevent from affecting or stopping from happening illness or disorder is always a wise person's life style. It is better to be always healthy and normal living rather than to swallow medicine to deal with the problem after it has generated. Regular urine drinking acts as a preventive medicine and avoids all possible common, chronic ills. Urine therapy is intended to prevent ailments that cause problems and health difficulties. It works out against occurring diseases.

2. Treatment

Human urine has an ability of therapeutic character, and its oral taking or massaging makes a user healthy again after an illness, It cures any bodily ailment. Even serious illnesses like T.B., psoriasis, sinus, skin diseases can be cured successfully. It is a natural medicine or medical treatment that cures an illness, there is no known cure but ailments can be treated. Urine is something that will solve problems of health situation. It behaves mysteriously in a particular way towards illnesses, gives a medical cure, or attention to a disorder, an injury, infection, etc. It uses its own chemical substances or elements and proceeds to clean, protects, preserves, treats in its own way, responds well to treatment in innumerable and incurable illnesses.

3. Immunity

The simple scientific principle working behind the efficacy of urine therapy is that, by drinking one's own urine one can develop immunity of the body which is the basic and urgent need for every person to be prevented from any disease. Urine contains many proteins, nutrients, minerals, hormones, vitamins, enzymes, metabolites. When these are introduced into the body they increase the immunity. Particularly it is very essential in the case of AIDS patients. So, it cannot catch on to be affected by a particular disease or illness.

One will eventually become immune to disorders. He will be protected from affecting diseases and therefore be able to avoid, the reaction of the body to the presence of an antigen of the body to the presence of an antigen or a substance that can cause disease to be strong.

An immune system, the system of your body that produces substances to help in fighting against infections, diseases or disorders, the human urine acts as a vaccine and provides longer immunity against any illness. It promotes the condition of being protected from diseases.

4. Auto-immune

Urine develops and preserves auto-immunity system. An auto-immune disease or medical condition is one which is caused by urine that usually prevents illness, disorders, and problems.

5. Healer of the Last Resort

Urine as a therapeutic measure that the people follow is called the last resort or first choice. In fact many people do not prefer urine therapy as first choice, but in case of dreaded diseases like cancer, asthma, etc., the patients are preferring urine medicine as last course of action that he should or can take in a particular incurable diseases, as a life saving measure patients come forward to drink as a last resort when all attempts, measures, therapies and pathies have failed. At the most basic level, what really moves us is our personal conviction and need.

So, it is natural to resort to or make use of sure-cure urine therapy as a means of solving the problem, because there is no other possible alternate solution. They feel obliged to resort to something discarded as waste. Prevention is better than cure. Instead of taking risk, wasting of time, money and efforts, we must make it a point to make urine therapy as our first choice. When all else fail the patient takes refuge in urine therapy.

6. Detoxification

When you drink urine, the urine inside the body undertakes biological function of detoxifying or removing all harmful substances or poisons from the body. It treats and keeps the internal organs of the body in order and keeps them pure, clean without dirty. Our responsibility is not just to dump stomach with food and non-food stuffs, but is also our bounded duty to keep the bowel, intestines and alimentary canal clean, neat and tidy. By eating and drinking indiscriminative food items, many harmful substances, gases and foreign materials get accumulated in the body and are deposited in different locations of the body. It is the function of the urine to remove all the dirty, poisonous things from the body that are unnecessary, unwanted and need changing and process of cleansing.

It makes you clean the inside house thoroughly, healthily and in good condition.

Urine is a cleansing agent. During detoxification and cleaning process, the excess mucus from the lungs bronchial tubes will go out.

7. Antidote

'Anti' means opposed to or against. The quality of being preventing, killing, freeing. It denotes that urine acts like an effective antibiotic treatment, for instance urine substances, for example like penicillin, it can destroy or prevent the growth of bacteria, cure infections.

Urine is anti-body, anti-infection, anti-bacterial, anti-septic, anti-viral, anti-cancer, anti-poison, anti-convulsive, anti-fungal, anti-neoplaston, anti-carlivogenic, anti-spasmodic, etc.

Substances that the body produces are deposited in the urine and in blood which fight against diseases is called anti-body agent. Many substances that enter the body and which cause diseases are called antigens. The body then usually produces antibodies to fight against the antigens. The human urine produces antibody medicine and fights against disease-causing substances.

8. Natural Vaccine

A vaccine is a factory-made substance that is put into the body or blood by injection, oral or by other means to protect the body from a disease.

Children are vaccinated against hepatitis-B.

Children are vaccinated against – Polio.

Children are vaccinated against – Measles.

To protect a person or an animal from a disease people are given immunisation especially by giving them an injection of a vaccine. In modern science, a new branch has emerged known as immunology, which is a scientific study of protection against disease.

Human urine acts as a natural vaccine, inoculation, immunisation, immunity refiller and its regular use prevents against serious illnesses.

9. Transformation

Urine is a medium of body transformer, reduces or increases the potential of physical strength or force. It changes the form and structure of a person. The physiological, biological and metabolic processes and reactions transform the body from defect base to disorder free physic. In due course of time, it completely changes the person's outside appearance, internal function and character of a urine practitioner so that he will be quite better than he was earlier. Its continuous process would transform a person quite differently. The way in which he looks would undergo a complete transformation over a period of time.

What is transformation? You wonder! You look different!

Urine when reingesting into the body means an act of putting vigour in a place or activity that needs it because of deficiency syndrome.

10. Deageing Tonic

One's own urine is a nature's elixir, most effective as deageing tonic ever known to mankind, but yogis of ancient times knew about this secret. The secret of longevity of life of *yogis* is the fabulous medicinal quality of urine. It makes a person remain fresh, or last longer than the non-drinkers of urine. Thus, a long life with both health and longevity can be achieved.

The number of years that a person lives without disease, decay, and figure change is possible if he practises urine therapy. Inspite of being old, old age symptoms do not appear. You do not look your age to seem as old as you really are but look young and fresh. Urine is as good as tonic as it builds vitality, vigour and strength.

For instance, the secret of longevity and exuberant health of Morarji Desai, the former Prime Minister of India, is his long practice of urine therapy. A centenarian, he lived for nearly 100 years healthily. One can live with full energy excitement and happiness being strong, young and youthful.

There are hormones in the urine which have non-ageing-properties, yet to be fully explored.

11. Restoration

Human urine assumes its natural biological functions and does the work of repairing and cleaning the body. Due to ageing the body is subject to lose stamina, strength and vitality. Its act of bringing the body back to the original status is a wonderful and miraculous work of the urine. The act of restoring from defects, torn out things to their correct place or keeping in original condition is the fabulous quality of the urine.

Drinking or external application makes you feel strong and the body light and healthy again. The restorative power of the intrinsic medicine is connected with treatment that repairs the body or organ or any part of it. It brings the body-situation or feeling back to that, which existed before.

Those who are taking urine are now fully restored to normal health. It makes damaged skin as beautiful as it was to be, so that it looks as good as it did originally. It is the job of the urine to repair damaged body. For instance, a scar that is left on the skin after a wound which has been healed, would also disappear.

12. Reconstruction

Drinking of urine as a regular habit has a useful and helpful effect on the body rather than being negative, unfavourable or with no purpose. Its work is involved in helping hyperactivity in people to use their energy more. Urine is encouraging all organs of the body to play their effective role in the reform process. The substances of the urine are properly utilised in order to improve the physical system by making changes, alteration, modifications and correcting defects. As reformer, it makes a constitutional change, far-reaching and sweeping reforms in the entire body.

As reformist urine assumes the role to rebuild, or make any part, organ, torn out tissues, dead cells, makes again that has been damaged or that no longer exists. The recycling, transmutation process of the body helps in changing or improving the condition, or the way the body works. The activity of rebuilding again that has been damaged, destroyed or defunct is a marvelous medicinal wonder of the urine. A medical treatment involves reconstructing parts of the person's body because it has been badly damaged or because the person wants to change his shape, form and colour.

13. Preservation

Regular practice of taking urine keeps the body's health, strength and keeps life force in their original state or in good condition. The extent to which the body would not change or damage by age, use, work, strain to which the body is subjected. It acts as self-preservation of protecting oneself in dangerous or difficult situation to which one is exposed. The practitioner who drinks will keep his body in his original condition long and prevents it from deterioration or early collapse. Urine contains such substances, compounds which prevent body from disease, decaying, figure change and premature death.

The solution contains nature's preservative and elixir. It makes sure that body is kept in a particular quality, figure, longevity, exuberance, safety from harm.

14. Natural Stimulant

Human urine is a drugless natural drug containing compounds that make you feel more awakened and gives you more energy. It is like tea or coffee which have mild stimulant. Urine has a natural substance which activates you more. In day to day social, economic and live pursuits, events, activities it encourages to participate more actively, makes everything more interesting and exciting about life events. The women are given fertility drugs, or injections from hormones isolated and extracted from urine to stimulate the ovaries.

It solves the problem of infertility of couples. It makes the drinkers feel enthusiastic, healthy as it works in sensory intellectual, auditory, sexual, verbal, visual, emotional as well as physical stimulation. It is a substance something like stimuli that produces a reaction in human beings like a stimulus agent.

15. Strengthening the Body

To do some work, the quality of being physically strong is an essential quality. To produce hormones, life-force, power a lot of time, energy, fuel and biological work is necessary. The life-force substances so produced are ending up in urine and being wasted by excretion. It may take a few hours or days for the body to produce them again. If you do not have strength to work, face force, hold heavy weight, or to do work the body gets damaged or weakened. The quality of work depends on the quality and quantity of strength. So, already produced force or fuel readily available in the urine should be conserved by putting it back into the body without wasting.

The strength of the body can be doubled by reutilising one's own urine. The power, strength, the life force of urine is very strong. The strength of the body is measured by how much physical energy is used by something, or work, effort, thinking, or emotion.

16. Specific Medicine to Specific Body

Urine is a specific medicine to specific body derived according to the individual's physical, biological and physiological characteristics. It is made and meant for him only, for his personality. It is just the right-medicine for the right person that what his body needs at a particular moment. The quantity and composition of urine often changes all the time according to metabolism. The biological and chemical analysis of one's own urine reveals a lot about the conditions of the body concerning general health and also specific medical conditions. A complete urine test is commonly used to diagnose the cause of his disease or disorder. So, one's own urine is the best medicine.

A diamond cuts a diamond, poison cures poison, likewise bodily diseases are cured by one's own bodily substances. All the systems and sub-systems of the body are interconnected, interlinked with blood flow stream and this means that the medicinal substances of blood will have a positive effect on all parts of the body.

17. Regeneration

The medicinal quality of the urine is that it has the ability to make any area, part, organ of the body develop and grow strong again which suffered adversely due to some illness, infection or disorder. The inherent-multiple substances of the urine like proteins, hormones, enzymes, etc., will be used to regenerate the lost one. It stimulates the cells of the body tissues and the skin to glow again and regenerate. If cells, skin or scar is left alone urine regenerate itself in a few months/days.

18. Resistance

The strength of the body of urine drinker is so strong, it usually refuses to accept something unfavorable or disorder and try to stop it from happening. It resists change to not be harmful or damaged by disease causing factors, a nutrient healthy drink would help your body resist from infections, flew, etc. It is the power of the urine as antibody not to be affected by something disorder. Drinkers are resistant to disease, urine is disease-resistant agent, not damaged by the antigen, a resistant agent, a resister.

19. Cosmetic uses

Urine can effectively be used for cosmetic purposes. It is a solution can be put on your face or body to make it more attractive. It improves the outside appearance of the personality. Urine is so intimately connected with medical treatment that it is intended to improve a person's appearance. No need to use costly cosmetic products or going for cosmetic surgery.

20. Moderniser

The dietary style, life style, living style and various other causes are responsible which make our body now outmoded, defected, disordered, as a result of which multi-organ malfunctioning leads to innumerable and incurable diseases. The physical structure becomes weak, delicate, and no longer useful to live healthy. Regular urine drinking modernises the body makes it fashionable and removes all defects and disorders. It eradicates all root causes of the malady instead of just suppressing the symptoms of the diseases.

21. Body Renovation

The medicinal secret of urine is a wonder whomsoever is the drinker, a child, young, adult, old. It has efficacy to repair the body to the extent damaged, so that it is kept in good condition and restore original status. It rebuilds torn out tissues and cells by strengthening them. Everybody needs renovation at the time of ageing.

22. Refilling Energy

We are spending everyday physical, mental and emotional efforts, using energy to do work, to think and to be emotional, Urine deposits continue to be regular source of power supply, life force supplying energy. It is like a fuel, used for driving a machine, a vehicle, providing heat or steam. So, it is important to store energy that is being refilled by additional intake.

The reintroduced urine has ability to put, spent effort and enthusiasm into an activity, work, thinking or emotion, It is not a waste product, but an energy product. A person who drinks urine will have always full of energy supply. Additional energy is produced by not wasting human excrement.

23. Rejuvenation

Internal or external application of urine makes one look or feel younger, or more lively resulting in rejuvenation of skin.

24. Urine–A Holistic Medicine

Natural human urine is considered as a whole medicine or being to be more than a collection of parts, Hence, urine therapy is recognized a holistic approach to the health or life of a person. As a holistic medicine, urine treats the whole person rather than just the symptoms of a disease.

Holistic is the measure of its ability to improve whole health and well-being. The urinopathic medicine usually takes a holistic approach where the physical, mental, spiritual, emotional and most often social well beings of an individual are treated. This therapy on the other hand is relatively focussed more not on any particular disease based on specific symptom; it considers health in terms of both physical and mental well-being.

25. A Panacea

The medical secret of human urine is that it has the character of efficiency and efficacy that will prevent, treat, and solve all human health problems of a particular body. It possesses the quality of being able to do wonders in the body in a confident and conspicuous way and that is the reason why that people find attractive, to think about and try a decide what is true, what will happen, why we should not practise as the last resort at least, but first choice preferable.

14

Quality and Taste

Quality

Qualitatively, human urine is quite different when compared with some other water solutions. How good urine is rather than how much of urine is there? There are many qualitative differences between water and urine.

What is the standard of the human excreta when it is compared to water like it? How good or bad is urine? Is good? Poor? Top quality?

Urine is a by-product of a blood, a thing that is a part of a person's biology, especially something good.

The qualitative analysis of urine reveals that it is:

Pure, clean, crystal, hygienic, mineral-based, transparent, clear, and filtered water.

As Good As Well or Tap Water

It is not mixed with any other unnecessary and useless things. Nothing is added 100 per cent pure watery solution.

Clean and not contained any harmful substances. Not dirty. Clean and tidy. It has a clean appearance, and clean surroundings, free from dangerous or unpleasant substances or materials. Clean drinking water.

Hence, drinking one's own urine is not offensive, not disgusting, no need to hate. By doing so, we are not doing anything that is considered immoral or bad or illegal or unnatural. It is not against law, not prohibited by any legislation, customs, practice and not unclean. As clean as a tap or well water or so called mineral water sold in the market.

The kidneys, nephrons undertake a difficult and complicated biological process to make urine from dirt or dust by washing or rubbing, to become clean. They remove things that are not necessary or wanted.

It is the responsibility of the kidneys, nephrons to remove all the things from the mixture particles of food and water we take that are thought to be unnecessary or needed changes to the body requirements at a particular point of time.

Easy to see through, transparent, that one can see through. So clear, we can see the bottom of the glass. Neat liquid.

It is hygienic because it is clean and free from of bacteria and therefore unlikely to cause or spread disease when reingested into the body. It is also prepared in the body in a very hygienic conditions and internal environment, clean in order to prevent illness or disease.

Urine is pure mineral water, because it contains substances that are normally present in the body, blood, such a water cannot be produced or duplicated in a man made factory outside the body except in the body.

Some minerals are also present in food, and water we take, and in the human body which are essential for good health and normal living. Mineral water as the people usually use in commercial market must mean water from a Spring in the ground that contains mineral salts or gases. A glass or bottle of mineral water sold in railway stations, but stations or drink shops are not truly mineral water.

It is filtered water because it is passed through blood filter process, but not a waste filtered in order to remove any material that are not wanted to the body nutrition.

Taste

Tasting, smelling or looking are pleasant and fresh urine has a clean taste and a lovely golden colour. A watery solution. You can notice in it is only slightly salty taste.

The taste of the urine normally depends upon the quality of food and water we take. If spices of various types of powders or seed come from plants and are used in cooking naturally the taste and smell are quite strong and bitter. Because spicy have a strong taste and smell. Spices such as ginger, cinnamon cardamom and others we all use variety in our diet for taste and flavour, they make urine strong and bitter.

When oils, fats, non-vegetarian items are added the urine slightly tastes variously. But using less salt, and proteins in making diet ensure your urine tastes and smells milder. A diet low in proteins and salt in general is essential for good health and normal living. Particularly fried and fatty foods definitely makes your urine strong, bitter and smells, tastes badly.

The smell and taste make people to vomit, when urine is of unusual taste, strong and unpleasant food and water from the stomach is brought back out through mouth. Sometimes drinking one's own urine is extremely uncommon and unpleasant. By practice the urine will quickly become thinner and taste more pleasant. But vomiting is not a sign as bad urine therapy practice. It is very common, vomiting cleans in a way the stomach no need to worry. Continue to do. Do not stop.

Urine is usually yellow and clear. It largely depends on a person's health and diet. It gives an ammonia-like odour due to the nitrogenous wastes. The type of certain unusual foods we take also greatly influences on odour. It has a slightly acid fluid.

15

Is Human Urine Poisonous–NO

There is a lot of misunderstanding and confusion in the minds of many people regarding whether urine is toxic? Poisonous? I think people are noticing that something bad is present, and that something may happen. Young generation people are more culturally, with family practices, environmentally not aware much more than their parents or ancestors.

There is the deep-rooted doubt in the minds of the people that is to be cleared.

Please bear in mind that "urine is not a toxic substance". Toxic substance, if at all exists, it is an insignificant quantity, for it is being removed from the body through liver, intestines, skin and through exhalation. When the blood is filled with nutrients it passes through the liver and at that stage only, the toxics are filtered. If we assume that urine drink is poisonous and harmful, we have to equally assume that it is harmful when it is present in the body, since it comes out of the body only. Therefore, the primary piss is not at all toxic. The amount of urea substance in urine is to some extent is poisonous that too when it is present in very large proportion in the blood. As against hundreds of substances found in urine, only the urea is poisonous that too when it is deposited in the blood.

One must understand the parts and functions of them to know whether urine contain poison or not. A liver is a large organ in the body that produces the bile and cleans the blood. In the process, its function is detoxification of blood. It removes all poisonous substances from the blood. They end up as bile in the intestinal canal, thus they leave the body, get rid of solid waste from your body through bowels called defecation.

Likewise poison-free blood alone flows to the kidneys.

There is no any scientific reason to believe that urine is a poisonous waste product. It is only an opinion of a layman, the belief is not based on fact. It has been scientifically proved that it is not poisonous and hence not harmful to drink.

I have already mentioned elsewhere in this book that urine contains mainly minerals, hormones, enzymes and many others which cannot be procured, produced or duplicated from outside the body. It is a watery solution with full of vital substances and only water, a healthy liquid which is filtered out of the blood stream.

What at one stage and time was part of the blood can turn to be the urine a split second later at next stage. Many vital substances are then filtered by the kidneys, with a complex process of nephrons and secreted as by-product . It is a raw material which can be directly absorbed by the body upon reintroduction into the body,

Any insignificant poison in our food and water we have taken, will be taken care of by the liver, intestines, skin and exhalation and sent out of the body. The poison will not enter into bloodstream. As well it is not the only function of the kidneys to remove poisonous substances from the body.

So, the food and urine we take form the urine we excrete which is poison–free and is a healthy diet. God has deposited in human body the most advanced and intelligent self mechanism by which the body makes selection between good and bad and makes selection accordingly. Only useful things are absorbed and get rid of solid waste from your body through bowels. The intestines also assume the function of selection, purification and cleansing.

Human urine is free not only from bacteria, but also anti-bacteria. In the body are present natural poison and bacteria, but they are not causing any harm at all.

As a matter of fact it is body made out of what we have eaten foodstuffs, liquids as such we will not die as if a person dies by taking poison. All the ingredients of the urine are being tested scientifically, and it is nowhere reported that urine is poisonous. The substances so far isolated and extracted are found to be more useful having medicinal value.

Urea contained in urine is toxic no doubt, only when it is in high quantity. The fact that urine contains very minute quantities of toxin. In average person's volume, it causes no chance of poisoning, it causes no one will die. Millions of people throughout the world are taking, not even a single case of death, nor any adverse side effects, after effects or ill effects are reported to urino-therapy.

16

Is Urine a waste Product–No

A Manna from Heaven–Urine is a By-product of Blood

One's own urine excrete is neither a waste product nor poisonous. How can the thing that is pissed out be of any benefit for our health? That is the question. In fact, urine is nothing but a blood product.

Urine is not toxic waste product. It is not only claimed by the urine practitioner, but also scientifically proved. Urinalysis by a chemist revealed that it is full of proteins, nutrients, minerals, vitamins, hormones, enzymes and metabolites, etc. It is explained in detail else-where in this book.

Scientific studies have proved that urine contains 95 per cent of water, 2.5 per cent urea, and 2.5 per cent of it is a mixture of valuable hundreds of substances nutrients chemicals and solubles.

Urine is a by-product of blood, but not the by-product of a waste material. If urine is a waste, blood is also to be considered as waste, but it is not the case. Urine is a blood derivative.

Now a days there is no a product which is said to be a waste. A product is said to be a waste product which is useless material or the substance produced while making something else. A body is not a waste paper basket, or a container for waste material.

Urine is said to be a waste, when any substance produced by it cannot be used or is no longer used for the well being of the body. It is not a waste but it can be used more than present. But we are not saving, conserving, recycling it, eventhough it could actively be used.

When urine is reintroduced into the body, the hormones, nutrients that exist in the urine are transpierced into the blood stream which is very useful for strength and vitality of a person. We can say that it is a waste only when it does not produce the results that you expected. It is needed for further use and therefore should not be thrown away. When it is not suitable for building or growing cells, tissues, vitality, strength and health, we can say urine is not useful and hence a waste product.

Urine excretion as a call of nature is not a process of getting rid of waste product. But it is an item not required by the body at a particular point of time or for the needs of the body. It is surplus or excess for the time being.

Hence, it is excreted. Urine is not like a household waste, industrial waste, toxic or radio-active wastes to be ignored or thrown out.

We have to see good from urine. Otherwise it is a situation in which it is not worth spending lot of money on food stuffs and drinking water since urine is a by-product of them. It is not used in a way that it should be. Something therapeutic value is there, it is recognised, not valued, or used in the way it should be. We are not making full use of our own useful and valid material.

Urine: A Blood filtration Not Waste Filtration

Blood Derivative

The efficiency and efficacy behind urine therapy is quite simple and persuasive because it has a therapeutic quality since it is derived by blood filtration, but not a waste filtration. As already mentioned it is a by-product of blood. In medical literature it is referred to as 'plasma ultra filtrate'.

It is a wrong notion to regard urine as merely a waste product rejected and excreted by the body. In fact urine is a by-product of blood filtration. All the substances usually found in blood are equally deposited in urine also.

Urine is a substance purified derivative of the blood which passed several stages from intestines, lever, processed by complex and intricate kidney system and cleaned by nephrons. What is blood at a moment, is at next minute turns as watery solution. It is like a factory which distils and bottles whisky, or alcoholic drinks. A body which makes urine, when the blood filled with nutrients, pass through the liver, the purified blood then travels to the kidneys where excess nutrients are eliminated from the body.

There is little wastage in the nature. Urine is a part of the blood filtered. Since it leaves the body by excretion, we consider it as waste. But medical science cannot assume it as a waste. For long we have neglected, hated, ignored it as a waste. We just feel as if you want vomit, you are assuming a feeling, a psychological weakness, as if you want to vomit. Simply because the smell of it nauseates you, makes you feel disgusted. Verily, blood contains many invaluable substances in excess or much more than requirement to the body. In such a situation it is the function of the kidneys to maintain balance between all the substances in the blood. So, kidneys remove by filtration process all vital substances and surplus water, which are present more than the body needs or wants at a time.

These vital substances and surplus water filtered out by the kidneys, subsequently form as urine. Such urine is composed of unused, not needed enzymes, minerals, proteins, nutrients, vitamins, hormones and other vital substances as found in blood. As a result, urine is found to be full of vital elements, which can hardly be called as "waste" product but the vital by-product of blood. Why kidneys filter? In order to save energy and bring back the blood into balance, the kidneys remove only the unused vital substances and surplus water. Urine contains many other waste products but in very minute quantities. They are called a waste but it does not mean that these substances are toxic or harmful. The function of the kidneys is not just to filter, but it has a regulatory, and balancing activity. Kidneys diligently retain, balance what is useful and dispose of everything else deemed dispensable and of no use.

The word "waste" simply means that the body does not require them at a particular point of time, and hence cannot absorb those so called waste, but are surplus substances at the present time. They are not left over from the blood as we have left-over from a meal. The body may use them later if they are again ingested into the body by the process of recycling and transmutation mechanism. So, one's own urine is not likely to be harmful or dangerous, as people believe, but it is likely to be useful or healthy if we use it again. Urine contains readymade valuable hormones, so it is an easier way, have medicinal use, to be introduced healthful urine into one's blood streams.

Urine excretion mechanism of the body is not the body's way of getting rid of things it does not want, and cannot contain harmful toxics. If food and water when they are too much not useful to the body, then the body will excrete excess. As the body does not want any more at present time, it is good to re-eat, or re-drink the same. Nothing will happen to the body when you consume your own urine. Very insignificant amount of toxics, if at all exist in urine are not abundant enough to be toxic to the body. Certain amount of toxics are needed to the body because they stimulate a cleansing process in the body and do motivational function.

The ingested urine does not go directly to the blood stream. It goes through a complex and intricate lengthy system of normal process of recycling and transmutation. When it goes into the digestive system, all ingredients are sorted out, classified, graded, recycled and all toxics are rejected automatically by the body at that lower stage only. It becomes more purified when it is recycled. Thus, the cleaner the blood and urine, the less is toxic effect on the immunity system.

This urine is not only non-toxic, but it is also anti-bacteria, anti-fungal and anti-viral.

Many other Blood Products

Blood is a red liquid that the body produces. It can be used in medical treatment. Human body produces not only blood, but also a number of other food, and medicinal by-products. In all countries, and therapeutic systems, either in civilised and uncivilised countries, blood and other blood products, by-products are used for nutrition and medicinal purpose without evoking the unpleasantness or smell. Milk products are put into packages before being sent to shop, stored to be stocked. For instance, prepacked milk and milk-based products though produce smell, we eat, using without evoking the repugnancy, disgust.

For instance :

1. Breast milk

The round soft parts at the front of a women's body produce milk when she begets a child. It is nothing but blood product. This milk is neither nauseating nor disgusting to us.

When a woman breast-feeds, she feeds her baby with milk from her breasts. Milk, the white liquid produced by cows, goats, buffalos and some other animals is their blood product only. It is a food for their young cows, goats and is used as a drink by the humans. Animals feed their babies. We and babies drink milk without showing a feeling of repugnance. It may be in the form of carton of milk, fresh, dried, powered milk, buttered milk, condensed milk, vaporated milk, malted milk, skimmed milk, etc.

2. Milk Products

The milk is a raw material from which a number of other milk products are made like milk chocolates, butter, cheese. Without considering their origin we eat and children eat. Cow's cheese is made from the milk of goat. Cheese is made from milk that can be either soft or hard and is usually white or yellow in colour. Similarly butter. It is a soft yellow food made from cream or milk. It is used in cooking onion which is fried in butter. Butter milk, the liquid that remains after butter has been separated form milk is used in cooking or as a drink.

3. Cells

The smallest part of living matter can exist in units. The blood is full of cells. The human body is made of cells.

4. Dairy Products

The dairy industry, dairy cattle, dairy farms have emerged to make commercial, medicinal, food products from milk. Dairy products like blue cheese are as sour drinks having bitter taste like the taste of lemon, of fruit, such as sour apples, a sour flavor eat like a thick white liquid food, made by adding bacteria to milk, served cold and often flavoured with fruit.

5. Bizarre Product

A number of very strange and unusual milk based products we make are considered to be tasty and delicious.

So, urine is nothing but a blood product. So, urine is a by-product which means that it is a substance, produced during the process of making a blood.

Cheese, butter and other milk products which smell much worse. What about beer, wine and other beverages? Are they not producing smell? Are we not consuming them?

17

Safety and Efficacy of Urinopathy

1. Safety

What is the safety and efficacy of urine therapy for practice? "Better safe than sorry" is a saying. It means that it is wiser to be careful than to act blindly and quickly. You should always be in safe hands. With urine, you are in safe hands as it takes care of you. It is safe to drink. It does preventive and curative activity in a careful way, involves no risk and, absolutely safe, not likely to cause any danger or loss to body. It does no harm, no damage.

Drinking one's own urine which contains numerous substances does not lead to any physical harm. It is a safe and effective remedy for human ailments. It is one of the safest, drugless healthcare systems in this world. On the other hand, the body is protected from any danger or harm. In practice and evidence for centuries, it is witnessed that there is no potential risk or harm to any patient of any ailment. It poses little or no harm to the individual. Urinopathic physician does employ no other modalities including minor surgery and prescription of some pharmaceutical drugs.

The safety issues in this health care therapy imply neither toxicity level of the therapy nor the competency of the drinker practising the therapy. No patient has so for reported health problems after following urine therapy. Problem, if any reported by the drinkers it means, who lacked sufficient knowledge of its usage.

Recent findings and literature show that the contents of the urine have not shown any harmful substances in human urine. However, any of the negative conditions reported after practising urine therapy must have occurred due to an interaction of the other drugs used. Some allopathic physicians, practising urinopathic modalities may prescribe both urine as well as drugs. In such cases such problems may arise. The drug-urine interaction may result in some troubles. Some research is needed to test the efficacy of use of both drug-urine therapies.

2. Efficacy and Effectiveness

Human urine has the inherent ability especially preventive, curative and immunity refilling power. It positively produces the results that are expected, wanted or intended. It possesses the quality of doing treatment well with no waste of money, time and convenience. It is a simple but highly effective treatment of producing results. It is effective even against degenerative disease like cancer, as scientifically proved. Urinopathic medicine gives the best possible results or benefits in comparison with money that is spent on modern medicine. So, it is a cost effective, and convenient way of fighting human ailments. A single substance, i.e., urine is effective for many illnesses, while allopathic drug is effective in treating some conditions but not others.

Urinopathic physician may use urine in treating multiple complaints. Each illness is associated with urine intervention, because the logic is that single urine contains multiple drugs of treatment.

How to Measure

The safety and efficacy of urinopathic medicine can primarily be measured through the following techniques :

Scientific study, research, clinical investigation and special studies.

The public opinion, experience of long practice of urine therapy for centuries available as oral evidence as household traditional medical practice.

The patients satisfaction level is high.

The public can rely on modern research findings and publication of studies conducted widely through-out the world.

The public can rely on findings published in mainstream allopathic, medical and pharmaceutical journals.

In addition, urinopathic medicine has its own reports in which studies, recovery stories are published.

Urinopathic field itself has its own platform of associations of drinkers, doctors, believers, crusaders, propagators, etc. ventilating their voice through their media.

One of the mechanisms with which the therapy seeks to develop is professional and urine drinkers associations. These organisations are often established with the objectives of furthering the interest of the members of the profession. They have close contact with the urinopathic physicians, drinkers and propagators. They have first hand reliable information about practice of this therapy, size, success stories and new development in this field.

In India, there is a Water of Life Foundation and many local, regional, national and international organisations. They often conduct conferences, workshops, seminars on topics ranging from practice, problems and policy implications. In India and Germany, international conferences on urine were organised.

Many associations have membership categories for drinkers, physicians, propagators and supporters of the efforts of the association. They offer various services to their members, including general practice guidelines and data-base.

In recent years, the growing interest in auto-urine medicine, to cure modern incurable and innumerable ailments of human race, has initiated new research directives in identifying, isolating and extracting hormones and other substances of urine in evaluating the safety and efficacy of urinopathic therapy for treatment of cancer, AIDS, CVD and infertility problems.

The results of research, treatment results have thus stimulated the public interest and attracted the attention of allopathic physicians also. The urine therapy has proven according to research standards and successful stories that it has a physical effect, given to patients has cured and they do not need other drug at all. But many in academic, medical communities are not showing interest, in conducting research in urinopathic medicine to establish that it conformed to the accepted methodologies in biomedical research which amounts to conspiracy.

Urinopthic medicine is a non-allopathic medicine, but an integrated part of allopathic medicine. But the former is a distinct paradigm. On the other hand, urine therapy is a holistic in nature than allopathic medicine, which could not stand to the test of effectiveness of holistic approach. As we know, holism is a belief that everything nature is connected in somewhere or other.

To review, to evaluate research to date on urinopathic medicine, we can conclude that it is a 'traditional alternative medicine.'

18

How Urine is Formed and Produced

The process of formation is very lengthy involving intricate and complex biological function. A series of steps are passed in order to produce a particular quality of urine. It is like a method of doing or making it especially one that is used in industrial manufacturing process. The food and water that we take is processed in some way to treat raw material food and water to change it by a process of elimination, filtration, adding in order to change the results in natural change, a series of actions and operations that are performed like mixing, cut up of food and water to produce fully proteins and substances filled.

Urine production process has to undergo by the following three precisely regulated and automatic process, they are:

1. Filtration, 2. Re-absorption, 3. Secretion.

A brief narration of these three series of actions and operations is given below :

1. Filtration

The first stage is a process of filtering liquid. In this blood is passed through kidneys and nephrons in order to remove any materials that are not wanted for the time being. It is like an air filter, oil filter, coffee filter, water filter, etc. A cigarette that has a filter at the end that removes some of the harmful substances from the smoke. On similar lines blood is filtered.

It is the filtration process where urine figuration and formation begins. It is a never ending continuous process in the body. The fluid containing both useful chemicals and dissolved unused materials soak out of the blood through membranes. A membrane is a thin layer tissue that connects, covers parts inside the body which prevents waste products from entering. The water, waste products, salt, glucose and other chemicals which have been filtered out of the blood is known as filtration.

Thus, the total rate of filtration for the whole body by all about two millions of nephrons in both kidneys is normally about 125 ml per minute. In other words about 125 ml of water and many dissolved substances, nutrients, etc., are filtered out of the blood per minute.

Per minute 125 ml,

Per hour 7500 ml,

Per day of 24 hours 1,80,000 ml, or 180 liters a day.

Now, we see that the amount of water that is removed from the blood each day is about 180 liters.

This is the first process of urine formation.

2. Re-absorption

The second operation in its series is the absorption. The urine formed in the first process is passed to or returns to the blood by the second process of re-absorption. It is an interesting and enjoying feature because it holds your attention.

The liquid containing the water and dissolved substances are again being taken in, that is called re-absorption. At this stages renal tubes involving the kidneys, capillaries which are smallest tubes in the body that carry blood start to function.

Tubules are shaped like tubes, parts in the body long a hollow through which blood moves from one place to another. So, the re-absorption is the movement of substances out of the renal tubules into blood capillaries. The substances which are reabsorbed are water, glucose and other nutrients, sodium and other ions.

As against 180 liters per day filtered, more than 178 liters per day are reabsorbed back into the blood stream. It means nearly 99 per cent of 180 liters of water that left the blood each day again goes back to the blood. The blood sugar, i.e., nutrient glucose is totally re-absorbed back into the blood. In the process, none of this valuable nutrient is wasted by being lost in the urine.

But the other two substances namely sodium and ions are only partially re-absorbed into the blood.

3. Secretion

Urine is expelled from the body, to force to leave the body. Bodily secretion is the process by which liquid substance like urine produced by the parts of the body passes out of the body. It is like insulin secreted by the pancreas, the secretion of bile by the liver, sweat by the skin.

The last and important process in the formation of urine is secretion. It is an action or operation by which substances move into the distal and collecting tubules. In this respect secretion is re-absorption in reverse. But re absorption moves substances out of the tubules into blood. Secretion moves substances out of blood and into tubules. It is where they mix with water and other wastes and converted into urine. The substances created are hydrogen, potassium ammonia and certain drugs, out of the blood and into kidney tubules, where they are eventually eliminated in the urine.

19

Role of Kidneys, Nephrons and Urine Bladder

The Kidneys are the two compound tubular excretory glands situated one on either side of the vertebral column. Each kidney is bean-shaped. They are situated in the lumbar region. The right kidney is slightly lower roughly half an inch than the left because of the liver on the right side. Each kidney measures about four inches length, two and a half inches breadth and one and a half inches thickness. In weight each about four ounces.

Each kidney receives its blood from renal artery. Kidney is an organ of the body, every one of us have two kidneys, looks reddish brown colour, bean shaped like kidney. The Function of either of the two organs in the body is to remove waste products from the blood and finally produce liquid urine.

Both the kidneys in the body carry out this essential blood cleaning function. It is the responsibility of the kidneys to pick up products out of the blood stream and send them along for final disposal. The waste products are filtered out of the blood system by the kidneys.

The blood circulates through out the body. The metabolism of the body is the chemical process by which the foodstuffs, water in living thighs that change food into energy for growth. It turns food into new cells, energy.

The waste resulting from the metabolism in the body cells are deposited into the blood stream. The unnecessary products so deposited are disposed off in the kidney process, so the blood is filtered to produce the urine by both the kidneys which carry out this important blood cleansing function.

Usually about 20 per cent of the blood pumped by the heart each minute will enter the kidneys for filtration. In medical literature, it is called Filtration Fraction.

The balance of about 80 per cent of the blood does not undergo through for filtering portion of the kidneys. But it is circulated to the rest of the body to serve the various nutritional, respiratory and other needs of the body.

Another important function of the kidneys to perform is that kidney tubule secretion play a crucial role in maintaining the body's acid base balance.

The blood cleaning work takes place not only in kidneys but also in particular in nephrons. There are about two million nephrons in kidneys, about one million in each kidney. The two kidneys, and two millions of nephrons put together actually form the urine. Urine formation takes place in the nephrons.

When we take food, water, liquid, etc. goes into our body, usually by swallowing, are destroyed, broken in a smooth, evenly at the end of a time or period in the stomach and intestines into extremely small molecules. Broken eventually into smallest unit, usually consisting of a group of atoms, into smallest unit, usually consisting of a group of atoms, into which the foodstuffs can be divided without a change in its chemical character. In the intestines wall there are tiny tubes, and these molecules are absorbed into these tiny tubes. Later they pass though these tubes into blood flow.

The blood moves around the body inside the system, carrying these broken foodstuffs in the form of molecules and many other nutrients, proteins along with critical immune defense.

In the blood circulation track, a number of elements are manufactured at different locations in the system of flow. The blood regulates a number of elements such as a red blood cells, white blood cells, antibodies, plasma, microscopic proteins, hormones, enzymes, vitamins, metabolites, etc.

The blood in its route of flow, passes through the liver. In the liver, toxins are removed and afterwards excreted from the body in the form of solid waste.

Thus purified blood goes to the kidneys. In the two kidneys, there are minute tubules called nephrons through which blood is pressed with high pressure, as a result filtered blood is produced.

In the filtering process, it removes excess amount of water, salt and other substances in the body, that the body does not need at a time. The used and unwanted water, salt and other elements are collected within the kidney system. This volume of collection is a purified, sterile watery solution, that is we call as urine. From this urine again many of the substances are reabsorbed by the nephrons and delivered back into the bloodstream. It is only the reminder part of the urine passes out of the kidneys into the urine bladder, and is then excreted from the body as urine.

Now, we must understand, the function of the kidneys is not only just to filter, but also to maintain balance between various elements in the blood. So, multiple quantities of substances of the blood that are deposited in microscopic manner in urine have enormous medicinal and therapeutic value. When it is reingested to the body, it improves the immunity system and has healing property.

In this way, urine is a natural drugless drug, self-therapy that nothing else does. Such a invaluable and intrinsic medicine we can not duplicate, or produce outside the body.

Urine bladder

A urine bladder is an organ of the body that is shaped like a bag in which liquid waste, watery solution called urine collects before it is passed out of the body. Like a gall bladder, an organ attached to the liver in which bile is stored, urine bladder in which urine is stored before excretion. It is one of human excretes, a liquid waste matter, as considered, passed out from the body. The bladder where urine is stored for discharge.

A bladder is a hollow viscus, which acts as a reservoir of urine, changes it shape and size according to its contents. When it is empty it has a base, an apex, a neck and three surfaces. The maximum volume of urine that can be withheld by the bladder is well over 1000 ml.

An adult may produce urine on an average ranging from one to two quarts a day, i.e., 1.14-2.25 liters. The bladder holds an average of about 16-20 ounces of fluid. But the average discharge is about half of that volume.

20

Urine Testing – Urinalysis

The liquid substance containing various natural drugs and chemicals provide a lot of information about the health conditions of the body. The expelled urine from the body is the raw data whose analysis indicates both concerning general health and also specific medical conditions of the body.

The process of biochemical analysis of urine is technically called "Urinalysis". The pathological examination tells about any disease caused by, or connected with urine, disease or illness or disorder. A doctor who examines the urine and from it he finds out the cause of disease. Urinalysis discloses to say exactly what an illness or the cause of a health problem.

A urine test is used mainly to diagnose root cause of variety of diseases. An accurate and right diagnosis is made after series of urine tests to identify the exact cause of an illness. For instance urine of a person is diagnosed whether he is a diabetic, creatine, etc. a high levels of urinary glucose in diabetic, and high levels of urinary ketone bodies in cases of ketonuria. Immunological analysis of urine is the basis for most pregnancy tests.

It is a detailed study of urine, done in order to examine the nature, structure, characters and composition of it to find out, recognise normalities and abnormalities in it, deciding cause of illness. The urine samples are sent to the laboratory for analysis using scientific examination.

Generally on the following items, urine is investigated to diagnose their respective characters. Urine for acetone, ketone bodies, urobilinogen bence-jones protein, urine for sugar, albumin, urea , creatinine, sodium, potassium chloride, uric acid, etc.

For each of the substances in the urine, the usual average level or standard is fixed scientifically, which every one would expect to possess under normal circumstances to lead a healthy or perfectly normal life. For instance, normal level of glucose, normal level of temperature, to live normally. If analysis reveals any deviation from normal level or standard, may be above or below normal, it is a case of abnormality concerning specific health disorder.

Normal is used to describe something that is what the body expects. Abnormality is a character in a person's body, different from what is used or expected, that is below the usual that may be harmful, worrying or cause of illness or disorder. This is an indication of surplus, deficit, or disorder in any one or two of urine substances of the patient. For instance, abnormality of urine glucose, abnormality of urinary ketone bodies.

To correct abnormality, doctors give medicine so that the body soon returns to normal, or to fitness, or make health fit a normal pattern or condition. It is called normalisation. If urine is healthy; you are healthy otherwise ill-health.

21

Why Should You Drink Urine

You are asked to drink because :

1. Urinopathic medicine can target a wide variety of mind-body-spirit health challenges without the use of drugs and surgery. This is the primary reason which rationalists choose to practise.
2. Drinkers want to integrate their medical treatment with naturopathic modalities as complementary and alternative measures to reap the best results offering as multi-therapy.
3. Today people look for alternatives because they are reeling under more newly emerging conditions which allopathic system of healthcare has proved failure.
4. what people realised today is to have a system that identifies the root cause of the health challenges and eradicate the cause of the malady rather than just masking symptoms with substitutes.
5. The aim of the therapy is to help the health feel better always, improving body's performance, without causing discomfort.
6. It upholds the truth that nature cures the disease, universal access, decentralisation, safety, acceptability, affordability and availability.
7. Today people of this generation are vexed with and resent modern medicine, human intervention, surgical and mechanical interventions which are sometimes more fatal than useful to common people.
8. Patients recently are increasingly realising the symptoms of the diseases are not the diseases or the cause of the diseases, this unknown therapy respects the expression of symptoms as the body's attempt to heal itself.
9. It assumes that all diseases are not always necessarily materially generated with evidence, and known risk factors, but urinopathic measure considers the complex interaction of physical, mental, emotional, genetic, behavioural and social factors as well when addressing human health.
10. Human urine is a bio-medicine, consists of a wide variety of biochemistry, naturally possesses the ability to determine the underlying cause of the illness and by refilling removes the obstacles on the way to optimal health.

11. An illness is caused by internal imbalance in the system of homeostasis, means between immunity, hormonal, nervous, detoxification and elimination factors. The power to keep balance lies in 'vital force' or 'life force', i.e., your urine. This is the central idea of drinking one's own urine substances to maintain optimal balance.
12. The yogis are first drinkers, in ancient times having history of more than 5,000 years. By practice they not only benefitted a state of perfect physical health, deageing, longevity, visualisation, tranquility, divine sight, physical immortality but also lived without disease, decay and death. [contribute to extend life span far beyond the usual expectancy]
13. Yet another strong ground to appeal to you to drink is that even today such drinkers are common sight every where, telling success and recovery stories from various disease. Such practice is passed from generation to generation, from parents to childrens and they are around us, it flourishes as long as human kingdom exists. But until recently it has been overlooked in general with the advent of modern medicine, is now once again gaining popularity in mainstream healthcare.
14. Why should I insist you is that it recognises the human body as an interrelated, interdependent, co-exist of sub-systems and it is a part of a tradition of medicine that emphasises finding and eliminating the disease causative factors and stimulates body's innate natural power of self-healing.
15. Many drugs typically proved ineffective in combating menace of modern ailments like cancer, arthritis, AIDS, HIV, proved only fewer results in respect of other conditions.
16. Indian people are poor and illiteracy is higher. Millions of them belong to the poorest sections of the poor, living below poverty line, and many are at average income brackets. When we look of all these encompassing factors, the trend of medical industry, the impact of high medical cost placing unconscionable burden on the poor. It is beyond the earning capacity to afford to expensive prescription drugs, diagnosis, surgical needs, the costly powerful medicine.
17. Finally, it eliminates your more common frequent, repetitive visits to your health care physician, because little or less manifestations are realised. Let your body enjoy health and protect it by nature in the future.

This is why you are asked to drink your own medicinal substance which proves so effective, where other systems fail.

22

Choosing Your Own Therapy

Selecting your personal therapy may improve your health, and wellness. Your medicine creates your health. The type of household therapeutic drug we use may describe our health situations and our lives are the way that we perceive our lives to be our perception then is the reality. When you say things are something in disorder or you are suffering from a disease, you are heading towards choosing your health therapy.

There is a long list of therapies which are in use, some are popular and some others are in use among limited number.

But the truth is that among traditional, alternative, natural therapies, urinopathy has a long history, wide known, has a growing number of people who not only swear that it works, but rely on it to live fuller and longer healthy. Increasingly, Indian 'urine medicine' is being put to the test by Western and European Scientists and results are not only miraculous, but also astounding.

The following is the list of various traditional, complementary and alternative therapies in use in different countries:

Hypno therapy	Ayurveda
Cupping therapy	Homeopathy
Magnet therapy	Urinotherapy
Acupuncture	Naturopathy
Yoga	Mind-body medicine
Meditation	Massage and touch therapy
Photo therapy	Detoxification therapy
Herbology	Traditional Chinese Medicine
Physical medicine	Behavioural Medicine
Nutrition therapy	Naturopathic manipulation
Life style counseling	Oriental medicine
Diet therapy	Light and air therapy
Mud therapy	Magnetism therapy
Reflexology	Colour therapy

Sound Therapy	Iridology
Kinesiology	Craniosacral
Aromatherapy	Polarity Therapy
Folk Practice	Gerson Therapy
Colostrum Therapy	Healing through Non–invasive Instrumentalities
Qigong practice	Culturally traditional healing practice
Anthroposophy	Healing through Fasting
Healing with food	Healing with sunlight
Healing with Sea	Juice therapy.

Traditional, complementary, alternative health care practices do not include surgery, x-ray, dispensing legend drugs, skin puncture, setting fracture, use of medical devices or manipulation of the spine or joints.

One Medicine for Multiple Problems

Urinotherapy is a proven treatment for a much wider variety of health conditions. One simple substances works for complex multifarious conditions. A natural therapy for virtually all common health concerns, but in recent times it is proved an effective medicine for treatment of even deadly complaints like cancer, cardio, HIV, AIDS, etc.

I am asked one question, what is the one solution for multiple conditions, there is only one supplement for many problems. What it would be? That is auto urinotherapy. Of all many natural therapies and medicines, we can safely narrow down to only one urine therapy for a much wider variety of conditions. Life style change also helps with many common health problems.

Why are you reading this topic

The word naturopathy encompasses a wide array of healthcare practices called as traditional, alternative therapies which are distinct from practices. Some forms are ayurvedic, *yoga*, meditation have been practiced for centuries, whereas others, as referred below, are more recent in origin. Urinopathy is a single, oldest diverse Indian traditional household medical and healthcare system, practice, product which is presently considered to be the earliest conventional medicine.

This therapy is now known as whole medical system, to be a separate category rather than other domains listed below. Urine is an energy medicine in the cure, mitigation, treatment or prevention of diseases. It is a body made drug based on patient's biological, circulatory and lymphatic system, without using any external materials like in a factory.

It is called as whole medical system evolved independently, naturally, to allopathic medicine. It reflects India's cultural system, is a belief that body has the power to heal itself, and that healing may involve techniques that use mind, body and spirit. It is to mean urine is a substance intended for the use of which may results in many benefits expected directly or indirectly.

Urine therapy has demonstrated efficacy in areas such as peace, mental health, disease prevention, treatment of communicable, non-communicable disease, improvement of quality of life for persons living with chronic diseases. Urinopathic medicine has shown great potential to meet a broad spectrum of health care needs.

What Type of Complementary Therapies are Used in Urinopathy

It incorporates other therapies also which are compatible with the basic principles of nature cure. The term urinotherapy is used to describe the mix of therapies associated with it to treat illness. Urinopathic medicine is practiced either as a primary system of medical care, or as a complementary to one or two therapies adjunct to natural treatment.

Urinopathic physicians have alternative options to use in combination of other therapies for prevention and curing the numerous and various complaints. The use of multiple therapies concurrently generates additional benefits for the patients.

The urinopathic medicine incorporates many complementary and alternative therapeutic modalities and hence it is called a medicine of comprehensive system. It blends other ancient knowledge of natural and non-toxic therapies.

It uses a wide range of alternative therapies which may include: Massage, Hydrotherapy, Ayurvedic, Nutrition, Dietetics, Meditation, Yoga, Culturally traditional healing practices, counselling, life style change, etc.

A brief description of these therapies is given below for general understanding:

1. Herbology or Herbalisim

A herb is a plant whose leaves, flowers or seeds are used along with urine as medicine for prevention and cure. A plant with a soft stem that dies down after flowering, called as herbal medicine. Urinopathic treatment originated as the use of herbs mixed with urine.

It is also called botanical medicine or phytotherapy. It is a corner stone of *Shivambu*, most of modern diseases are cured with medicinal plants and urine mix. *Shivambu* recommends several medicinal plants and their products to be used mixed with urine for curing many ills of human race. Modern scientific researches have substantiated many of these plants having medicinal values. In ayurveda also, they have increasingly found ways to use along with urine in treating modern complaints.

Herbs are characterised by their low toxity and lack of accumulation in the body. Urine-herb based medicine is a means of providing affordable primary healthcare. A particular herb is appropriately selected for a specific disease mixed with urine. Urinopathic medicines offer powerful, safe and effective approach to healing with no or little side effects. So, it is advised to acquire dried herbs to keep at home and can be used for many years.

Herbs have also medicinal properties, when used mixed with urine treating many today's incurable human ailments. Used for centuries and valued in ancient societies adds to good health. The amazing herbs have healing properties, live naturally with urine and herb.

Shivambu recommends some of the following herbs such as: gaduchi; tinospora, londifolia, harade, terminalia, chebula, Kostha, belavica, phylonthus, embica, etc.

2. Dietetics

It is the therapy which deals with the scientific study of diet and healthy eating. A dietetic study of diet and healthy eating. A dietetic advice and principles are also followed in urinopathy. Here a patient is advised on what kind of food he should eat to keep healthy.

3. Hydrotherapy

It is also called as water therapy which means the treatment of disease by doing physical exercises in water and drinking. It may use hot and cold water application. One can stay hydrated with the power of water solution. It is true the dehydration is a common problem. To say, as much as 75 per cent of the human body is water. Its maintaining levels requires one to three liters of water daily . Use of Urine is a natural remedy, to treat many ailments.

4. Nutrition

Many people suffer from a serious nutrient deficiency. It is one of the serious cause for affecting a disease. One should take always nutritionally balanced diet to restore health. People must take food necessary for them to grow and be healthy. The biological relationship between diseases and nutrition cannot be overlooked. All health conditions can be improved through changes, and maintenance in diet alone. A proper balance and supplementation of specific nutrients are equally necessary. Clinical nutrition is a major component of urinopathic treatment. Besides human urine contains valuable natural nutrients, made by the body. Retaking our own urine develops optimal wellness and enhancement. Nutrition is a real paradigm in maintaining good health.

Malnutrition is a devasting problem in India, world wide epidemic. Many suffer from this deficiency. It is one of the single biggest reasons for AIDS/ HIV positive. Rich nutrients of urine offer a powerful vitality to overall health at a very low cost, complete nutrition prevents from many aliments.

5. Meditation

The art of meditation is one of the natural therapies of urinopathic medicine. The exemplary life style of the yogis shed light on the mechanisms of meditation.

The daily practice of the art of meditation is to supercharge your mental abilities and not just to become a monk. The meditation offer many benefits to the practitioners like to enjoy relaxation, increased attention span, better cognition and other health benefits.

6. Yogic Therapy

Yoga is a 5,000 years old indian tradition that offers many health benefits. There are today many *yoga* schools, centres that impart yogic training. Most *yoga* practices include postures, breathing exercises is being practised world wide. New research studies reveal that *yoga* is better than allopathic medicine for many common ills.

Yoga improves mood, reduces inflammation, and relieves chronic diseases. As people think, *yoga* is no longer just a gentle stretching for aging hippies, as an ancient ritual it improves, mood, prevents diseases, reduces inflammation, rebuilds immunity system, balances nervous system, counteracts fibromyalgia, makes to work the detoxification and elimination process effective. It is a common knowledge that *yoga* improves peace and shrugs off stress.

7. Counselling

In cases of complaints like chronic, acute conditions such as intestinal upsets, chronic illnesses, such as migraines, musculoskeletal pains, arthritis, heart disease, degeneratives infections like AIDS/HIV, VDS, mental and emotional problems and physical problems consulting a urinopathic physician if available is desirable for quick and effective results. He will give professional and expertise piece of advice towards lifestyle, dietary style counselling and modification.

The success and popularity of this therapy is low because lack of urinopathic counseling and physicians. The cornerstones of urinopathic philosophy are prevention and responsibility for one's own health. The curing process, is based on assessing risk factors connected with the patients life style, dietary style, etc. Treatment procedure requires removal of obstacles to the health.

It is a sort of life style counselling and practice of urine drinking. Health counseling from urinopathy wherever they are available for a problem is necessary.

The underscore of urinopathic philosophy is prevention and responsibility for one's own health. It is based on analysing risk factors connected to the patient's life style, diet and environment. These and other factors are taken into consideration when designing a treatment plan with a patient. The aim is to remove obstacles to the patients' own state of optimal health.

8. Massaging

Massaging with urine and touch therapy have many health benefits. Today this therapy with urine is practiced all over the world. But massaging with fresh urine may be avoided. Urine is beneficial for many ailments. Particularly the following benefits can be obtained from massaging :

1. Relieves from migraines and stress,
2. Improves blood circulation,
3. Rehabilitates physical functions,
4. Loosens the tense muscles,
5. Urine enters into the body and then begins the healing process,
6. One can avoid paid medication,
7. Improves the conditions of the skin,
8. Boosting immunity system and blood pressure control,
9. Decreases itching, anxiety, depression, pain and tension,
10. Patients who are suffering from cancer are benefited much.

9. Happy People Live Healthier

Urine drinkers are happy people who live healthier, longer lives. They have an advantage over unhappy ones, because they may be healthier and may live longer. The lives of the people living with urine indicates that high subjective well being, it means life satisfaction, optimism, positive emotions, causes better health and longevity. They are the people of discontent over modern day medical care. A better way to health is to make sick people heal with urine.

These complementary and attractive methods long have been respected throughout the human evolution.

10. How to Use

Urinopathic medicine is explained by its fundamental principles, the methods and modalities. They are selected and applied based upon these principles and its bedrock philosophy and depending upon its relationship to the individual needs of each patient, type of disease like internal, external, hormonal, etc. The patient is advised to practise nutrition, dietetics, therapeutic fasting, medicine of, minerals, hygiene, hydrotherapy.

The scope is dynamic in nature, select one or two or combination of use of variety of methods which best serve the patient's condition. The competent urinopathic physician can evolve their manner of practice of healthcare to provide enhanced or new benefit to their patients. What type of modality is needed including immediacy, common, acute, chronic, long, short degenerative or opportunistic infections, etc. are considered before selecting a method. The patient's willingness and preparedness are also assessed by the urinopathic physician. The cure process is the patient's own body medicine, the decision for its utilisation is ultimately also the patient's.

The methods by which prevention and curing of illness, and maintenance gives ample scope to employ a variety of urinopathic-intervention to achieve optimum health, the method of using is that which is more appropriate in every case, can be modified to suit the condition of the case and progress.

23
Urinopaths

A group of people practising *yoga* and naturopathic medicine as a traditional and complementary health care system, with particular specialisation with auto-urine therapy. Like medical courses and degrees they do not possess any formal educational qualifications undergoing four-five years programme.

The practitioners, crusaders, propagators with their long practical personal experience and background knowledge promoting awareness including the habit with a sense of self-health responsibility among the public, some members call themselves as urinopathic doctors, urinopathic physicians, and even as urinopaths.

Elsewhere, the members of these groups as designated urinopaths may also be called naturopaths, urinopaths, traditional uropaths, urinopathic practitioners or counselling urinopaths. The claim is most traditional by practice locally. The use of the word doctor, physicians does not imply a more formal with systematic background of course of academic discipline.

It is a more general term, because it values its traditional medical freedom more than standardization and formal. Sometimes they are senior member of the family following the tradition of urine drinking from generation to generation as an early form of household practice which later became popular with more modern English word as urinopaths. It has a long history of ancestry, i.e., the family or the race of people who are descended from.

It is more common to call them as such, because it values its traditional medical freedom more than scientific knowledge. By tradition and belief, public is making its own decision to seek medical advice from urinopaths for long. In those days it is their right to access to them as it is a non-invasive.

Urinopathic physicians voluntarily educate and encourage locals as the only remedy of the days and self-healing abilities of the body as teachers and counsellors than by the name doctors. Urinopathic physicians blend centuries old knowledge of self-healing power of the body, herbal, non-toxic, drugless therapies known as natural, complementary and alternate therapies with current advances in the understandings of health and anatomy.

Urinopaths, in their profession typically adopt a wide range of alternative therapies and pathies including herbology, massaging, hydrotherapy, *yoga*, meditation ayurveda, nutrition as well as dietary practices, without surgery. So, urinopath is a person whose job is to advise people the medicinal benefits of auto-urine to keep healthy.

24
Model of Care

Urionapthic medicine is based primarily on a model that autogenous has medicinal properties like curative efficacy, strategy of preventive maintenance, care, as well as health promotion. It respects the urine's natural healing process and its model is for both common, acute, chronic degenerative, opportunistic infections, injuries and natural tendencies. While the emphasis is on the natural healing capability of the individual body. Urine drinkers are also to blend hydrotherapy and herbal measures. Urinopathic physicians offer a unique set of natural, ancient practices and services to the willing drinker, that may range from integrative medicine to life style, dietary style, occupational styles education, *yoga*, meditation, regimentation depending on the practitioners and complaint.

The counsellors choose urine as medicine as their primary form of healthcare instead of allopathic medicine except recommendations in exigencies and minor surgeries and obstetrics in emergency situations. Sometimes urinopathic and allopathic physicians or allopathic physicians practising urinopathy work collaboratively to treat the exceptional conditions of the patients for specific diseases. Urinopathic physicians most often see clients, patients with chronic aliments like cancer, asthama, sinus, cardio, and acute conditions such as constipation, infertility, bronchitis. Urniopaths view themselves as general family practice physicians.

As regards urinopathic physicians, and drinkers are concerned their size and number, no detailed, recognised and authoritative statistics, records are available. Information is not available on the sex, nor data available on racial, ethnical identification of physicians and practitioners as to cultural acceptability. While the actual number of individuals or families practising the therapy is unknown, as a matter of fact this therapy is an ancient traditional household medicinal practice. No estimate nor collection is possible. But approximate number of individuals drinking, physicians guiding and encouraging could be located throughout the globe, through national, regional and local urine drinkers associations, groups, formal gatherings and their reports.

As there are no state licensing bodies, regulatory authorities for urinopathic medicine, for controlling, supervision, registration and to obtain licenses for practice, collection of data and reporting.

Another element of this sector to know is the pipeline of predecessors, family heads, crusadors, propagators, foundations, believers, practitioners, followers, people promoting awareness to various levels and individuals.

25

Checklist Towards Auto-Urine

1. A drugless drug, priceless, natural, divine and self-therapy.
2. An intrinsic, invaluable, holistic, ancient, universal household traditional medicinal practice.
3. First do no harm, self-healing power of the body, addresses the cause of the disease and treat whole of person, nature-friendly
4. Individualised, customised, decentralised, private, personal, confidential and no use of prescription drugs or non-presctiption drugs.
5. A peculiar therapy locates the root and really cures rather than simply suppress or masking the symptoms.
6. No unclothed examination, skin puncture, surgical procedure and use of mechanical instruments.
7. What you eat and drink at a movement, in the next minute they turn into blood and urine ?
8. One simple solution to multiple complex conditions, challenges of wide range of aliments of human race.
9. A therapy stimulates the natural healing power inherent in each individual.
10. Prevents, cures, refills immunity, promotes, maintenance, optimises health of an individual by inspiring rational hope and encourages self-responsibility for health.
11. It protects the quality of naturality from being adversely affected by modern medical practice.
12. It recognises the role of trinity that you are a patient, drug and physician.
13. Replacement of 'disease' with 'ease' condition with 'easier', 'real' healer inside. Your own body made perfect medicine.
14. You have not only physical but mental, spiritual, emotional as well as psychological illnesses.
15. Urine is a *manna* from *heaven*.

26
People are Shy

We just follow the foot steps of parents, and ancestors, who have considered urine a waste product. We, too, consider it a waste without rational thinking and reasoning. Because they showed as a strong feeling of dislike or disapproval to drink urine, you too consider it unacceptable, or for the reason that it looks or smells unpleasant. People refused, wrinkled nose in disgust at the smell of urine, that is all the reason.

The urine disgusts you. It makes you feel shocked and wonderstruck how it is a medicine? And it becomes almost abominable because it is so unpleasant to drink unacceptable and dirty.

You refuse to drink urine even when a practitioner advises. You also hate those who practice it, whom you know the way they always drink. You would prefer not to have it. You hate urine–awareness-campaign also. You hate it because primarily you dislike it. The idea of curing, presenting with urine against deadly diseases of their own is also hateful to you. You feel nothing short of hatred for this practice.

On the other hand, drinkers of urine also feel guilty, embarrassed and hesitant to tell other people about its merits . It is because he is a shy practitioner. Don't be shy.

Some others feel shy to ask anyone about urine therapy for seeking advice and help. Someone is not generally willing to come near the urine drinking people. But there will be a typical man who had never been shy of saying or advising others.

We are shy because we have not understood it in true spirit.

In shot, urine is a substance that is being produced during the blood-filtration process.

27

How Can You Overcome the Barriers to Drink Your Own Urine

In this topic are given to you step by step instructions as lessions useful to the beginners, to overcome any initial aversion towards urine dinking.

Very briefly, please follow the guidelines given below explaining what the beginner's job is and how to start therapy and overcome the barriers. Get prepared to deal with urine. Here are introductory lessions that are suggested to do urine therapy. But this is in no way force you to use the therapy but simply instructions that are given telling you how to do with it, something that can be used to help you make a decision or form an opinion to begin. Many people are inexperienced, unaware and need a guided hand. Here is a guiding force having a strong influence :

1. First start smelling your own urine that can solve your problem of disgust which is a main barrier to this therapy.
2. A second step forward is touch, sense and then start rubbing some drops on your skin.
3. A regular bathing, massaging of urine into your skin, body is also a good measure to be accustomed with your own urine.
4. The easy method to overcome the barrier of repugnancy is putting a drop. Then drink urine by taking a very small amount each time, like a sip of tea, beer, wine. By this way your body, mind and soul get accustomed to this divine nectar.
5. Have a strong feeling of liking, or pleasure but not a feeling of dislike or disgust. After your initial experience for one or two days you will be able to like and love it.
6. To let go of the idea of smell mix your own pure urine with fruit juice, honey, water, cardamom or any other your liked flavour.
7. Gradually avoid mixing water and drink pure fresh urine.
8. Anyone who persists and overcomes the difficult of disgust or smell, one can enjoy the eventual happiness of healthy life and long living without disease and decay. You can with a few drops.

9. To begin use one-five drops on the first day, followed five-ten drops on the second day, five-ten drops also on the morning and evening of third day.
10. Dilute if necessary the urine with water and this diluted solution may be taken up to reduce smell or thickness.
11. Place two or three drops under the tongue to taste and to get familiarity with it.
12. The intake of urine dosage can be progressed by increasing the quantity to ounce or ounces.
13. Gradually increase up to one glass a day. Take full urine of the day in case of chronic diseases, regularly, it prevents you from diseases.
14. As a way of life activity just like brushing, pissing, or going to toilet every morning it should be made as our daily routine.
15. Before being initiated into a urine therapy you must get mentally and psychologically prepare and decided.
16. The idea of drinking your own urine is something repugnant should not be conceived. Drink as if you are taking medicine solution, or liquor. Do not woke the repugnance associated with urine.
17. Drink urine, taking a very small amount each time, take a sip of urine, like sipping tea and coffee, don't drink like water.
18. In case of complaint like cancer, AIDS etc. drink full day urine. In practice for preventive maintenance, drink at least one litre per day without missing morning urine.
19. Avoid drinking urine to be passed during the night before two am.
20. Ensure the purity and quality of urine.
21. While collecting sample it is necessary to wash the genital area thoroughly.
22. Before taking urine into the body morning first urine, it is desirable to take with fasting.
23. After taking the urine into the body, the practitioner should refrain from taking any food for at least nearly one hour. Avoid taking when the stomach is full, or after taking food.
24. As far as possible preferably drink your own fresh or old urine. It is a self-medicine, holistic and you are pleasant with it.
25. After drinking urine, please give a gap of at least 30 minutes, don't eat.
26. Full day urine can be taken in the case of any treatment for a specific ailment.
27. After taking foodstuffs wait for at least one hour before drinking urine.

28
Science Validates Urinotherapy

You will be pleased to know that several studies are undertaken, findings are published in leading medical journals, books are showing outstanding results from urinopathic treatment. Well-designed high quality scientific studies have confirmed the real benefits of urinopathic medicines as a distinct from placebo. For some ailments, the drug have beneficial effects.

Lakhs of people who suffer from cancer, AIDS/ HIV, will be pleased to know that several studies published in leading medical and other journals have found outstanding results. Science validates urinopathic medicine.

Scientific Basis

There is a small, but growing body of scientific research into the clinical effectiveness of urinopathic medicine and the modalities commonly used in auto-urine therapy. Much of the clinical practice of urinopathic medicine is based on ancient textual evidence, traditional empirical evidence, household and hearsay evidences, expert opinions, current best practices, individual therapeutical trials and recovery stories.

There is a growing interest and resources, bibliographical references, citations, fields of further research are identified in uropathy system. Due to the individualised treatment approaches and multiplicity of therapeutic applications, however designing rigorous clinical trials is challenging, requiring institutional effort and will.

Urine Therapy : a Medical Science

Urinotherapy is a science, an integral component of medical science, connecting with ways of preventing and curing illness, a branch of human science. It is a therapeutic system of organised knowledge about human health, an exact science.

Today, it has come to be recognised as a medical science. Prior to this, the knowledge of practice of therapy was not well organised, opinions and public experiences were the only way to know about it. This organised body of therapy has its own distinct boundaries and fields of activities. Its research, clinical investigations helped a lot in gaining a rational approach to extract the substances of urine for curing many modern incurable diseases.

That is why, urine therapy is called a part of science.

A science is a systematically organised body of knowledge on proper findings and exact principles and is capable of verification and the principles are universally acceptable and applicable. Its medicinal value is a reservoir of fundamental truths and its findings apply to all people, in all places, in all countries, races, religious. The generalisations are made on the basis of empirical studies and so they may be applicable in future also. Any therapy which is preventing and curing any disease scientifically and by practice and public experience is a science.

In order to reconsider a therapy as a science, it should have the following characteristics:

1. To have a systematic body of knowledge including concepts, principles and theories.
2. To have a formal teaching.
3. To have a method of scientific enquiry.
4. To establish cause and effect relationship.
5. To have the principles to be verifiable.
6. To ensure predictable results.
7. To have universal application.

Urine therapy has satisfied all these features to be called a science to support.

1. It cannot be denied that this branch of medicine has a systematised body of knowledge pertaining to its field. It is a part of medical science.
2. The therapy knowledge can be communicated to the aspirants in the profession, through formal teaching. This therapy, too, satisfied this character.
3. Its medical properties are scientifically enquired with empirical evidence. An innumerable special studies, clinical investigations and scientific researches, tests were carried out over several years in USA, Japan, China, Switzerland and many European countries.

   It has been conclusively proved, and discovered that there are many substances in human urine, like hormones, antibodies, vitamins, pigments, carbohydrates, enzymes, etc. will be discovered, isolated and extracted as very useful to cure many diseases ranging from common, acute, chronic degenerative, opportunistic infections, etc.
4. The medical secrets of human urine have been verified in many countries and practical case studies.
5. Its clinical application resulted a miraculous preventive and curing properties of many diseases.
6. It proved itself as a successful universal medicine.

Now, from the above arguments we can positively conclude that urine therapy does satisfied essential characters required to call as a science. But now a days urine therapy is a mass household traditional practice. Modern science is not an exact science but urine therapy is an exact science. There is a lot of difference between life and death likewise there is between public experience and science support.

Scientific Research Finding and Evidences

The therapeutic use of urine has been known for many centuries, and it is an age old traditional household practice in India. But during the past few decades, a number of special studies, researches, clinical investigations have been undertaken particularly in other countries on the medicinal properties of the urine, substances and its impact on various diseases.

The findings of the studies have revealed the fabulous curative modalities of urine as a drugless drug, self-therapy for prevention and curing. In recent years, the interest in the urine therapy and its effects on various diseases has vastly increased due to emerging new ailments and incurability of certain degenerative diseases like cancer, Aids, etc. As a magic liquid, it seems urine possess power that appear supernatural to the new entrants.

Several research laboratories all over the world have undertaken research today, investigations directed in finding the medicinal, therapeutically valuable hormones, substances contained in human urine. They are actively involved in isolating and extracting drug substances most useful in curing most of the emerging incurable modern diseases.

There is a strong possibility of their being several other medicinal hormones, other substances not yet known to science, but blind belief and practice are preventing and curing many modern incurable human ailments.

There is a lot of scientific findings, documentary evidence that fills volumes establishing the fact that one's own urine has medicinal properties and therapeutic value.

1695: Salmons, English physician, finds that urine is serum, varing medicinal, curative properties useful for dissolving, cleansing, resists putrefaction, liver, spleen, gall, dropsy, jaundice, heals, dries up, dandruff, scrub and many other ailments. He is an English physician writes the prophylactic and healing properties of auto-urine.

1700: Aristocratic French women in the seventeenth century reportedly bathed in urine to beautify their skin.

1800: The eighteenth century French dentists used to recommend rubbing one's own urine on the teeth and gargling with it for the treatment of various dental disorders. In the eighteenth century it was much extolled as a valuable mouth wash by Parisian dentist (J.W. Armstrong).

1912: Subcutaneous urine injections was practised by Duncan.

1927: Auto-urine therapy for urinary infections, Cimino from Palermo reported.

1931: Rabinowitch, described this auto-urine therapy for gonarthritis.

1933: Jausion, et.al. used this therapy for desensitisation and endocrinological problems. They treated with auto-urine therapy injections for patients who suffered from migraine, pruritus, asthama, urticaria, eczema, psoriasis etc.

1934: Teberi, R, value of auto-urine vaccine therapy in acute hemorrhagic nephritis, Ladiagnosi, 14(119/34): 183-196, 1934.

1935: Garotesw, M, treatment of calibacillary cystitis with auto-urine therapy, Romania Medicala, 1935.

1936: Day, treated patients with acute and sub-acute glomerulonephritis by injecting of an autogeneous urinary tract.

1938: Sandweiss saltzstein and farbman, an extract from urine of pregnant women has a prophylactic and therapeutic effect on experimental ulcers in dogs.

Shortly thereafter, the same group noted that an extract from urine of normal women has similar beneficial effect.

1940: Knebs, M the use of convalescent urine in the mitigation of acute infections.

1941: Sandweiss, D.J. et.al., the effect of urine extracts on peptic ulcer, *Journal D.D.* October 1941, 371-382.

1943: Thompson, J.H.H. for cancer. The study found that H-11 is an anti cancer urine extract. This study claims that more than 300 doctors and researchers have found that " H-11 was clinically effective in inhibiting the growth of malignant cells in humans".

1944: J.W. Armstrong, USA *The Water of Life*, published in London. A medical practitioner, followed urine therapy and cured numerous patients of several diseases like including cancer, proved about the efficacy and harmlessness of auto-urine therapy. He restored the credibility and prestige of auto-urine therapy.

1951: Bjurnesjo, K.B., on the effect of human urine on Tubercle bacilli – II : The Tuberculostatic effect of various urine constituents, Acta Scandinavia, 25(5): 447:455, 1951.

1958: Normal human urine has been found to contain a powerful artery dilating agent resembling nitro glycerin in the ability to increase the coronary blood flow to the cardiac muscle used for the relief of "Augina pectoris", Science Digest, july 1958.

1958: Report presented at the annual meeting of the Federation of American society for Experimental Biology in Atlantic city, USA under the heading "Bringing Cancer Cells into line".

Two researchers found that unexpectedly that the urine extract which they call it as "Directin" when added to the culture medium causes the cancer cells on which it has been so far used to align themselves end to end into straight rows. *Science Digest*, July 1958.

1961: Dr Novak therapeutic results of the use of an auto–urine extracts on malignant tumors, zeitschrift Innere Medizine, 1961.

This is the report from a German doctor who employed with much success injections of natural extracts of patients' own urine to treat cancers of breast, colon, lungs, uterus, lymph, nodes and stomach.

1962: Lerner, A.M. et.al., Neutralising antibody of Polio viruses in Normal Human Urine of Clinical Inestigation, 41(4), 805-815,1962.

1963: Hegyeli, A.et.al., Preparation of Retine from human urine, *Science*, 20:15 71-1572.1963.

A fraction of human urine was isolated and named retinene. It was tested on mice with artificially induced skin cancer and was found to inhibit the growth of tumors, larger doses were shown to cause the regression of tumors.

1965: Tsuji, S.et.al., Isolation from human urine of polypeptide having maked tuberculosatic activity, *American Review of Respiratory Diseases*, 91(6):832-838,1965.

1967: An extract from human urine shows great promise for treatment of certain deadly diseases caused by formation of blood clots. At the Scientific Sessions of American Heart Association, the research physicians disclosed that: "The extract is called urokinase, activates substances in the blood stream that dissolve the clots. Experience has been obtained from about 200 patients with pulmonary embolism. It is the most common Lung disease pointed out by Dr Sherry. *Science Digest*, July 1958.

1972: Dr T.M. Shiva Samudram, Karnataka. He succeeded in giving relief to the Asthama patients by injecting their own urine. Published in *Integrated Medical Association of Karnataka State*, India.

1973: Dr Hamao, a Professor at the Medical University, Kyoto, Japan. He isolated and extracted a substance from urine which is beneficial for the treatment of cancer, The Illustrated Weekly of India, 26th August, 1973.

1978: Dr K.K. Data, a renowned heart specialist stated in March 1978 issue of the journal '*Auto-urine Therapy*' that adventurous Himalayan mountaineers drink their own urine to maintain their energy, vigor, resist adverse atmospheric conditions. The famous mountaineer Morris Wilson testifies this fact.

1983: Wilson, C.W.M et. al., Auto-Immune Therapy against human Allergic Disease: A Physiologic disease, *Medical Hypotheses*, 12: 143-158, 1983.

1990: Dr S.R Burzynski, M.D., he isolated and extracted from human urine a substance known as Antineoplastons as an anti tumor agent capable to make malignant cancer cells revert to normal. *Oncology News* (Vol.16, No. 4) Academy of Professional Information Service.

1991: Ken Hashibara, President of Hashibara Laboratories, Japan, in his letter addressed the then Prime Minister of India, Morarji Desai, wrote about research finding as under: "On research I discovered that cancer and other incurable diseases can be treated with leucocytes found in urine. AIDs and Hepatitis can also be treated with urokinase, an enzyme found in urine while thrombosis can be completely cured by it".

1991: Mills and Faunce, New Castle University, Australia, found that ingestion of morning urine into low PH gastric acid would cause deconjugation of its esters back to the active form of melatonin.

1997: J. Eldor, M.D., Urotherapy for patients with cancer, originally published in *Medical Hypotheses* 48(4th April, 1997).

2000: Yang Liansheng, a professor from the liaoning Institute of Traditional Chinese Medicine, " Urine contains no bacterium and is more sanitary than blood".

- Shri Ravjibhai Patel, Dr Paragji Desai, India, cured innumerable patients by means of auto-urine therapy.
- Shri Morarji Desai, the Ex-Prime Minister of India, was a strong proponent of this of therapy. He is a shivambu rishi, sage, great devotee , propagator, practitioner, centenarian. He boldly and emphatically declared that was the secret of his longevity and exuberant health. It accorded a world recognition, glory and greatness.
- Dr Jivraj Mehta, Former Chief Minister of Gujarat, India, was also one of the adherents of urine therapy.
- Dr Maganbhai Salaria, Ahmedabad, India, he has given injections of the patients' own urine before surgery. This helps in maintaining the efficacy of the patients heart and prevents post operation complications.
- Dr Morris Mezel, Chicogo, USA, a chief surgeon of Edge Water Hospital, he discovered a substance in urine called urokinase, isolated and extracted which dissolves blood clots. His findings are such that there is no substance more efficacious in the treatment of heart disease than urine.
- Dr Beatrice Barnett of USA, is a practising urine therapist, in his writing '*Miracles of Urine Therapy*', he covers treatment of AIDs and given details for the successful treatment of many AIDs patients with urine therapy.
- Lars A Hanson and Eng M.Tan at the Rockfeller Institute, Newyork, his studies showed antibodies for cholera, salmonella typhi, dyptheria, tetanus, taxaid and polio are present in human urine.
- Dr. Alexander N Glazer and Stocker, University of California, in their study they discovered the yellowing dye responsible for jaundice present in urine

which was previously considered as valueless bodily waste till now is very much useful to reduce tissue damage in cancer, aging, inflammation and heart disease.

- The Noble laureate, Albert Sczent Georgyi. He has conducted a number of research studies on one of the ingredients of the urine called methyl glyoxal, and its application, effects on cancer patients. He succeeded in several cancer cases.
- Dr Dharmadhikari, Pune, Maharashtra, India has applied urinotherapy on more than 200 patients and carried out many scientific investigations. He succeeded in curing many diseases and disorders.
- Dr Vasant P. Mehta, Mumbai, India, teaching medicine and surgery in a medical college, had experimented and expressed that urine therapy has played a major role in his recovery from throat cancer.
- Dr John F.O. Quinn, USA., Urine Therapist, author of *Urine Therapy : self-Healing Through Intrinsic medicine*, President of Life Science Institute. "I predict urine therapy will be the only cure for horrible AIDs".
- Dr Manu Kothari and Dr Lopa Mehta, India authored a book "*Cancer Myths and Realities About Cause and Cure, writes* that "If any cancer patient takes routine allopathy treatment his/her life is shortened and death becomes painful where as those who don't opt for the treatment they survive longer and their death is painless". Dr Kothari had neither done biopsy nor given any treatment to his parents suffering from cancer.
- Dr T. Wilson Deachman writes that "What cannot be cured by the forces of the body some other useful studies cannot be cured by the forces outside the body".

1. Dr G.K. Thakkar, *Wonders of Uropathy*, India.
2. Beatric Bartnett, Margie Adelman, *The Miracles of Urine Therapy*, USA.
3. Martha Christy, *Your Own Perfect Medicine*, Mumbai.
4. Martin Lara, *Uropathy: The Most Powerful Holistic Therapy.*
5. Flora Pescheck Bohmer Therapy, *Urine Therapy Nature's Elixir for Good Health.*
6. Coen Van der Kroon, *The Golden Fountain.*
7. John W. Armstrong, *The Water of Life*, U.K
8. Plesch, J., *Urine Therapy*, Medical Press (London), 218:371-382,1947.
9. Dr John, F.O. Quinn, *Self-Healing Through Intrinsic Medicine*, USA.
10. *Auto-urine Cure, Arthur Lincoln Pauls*, USA,
11. Linda Clark, *Get Well Naturally*, USA.
12. Harald W. Tietze, *Urine the Holy Water*, Australia.
13. Dr Chanchalmal chordia, *Uropathy*, India.
14. Dr C. Mithal, *Miracles of Urine Therapy.*
15. Navneet Publications, *Auto-Urine Therapy.*

29

Rise and Fall of Urinopathy Movement

The modern medicine called industrial medicine, or allopathic medicine, or drug medicine is 200 years old only. Whereas urinopathic medicine has been the primary medicine used by the human community since time immemorial, has history of 5,000 years. After advent of allopath, antibiotics, brufin, aspirin, painkillers, symptoms treatment drugs, advanced surgical technology created a belief among the public against urine therapy.

A renaissance in nature cure began in recent years. People, institutions experts became aware of the limitations, dangers, harmful effects of antibiotics, painkillers, surgery, suppressive drugs, science and medical technology. A growing public interest, awareness in natural medicine to maintain, prevent and restore health has led a resurgence of belief in the urinopathy, diet, lifestyle towards ideal health. This validated the original philosophy and principles of Shivambu.

In recent years, many are no longer happy and are feeling enthusiasm with what had become modern medicine, people are not believing it as holistic medicine good or worth doing, people are becoming disenchanted with the drugs causing harm to the natural body.

Patients very greatly felt or experienced very strongly, gained great knowledge and understanding of its :

1. Clinical limitations,
2. Prohibitive cost,
3. Side effects,
4. Reactions of prescription drugs.

They all put together out weighted their benefits. As a result millions of people throughout the globe choose to look for options and alternatives. Urinopathic medicine, and all of complementary, natural and alternative medicine began an era of rejuvenations.

Today, more people than before are seeking urinopathic medical care. Auto-urine awareness programmes are growing at rapid rate to inculcate interest and increased demand for urinopathic knowledge. In some states, government authorities, institutions, doctors, researchers recognised the urinopathic therapeutics. It is driving force for the therapy.

This book is instrumental in the development of the therapeutic knowledge, and practice, and in the expanding awareness of vital of urinopatic medicine has to play in the future of the healthcare system of human race in this country and outside. As we entered the twenty-first century with innumerable and incurable human ills, people are at healing crisis, and cross-roads. Urinopathic medicine finds itself well recognised widely for a new era in healthcare.

Besides, more and more scientific research findings, studies and result are supporting the therapy, it is hoped that the auto-urine medicine is poised to make the transition from a 'shy' practice to truly mainstream medicine. With expanded educational programmes, awareness, it is witnessed an increased interest in the holistic, traditional, drugless drug urinopathic medicine, and alternative healthcare awareness, urinopathy experiencing a resurgence of interest.

In the past a few decades, urinopathic medicine experienced dramatic growth with special scientific studies, research findings, clinical observations on safety and efficacy, expanded applications to emerging new conditions, diseases, degenerative diseases like cancer, cardio, and opportunistic infections like AIDS/HIV positive.

Urinopathic medicine is well recognised scientifically as a distinct holistic system of primary healthcare that use human urine, and its substances to support and stimulate body's self-healing process with prevention, maintenance and curative capabilities. Today its use is widespread throughout the world.

Today urinopapthy is also practised in USA, Japan, China, France, Great Britain and other countries.

The past a few decades have witnessed extraordinary recognition, increase in number of drinkers and awareness for safe, effective and cost effective natural healthcare. Accordingly, urinopathic medicine has emerged as the healthcare product best suited to meet changing socio-economic conditions of life. Although the therapy almost disappeared in the mid twentieth century because of popularity of drug, surgery. Urinopathy now offer an effective natural practice as a vital part of the healthcare system of twenty first century.

As a matter of fact, it is evident that there is an increasing global recognition of the value and relevance of urinopathy which has in part arisen from a growing awareness of the practical and usage limitations of modern medicine. Furthermore, urine therapy entails both the preventive and therapeutic dimensions of urine.

An important element in the world-wide trend towards urinotherapy has been the prominent emergence of tech-pharmacology being most prevelant–in the industrialised countries.

It is generally deplored that use of natural agent, i.e., urine is nothing but relooking of outdated, unusual and exciting thing which is not relevant for industrial medicine. This view is backed by conducted many extensive research studies. But it is also identified that in general the therapy represents a still poorly explored field of research. There is nonetheless a compelling basis for recognising the global relevancy of research and development in the field of traditional healthcare medicine. Only a little, compared to allopathic is actually known about urine as a source of medicine and nutrition.

So, it is that out of hundreds of hormones, substances of urine in minute quantity, but multiples, each of which is a powerful medicine for treating many modern human ailments, only a few have been adequately investigated by medical science. This meagre understanding of urine is particularly acute in India, where nothing at all is known about bulk of our urine.

But known people are blindly using and producing good recovery result. It is thus being increasingly acknowledged, the utilisation of urine as medicine by household people, remains as the most and timely means of potential value. But literally, many of the people are still remain totally unknown to the science of urinopathy. In the recent era of natural and traditional renaissance, the awareness of urinopathic medicine by western and European communities has been steadily increasing particularly over the past two decades. The urine drinkers are not discussing and disclosing their practice with others or physicians.

During the past few decades there has been an increasing interest and awareness in the industrialised nations and modern scientific world about the medicinal properties of human urine. Sources of details are indigenous knowledge, research findings, scientific literatures and other documented sources.

Inspite of its potential for the development as main stream practice, but it has not received significant inputs and encouragement from the government. This is more revealing when compared with what research is going on in many other developed countries. The therapy as feared, may deteriorate primarily due to the lack of concern and at times due to apparent ignorance on the part of medical authorities in responsible position. All healing practices involving urine medicine in many counties continue to be limited to the household sectors. This fact alone contributes to the isolation and subsequent non-recognition in the national health system. Today healthcare system is almost exclusively based on the concept of modern medicine.

Many people of modern days do not have adequate knowledge and awareness of urinopathic healing system. Inspite of the voluntary efforts of the public, little has been done by medical industry in recent decades in India, to embrace and develop the beneficial aspects of urinopathic medicine, including related awareness programmes and to bring into as main stream medicine. This calls for an urgent action to document and preserve the ancient medical knowledge before it disappears from the country. Everyone must firmly support and encourage this practice as a part of national heritage. Urine drinkers are there at every level. Efforts have to be made in coordination with them for wider implementation at the community level. However, recently efforts are made at national and international level to expand and encourage its utility. Hopefully, these are similar efforts by research organisations will help to change prevailing trend.

There is also a need to shift the widely held notion by the medical community that research on modern medicine is more significant and considered as prestigious than that devoted to urinopathic health system. The relatively small amount of research, few studies devoted to urine medicine is a striking feature. From the side of allopathic physicians very little efforts have been made by them to understand the true power of its healing. They seem to think that there is no logic to whatever urine therapy do and they remark as mockery.

In addition, today there are regional, national and international associations with members of urine drinkers, doctors, researchers, crusaders, propagators with strong federal structure. They are giving consultations that provide clients with the necessary information. In the post industrial, and electronic age, recently people increasingly realising the impact of modern medicine's side effects, after effects of drugs, antibiotics, painkillers.

Today, a new group of medical professionals have entered the healthcare industry. They are called as "Medical Urinopaths". It is a strange combination, originally by profession they are allopathic physicians practising drugs and surgery based medicine, and now shifted to urinopathic, practicing holistic, non-drug urine medicine. They are vexed with drug, as certain conditions cannot be cured by prescription drugs.

30

A Note About Doubts On Urinopathy

The topic is about some thoughts on sceptics of urinopathic medicine. In all small or large group of cross sections public interactions, I have experiences that many people having doubts about the claim, whether the therapy is true or that this will cure? Many have sceptical. Many are unable to convince the sceptics in the audience. The attitude of doubting is as old as its evolution.

The incidents of expressing disapproval of the therapy and opinions about its faults or bad qualities are heard even today. To say, what you do not like or think is wrong about it is not universal. But there is a widespread criticism of the handling of the therapy by the government, institutions and medical field.

Doubts about the urinopathy like doubts of any alternative therapy can be unhealthy when this is based on ignorance of it. Similarly, it is unreasonable when one blindly maintains, argues with closed mind or denies good scientific evidences. Sadly, the vast majority of people who express doubts about urinopathy do not maintain a healthy criticism, but they tend to be uninformed, misinformed, unaware, not based on personal experience. They blindly deny about auto-urine therapy and the latest lot of evidence that confirm its efficacy and benefits.

Unfortunately it is very small ironic comment to oppose of what they are saying. Besides those people who hold themselves out as defenders of science validated system tend to have such an unscientific attitude towards uropathy. They exhibit themselves their ignorance and arrogance about their view-points only. They have no or little thought for other methods, behave proudly and in an unpleasant way. Those people who are allopathic physicians knowing well, intentionally attack uropathy on argument that there is no scientific evidence that the therapy works. Infact they make this assertion so often, and they support their own therapies and pathies and oppose others.

Needless to say any one who says that urine is poisonous and harmful to health and that there is no scientific evidence that urinopathic medicine works is simply proving ignorance of the bio-chemistry of this subject. As this book on this sensational issue validates or verifying its propensity for misinformation.

The fundamentalists of allopathic physicians believe that what they have studied, and that the allopathic medicine is the only completely true and universal subject also like to assert that there is no physical evidence and mechanism for how urinopathy medicine works. Such opinions speak about a serious ignorance of medical history and bio-chemistry.

As a matter of fact, they do not properly and adequately understand the mechanism of action, reaction and side effects of aspirin, painkillers, antibiotics, surgery except abuse of over prescription of drugs. Urinopathic physicians, practitioners, propagators where-ever, made reference to many clinical research studies that support and verify the efficacy of uropathy, the deniers ignore as insignificant. They have not taken up any initiative for deep study to show that urinopathic medicine do not work. The only study in which they have been keen is in prescriptive medication. Sadly, there is a silent open secret as to anti-urinopathic movement, simultaneously there is understood wide practice of auto-urine therapy as household and personal practice.

On the other side of the coin, these fundamentalists are not willing to take risk or to do innovative studies enough to prove that evidence to evaluate to prove that urinopathy shows no benefit.You know the physical proof of electricity is the shock to feel. No study so far has shown weight of evidence that urinopathic medicine has failed.

Urinopathic medicine is a medicinal substance obtained from human drug urine like 'pencillin' substance obtained from mould used as a drug to treat or prevent is proven everyday. And yet believers, drinkers likewise are saying.

Urinopathy is proven everyday by millions of users world-wide since centuries. It includes many of the most respected statesmen, monks, scientists, physicians, political leaders, yogis, clergy and spiritual leaders, literary greats, sports stars, mountaineers, soldiers, discoverers, voyagers, adventurers, many unknown and everyday average people.

However, newspapers, magazines and even some books in medical field ignore importance of showing efficacy of urinopathic medicine in treatment. This ignorance occurs despite evidence of its significant efficacy as verified in several studies published in medical journals. In addition to the scientific evidence, for urinopathic treatment, public opinions tend to show that urinopathic medicine is one of the more popular traditional treatments used by people as household drug.

The practice of urine is based on traditional empirical evidence, documentary evidence, public opinions, individual therapeutical results. The bottom line in a vast society, there will be always a group of 'denialists' who tend to establish a social view point of refusal to accept that the therapy is unpleasant or painful is true. They don't understand the real fact nor evaluate whether the therapentic value of medicine for the disease.

A group of patients who are cured with urine, if brought on one dais to ventilate in one voice their recovery cases, these denialists will not accept and they say it is mockery or ridiculous. People are still sceptical about urinotherapy might benefit even from observing of people, listening their practical success stories.

Because history, reality confirms that allopathic physicians are the first line of threat to urinopathic medicine for their not coming up and popularity of the therapy. Many of the drinkers who are practicing, spreading awareness are facing cut-throat discouragement from allopathic medicine.

Its traditional practice, popularity received strong opposition, and discouragement from allopathic medicine, which labeled urinopathic medicine as "quackery". Hence, the urinopathic medicine experienced a significant decline in popularity from industrial era, as most health care at that time centered on the allopathic medical model and the rise of painkillers, antibiotics and suppressive drugs. Most of our doctors have severely misinformed the public as well as most of the medical profession, also believes that it is not based on sound scientific principles and it generally does not work. What a pity, these opinions are not even remotely correct. The therapy has been around us for a great deal longer than any of medical course. Power and greed closed their mind with tremendous ignorance. It is many thousands of years old, but proper training in this field is not given in their curricular of many years of intense study.

To quote Abraham Lincoln:

"You can fool some people all of the time, and all of the people some time, but you can not fool all people all the time".

Finally, it may be appropriate for the readers to recollect invaluable sayings of great people:

Diamond cuts the diamond.
Poison kills the poison.
Bodily substance heals bodily ills.

Dare to taste, to experience,
The taste is in pudding,
Try it yourself and see for yourself,
All great truths begin as blasphemies.

31

Benefits Conferred By Shivambu

Shivambu Kalpa confers numerous health benefits and medicinal secrets of auto-urine. It is a heavenly nectar, which is capable of destroying senility and diseases.

Lord Shiva expounded to Parvathi the following actions of auto-urine therapy :

1. Drinking *Shivambu* for a period of one month, he will be purified internally.
2. Drinking it for two months stimulates and energises the senses. Five powers of senses are sight, hearing, smell, taste and touch.
3. Drinking urine for three months destroys all diseases and frees one from all ailments.
4. By taking it for five months, one acquires divine vision and freedom from all diseases.
5. Practice for six months makes the drinker highly intelligent and proficient in the scriptures.
6. If the duration is for seven months, the practitioner obtains extraordinary strength.
7. Regular practice for eight months, one acquires a permanent glow like that of gold.
8. One is freed from tuberculosis and leprosy if it is practised for nine months.
9. Ten months of this practice makes one a veritable treasury of lustre, feel an extremely strong, especially sexual, desire for something.
10. All the organs of the body are purified if urine is taken for eleven months.
11. Practice for a year becomes equal of the sun in radiance.
12. Continued for two years, one conquers the element of earth.

    Continued for three years, one conquers the elements of water.

    Continued for four years, one conquers the elements of light.

    Continued for five years, one conquers the elements of air.

Continued for seven years, one conquers the elements of pride.

Continued for eight years, one conquers all important elements of nature.

Continued for nine years, one frees one from the cycle of birth and death.

13. Those who practise for 12 years will live so long as the moon and the stars exist.

    He is not troubled by dangerous animals like snakes and no poison can kill him.

Benefits of Urine Mixed With Variants

14. Auto-Urine mixed with powdered amrita (guduchi, tinospora condifola) and taken habitually for six months, one is freed from all disorders, and acquires happiness.
15. He who takes powdered *haritaki* (*harade*, terminalia chebula) in combination with urine taken assiduously destroys senile degeneration and all diseases. If it is taken for a year, it makes one exceptionally strong.
16. One *masha*, nearly one gram of sulpher along with *shivambu*, if taken every morning for three years, he will live as long as the moon and the stars last.
17. The powder of the *koshtha* fruit mixed with urine and practised for 12 years, the body will be free from the ravages of the old age features like wrinkles on the skin, whitening of the hair, acquires the strength of thousand elephants.
18. If the powdered pepper and *trippal choorna* mixed with urine is taken regularly one acquires a radiance Gods.
19. The essence (*bhasma*) of mica and sulpher mixed with *shivambu*, with a little water cures all digestive problems caused by malfunctioning of the digestive system and disorders caused by the *vata* humour. One becomes strong, acqurires a divine radiance.
20. Taking *shivambu* daily and excluded salty, sour and bitter food from diet, acquires divine accomplishments quickly, freed from all ailments, possessing a body comparable to that of Shiva himself, disports like the Gods in the universe for an eternity.

32

Urine is a Life Force

Human urine, as an energetic medicine supplies power and strength within the body, and as a self-therapy it effects energy fields of the body. It is almost impossible to explain, describe its measurement.

The distinct therapy is based on the concept that the human beings are by nature gifted with a subtle form of energy.

This is known as vital energy or life force. This force is understood to circulate throughout the physical human body. As an intangible power, it has not been unequivocally measured by means of modern medical instrumentals. But urine therapists or drinkers claim that they treat a particular type of illness or disorder with the subtle energy or life force.

They see, touch, smell, rub, drink with their own senses and use it to effect changes in the material body and influence health. This energy flows throughout the body touching all the bio-fields or subtle energy fields.

Further, urine drinkers believe that illness results from fluctuations or disturbances in these bio-fields. For example, more than 5,000 years ago, the first practitioners of urine the *yogis* postulated that the flow as well as the balance of life forces is necessary for maintaining health and also described the procedure discipline and diet to achieve the result. They believed in correcting imbalances in different internal bio-fields by reingesting the urine to reinstate health. Some therapists practised vital life force transfer from emitter to others suffering illness to restore health.

Finally, I am bound to say that the life force has inherent power to build or refill immunity system which prevents the body from getting a disease or infection.

33

Urine – The Unknown Medicine

In all hopeless cases and incurable diseases, it proves its efficacy and gives wonderful results, a panacea to health.

1. For innumerable human ailments, there are many drugs. The question is where will it all end ? For each ill a seperate drug, separate side effect ! In modern medicine for every small imaginable type of ailment, separate new drug, vaccines, inoculations for many diseases are also recently designed. Like this, it may go for all diseases. The question is what is the state of the human body, blood after it has been inoculated with all these poisonous preventives. Benchetrit pointed out that vaccines and *sera* are to be chiefly responsible for increase of these two really dangerous diseases; cancer and heart disease.
2. Urine drinkers are less prone to cancer, AIDS, CVD, Asthma and other chronic and acute diseases.
3. Also, this therapy does not require services except very rarely, of all or any assistance towards diagnosis to whom modern medicine now a days resorts. It advocates large scale preventive assurances against one or all of these diseases, preventative against all such modern deadly diseases, is a heavenly nectar.
4. The name diagnosis and cause of the ailment is not fundamental, for the selection of treatment, doses, course etc. It corrects the root cause of the disorder, imbalance, or deficit, this is the one of the merits of urine therapy. It is our just duty to give urine a chance to do the work, it knows the nature of the body.
5. The wonder of the therapy is that the treatment for all diseases is virtually the same procedure almost. To do its work to cure his or her aliment the only prerequisite is to reingest autogenous urine into the body. No need to have any intervention in it. The urine must be left free to play its role of curing, it heals, rebuilds, reconditions the vital organs including repairs. Hundred per cent curing is attainable.
6. A urine is not a manufacturable product outside the body by processing raw materials, chemicals, etc. It is a natural commodity, like elixir, made by the intelligent mechanism of the body. So not harmful. There is no

trade, exploitation of innocent unwary, no sale, no profit, in auto-urine self-therapy. No one can duplicate, or produce the same urine sample outside the body. This is the medical power of the urine.

7. This being a fact, I am optimistic enough to forecast, that in the not too distant future where all incurable diseases will be treated with urine only. This will be the only future medicine to ailing human race. Why cancer and other patients are destined to die on the dictum to be incurable, as when it is possible to cure with urine. Urine therapy can never be unpleasant as in a situation of survival, life and death. As many doctors, research findings, special studies themselves are now as much in favour of urine therapy and recommending. A reform and drastic changes have to come in medical profession.
8. Human urine is the only preventive modality against all these human health problems. The immune system of the body will collapse when a person goes for vaccine, immunisation against all the diseases. There is hardly any preventable and treatable human disease which cannot be controlled or cured with the substance of urine.
9. The underlying rationale for the effectiveness of urine therapy is based on the basic principles that urine contains numerous medical substances that possess therapeutic properties.
10. The urine excretion of each person contains a unique set of drug properties specific to that individual, particular and peculiar to the constitution of the body. These customised properties have medicinal character of curing body's ailments.The urea, nitrogen component of urine of everyone possesses several therapeutic effects.
11. There are many schools or therapies and paths like osteopathy, herbalism, homeopathy, naturopathy, bio-chemic system of medicine, ayurveda, traditional and complementary therapy, hydrotherapy, acupressure, magnetic therapy, healing with food, healing with fasting, healing with sea, healing with sun-light, mud therapy, healing with hives, serums, vaccines and many more. Among them urine therapy seemingly cured, prevented not only in this country alone, as well as outside, lakhs of patients who had in vain who sought relief at the hands of allopaths or other paths.
12. No two people are exactly alike. Likewise there are no two urine samples that contain exactly the same volume of substances, quality and quantity. The medicinal contents of the urine of each one is quite distinct both in colour, taste, substances, volume, etc. Varies according to their body constitution and physiological and biological function of individual.
13. The product urine that targets your health working on circulatory system, digestive system, lymphatic system, muscular, skeletal system,

endocrine system, respiratory system, reproductory system, cardio-vascular system. Urine therapy is based on ancient bio-energetic life force principle and the most complete method available to assume a full body treatment. Urine works on the entire organism, no part of the body is left untouched by its healing energies, hence called as holistic medicine.

14. Urine is the only known body excrete that contain all bio-chemical, substances, nutrients, hormones, enzymes, mineral compounds, etc. that body reabsorbs its own original substances with more concentrated healing potentials, than external drug supplement. This is the medicinal secret and used by the *yogis* for thousands of years to maintain and optimise health, strength, stamina and longevity.
15. The curing power is not just to suppress the symptoms of ailments but works on the root cause of the disease. It acts on complex bio-chemical reactions, which directly influences, the very metabolic process at cellular level.
16. Many scientific studies, clinical investigations have shown that substances of urine have medicinal properties, a therapy for treatment of asthma, arthritis, allergies, acne, cancer, indigestion, migraine, wrinkles and host of other conditions. Many research studies are under way to investigate the potential of other urinary substances to treat infertility and specific form of cancer.
17. Bacteria are often a cause of many diseases today. Human urine possesses bacterial properties, has the capability to destroy the disease causing bacteria in the body, particularly, those infecting the digestive tract.
18. Self-healing principle of urine helps body to overcome virtually any illness. It has been used for centuries to heal the sick. Healing with self-urine is the India's most ancient and natural healing mechanism. When once urine is reintroduced into the body, it knows how to heal, repair itself, build auto immunity.
19. Multiples of many compounds present in the urine in very finely divided and highly potentised form. They are present in a very small quantities but are of substantial benefit to the body for treating many ailments of human race.
20. It is a drugless universal medicine. It costs nothing and can be used by poor and the rich alike.
21. A large number of people having little or no money, poor and rupee-less are treating themselves with their own urine in their own homes, cheap immunity building tonic and the healing does not cost them a rupee.
22. Any ailing patient of any disease can proactive this therapy without any blind risk to themselves. The medicine is always with you and in you, a personal doctor.

23. The practitioners of urine therapy are not visiting hospitals for treatment, or a less than the number of repetitive visits for new complaints than the number under allopathic treatment.
24. The medical data that urine contains therefore cannot be duplicated or derived from any other source.
25. One must not lose sight of the fact of high probability of presence of many substances in urine which are as yet unknown to science, not yet discovered.
26. Regular practice of auto-urine therapy makes the body to absorb more oxygen from external source, motivates metabolic, biological reactions.
27. Urine has the efficiency and efficacy to supply to your body full of life force with energies they need to restore and maintain health.
28. It restores substances, balances the damaged cells, torn out tissues and neutralises. It comes from blood extract and is the most important natural remedy of traditional medicine.
29. Traditionally considened by the yogis, as a panacea a strong holistic non-tonic enhance the energy, life force responsible for your health, sexual, cosmetic, spiritual, stress, anxiety, emotional and behaviour.
30. Any ailment, disease or illness is a symptom of one or more body systems, tissues, cellular disorders. The cause is known from health data of urine. It gives your body nourishment, medicine, to resist, repair, rebuild to achieve optimal health.
31. It should not be forgotten that urine is not at all harmful to the body. Scientific research investigations relating to this area has proved this.
32. The body creates and provides us with a intrinsic and elixir drug most advanced and intelligent system for regaining, rejuvenating, superb human health and beauty.
33. Healing urine is renowned to have medicinal secrets, has been used by indigenous cultures since before recorded history.
34. Urine is considered as nature's own best medicine for its body ailments, supplies nutrients, proteins to the living cells and tissues. Most powerful natural drug known.
35. Urine is a type of antibiotic, substance extraction from blood, a serum used as a drug to treat or prevent infections caused by bacteria. An antibiotic drug, effective antibiotic treatment, like penicillin that can destroy or prevent the growth of bacterial and cure infections.
36. One's own urine is best but in a critical and survival situation someone else's urine can be used as a treatment or cure for a variety of ailments.
37. Auto-urine therapy is an ancient holistic healing system in India.
38. Urine is a body's natural elixir, a human nectar. A medicinal tonic that makes you feel stronger, happier, healthier especially when you feel

tired. A herbal tonic, strengthens the body. A tonic water, with a slightly bitter taste.

39. It confers longevity, long life with good health. A life of physical immortality, a state of health and longevity.
40. Human urine is a anti-poisonous. Urine as a medicinal substance controls the effects of a poison, acts as a antidote to the poison. It is an effective antidote against the harmful scorpion, snake bites. It cures a wound that you get when a poisonous creature bites you, and functions are improved and speeded up.
41. The imbibing of one's own urine would definitely increase in the number of red blood corpuscles in and the hemoglobin content of the blood.
42. Urine reabsored by the body would bring substantial changes in the body functioning.
43. Urine adds the essentials nutrients, proteins, vitamins and other foods eaten in addition to what you eat and drink. It supplements and builds up the deficiency of any substance, minerals in the blood.
44. Enzyme, a substance present in urine which plays a chemical change happen or happen more quickly without being changed itself which a substantial benefit on the physiological reaction taking place in the body.
45. Body needs 12 types of biochemical salts, any deficit in them leads to concerned disease. Human urine contains valuable salts necessary for good health and normal living.
46. Urine increases natural power, resistance to disease.
47. The therapy is based on a fundamental principle of one drug for multifarious diseases rather than modern medicine of risk of selecting from out of thousands of drugs for several diseases. A simple solution for complex problems.

34

Urine Urea : A Natural Drug

Urea is a colourless chemical substance containing nitrogen that is found in urine especially in multiple quantities. Natural urea is deposited in human urine is a natural drug, having medicinal quality has much commercial therapeutic value in curing many incurable modern innumerable human ailments.

The figuration and formation of urine in human body begins with the process of filtration. The filtration consists primarily of water, excess salt, glucose and a waste product of the body called urea. The substance urea is formed in the body to eliminate the very toxic ammonia products which are formed in the liver from amino acids. The interesting feature is that humans cannot excrete ammonia. So it is converted into the less dangerous urea and then filtered out of blood. Urea is the most abundant of the waste products that must be excreted by the kidneys.

Urine consists of 95 per cent of water, 2.5 per cent urea and 2.5 per cent is a mixture of minerals, salts, hormones, enzymes. The critical nutrient urea is produced to the extent of 24.5 milligrams per day. The average quantity of this substance in 100 millilitres of urine is reported of 1,459 milligrams, and 682 milligrams of urea nitrogen.

So, urea is second main constituent of human urine next to water, which has some well known commercial and medicinal use.

Urea is an organic, means carbon based compound whose chemical formula is $CON_2\ H_4$ or $(NH_2)2Co$.

It is also known as carbamide. Urea in urine is derived from ammonia and produced by the domination of amino acids. Amino acids is of any substances which combines to form proteins. The amount of urea in urine is related to the quantity of dietary proteins. Urea is produced when the body tries to balance the ratio of sodium chloride with water.

The medicinal secret of urine urea is anti-fungal, anti-bacterial, anti-viral agent. It has the ability to kill bacteria and restricts inflammation, it is often used in ointments and lotions. It is an excellent scarce cosmetic cream and lotion.

Urea when reintroduced into the body by urine it purifies, cleans up excess mucus and performs a number of other medicinal functions. Urea when recycled by ingesting will be converted into essential amino acids, substances which combine to form proteins. It is one of the chemical components of urine. It has some well known commercial medical uses. The principal ingredient of the nitrogenous wastes in urine is urea, it is a product of protein decomposition. Among other things, urea is a diuretic, means a substance that causes an increase in the flow of urine.

According to some scientific study, that 25 per cent of urea in an adult finds its way into the intestinal. In them, urine is decomposed into ammonia by intestinal bacteria. Some of its quantity ends up in the liver, where a part of it is converted into urea, and another part is converted into glutamine. It is an extremely useful amino acid.

In has healing effects on ulcers and wounds in the intestinal canal.

Glutamine is essential in the :

Maintenance, construction of specialised tissue;

Growth and activity of the mucus membrane of the intestinal canal;

It has the ability to strengthen the immunity system;

It is used in the treatment of cancer, like breast cancer, liver cancer, several other kinks of cancer, liver enlargement.

Urine urea increases the efficiency of the functioning of the kidneys.

35

A Traditional and A Nature Cure

Human urine is a natural medicine, having a natural ability, healing property and a method of intrinsic ability to cure, by which practise a person lives healthily. No need to take any external drugs. A natural elixir that is produced in the body and that can be used as a medicine. The theory that the Creator has taken care of health of His creatures and inbuilt medicine, and life is based on laws, natural elements, causes and laws and not on drugs to be made in factories with external chemicals without special treatment, help or drug, naturally occurring medicine. It is called natural living.

Like earth science and life science, urinopathy is a science concerned with studying the bio-chemical drugs. Living naturally is a process by which human kingdom that can adapt body nature and survive. Urine is a body made substance not found in nature or outside the body. It is the way that body produces, on which man has no control.

Law of the nature of the body. Nature takes its course of action. Body illness is the nature's way of curing. When we consider it as a life force, that effects the human beings. The feature of it is its extreme simplicity as any one can practise without telling. It is not a specific drug for a specific complaint, it is a specific for whole body, for health, a holistic drug.

I do not exaggerate when I say against many therapies and pathies in the world, now known from experience that there is nothing equal to urine for large number of afflictions. We are ignoring and neglecting the nature, not believing its power, if we give a chance it will do its work honestly. It will cure in her own way. We have to understand the mysteries of nature. Trust and see the results. We are not allowing the nature to interfere, we have designed our own ways; we have failed.

Urine therapy is a nature-cure in the real sense of the word, to the natural body. But we are adapting drugs which are against the nature; hence we are unsuccessful to find a preventative and holistic drug.

Urine therapy is the outcome of ancient layman's experience and experiment. Any practitioner who knows body's medical history also knows that layman's opinion and long inheritance practice contributed much to the survival of drugless medicine. He is not a doctor, nor a chemist, druggist but merely natural animal.

We have to learn many lessons from urine way to nature. Live with nature, she will co-operate. We are all born as a group of human kingdom, a part of nature, let us try to be humane and nature. When the nature has provided us with such an inbuilt simple, easy therapy body tight cure and even prevent from diseases, we all must understand and follow the secrets of the nature, body secrete and the life style. Today we are looking at this therapy as the last resort instead of the first choice.

Try this therapy once for any of your common disorders or for external application sincerely and you can find an amazing and wonderful results. Thus you will become your own doctor, your own medicine, for your own disease and a firm believer in your good health is in your urine. An immunity system is built in your body. This wonderful system will protect you from all diseases. The principle of any medical system is to work on the cause of the malady and its removal rather than just to suppress the symptoms of the disease which is the aim of the allopathy system.

Dear reader, you are aware that urinopathy is a drugless, priceless natural substance, body made and self cure as designed by the Creator. Moreover, it is not dangerous, it has no side effects, after effects, nor ill effects.

For many years, mankind has recognised the relationship between health and nature. This is not an entirely new concept as natural healing is still used in many cultures, but perhaps one that has been temporarily overlooked in our own culture since the onset of modern medicine.

Slowly, the case for urinopathy type of healthcare becomes stronger. The wonderful achievements of urine medicine have brought health to our society but perhaps some have forgotten the origin of the natural therapy to disease treatment.

36
Drink Mid-Stream Urine

Drinking the mid-stream urine of urination is the best sample to practise. The part of the urine we are passing at a particular time, is not exactly equal from starting to end point drop. A stream means urine flowing from the bladder, or poured out in a continuous flow freely after starting, collect the middle stream of the steady and continuous movement of the morning first urine. A little quantity at the beginning and ending of piss should not be collected.

The reason why one should not drink the first part means, it removes dirt, impurities from the genital urinary track or passage by washing the track with the same urine. It rinses the way out before so that the rest of the urine will be sterile, clean and free from impurities.

In the urine bladder at the bottom solid material like dust, impurities, mud, stones in small quantities would settle. So, the last part of urine flow contains these sediments and is of little use, better to leave.

The ancient Hindu and yoga texts mention that in auto-urine drinking only the mid-stream samples to be used.

According to *Shivambu Kalpa*, it is wise, one should leave out the first and the last portion of the urine excretion, and collect only the middle portion. This is considered to be the best procedure and practice.

In another verse, the text states the reason why should one to take middle urine only. The answer given is that just as there is a poison in the mouth of the snake and the tail of the serpent; it is even so in the case of the flow of *shivambu*.

37
Drink Morning Urine

The entire urine that you pass in a day is a drinkable good quality of urine. But the urine you excrete between four-six in the morning is preferable. *Yogis* who follow nature and live naturally prefer the early urine. It is because of the fact that the hormones released during the night are propitious in inducing the meditative state of mind. That is likely to produce a successful results.

Either for internal or external use, it is beneficial to collect the morning's first sample. The first urine of the day is considered good both by traditional literature as well as scientific findings.

The ancient yoga texts that mention auto urine drinking, require it to be practised before sunrise.

The *Shivambu Kalpa* also says that after cleansing the mouth, and performing the other essential natural morning functions, one should drink one's own clear urine, which is the annihilator of senillty and diseases. Further, it states that the practitioner of *yoga* should take it before proceeding with his other rituals.

The sagacious practitioner should get up when three quarters of the night has elapsed and should pass urine, facing the east.

It is the custom of the yogis to take morning urine, because hormones are active at night, something wonders happen during the night. Morning urine contains pineal hormone called Melantonin and its different forms of esters in significant quantities. The pineal gland, at the right side of the head, produces a liquid substance hormone called Melantonin at about two am. when eyes which we expose to bright sunlight in the morning, the gland stops producing the Melantonin hormone. It is found in research that when the urine reintroduced into the body by oral taking or given intravenously it causes a particular reaction of tranquility and heightens visualisation. Mills and others, New Castle University, Australia, 1991, suggested that there is high concentration of Melantonin hormones in the first morning urine.

This, they opined, might restore the colourless part of the blood in which the blood cells, etc. float night time Melantonin levels, So, oral pre-dawn consumption of auto-genous Melantonin slows down brain wave activity. This is the scientific reason behind alleged benefits ascribed to auto-urine drinking by ancient texts of yogic religion.

The first flow is the best, and the best time of the day to drink it is between three am–four am. According to *Shivambu Kalpa*, the sagacious practitioners should get up when three quarters of the night have elapsed, and should pass urine facing the east. They should take it before proceeding with their other rituals.

Don't Waste Morning Urine

Urine passed throughout the day is useful, can be drinkable, but first morning urine should not be left over. At night, when you sleep well, you are calmer and less worried, muscles relax completely, all senses relax and sleep, A sleep is a sort of resting and enjoying yourself, something pleasant, clam and not anxious or worried.

A good quality and higher level hormonal discharge takes place at night when you sleep and relax. So, the first morning urine contains the richest in vital substances like hormones, vitamins, proteins, nutrition, minerals, enzymes, metabolities.

Early urine is not poison. Some amount of poison is necessary to the body to stimulate.

When it is taken in morning hours on an empty stomach, it acts as a natural medicine that makes bowel empty, due to the laxative action of hypertonic solution of urea which is present in the urine.

The use of first urine after sexual intercourse is also recommended by urine therapist because during the process of sexual stimulation certain hormones are released in the higher endocrinal glands which have regenerative effect on the body both for men and women.

So, even the slightest reabsorption of morning hormones may well have a powerful effect on our state of health. For instance, Melantonin is a urine which has a calming effect. Urine is a tranquiliser drug which reduces anxiety, makes a person clam or unconsious, a fast acting tranquilising drugless drug, makes a person quiet and peaceful.

Yogis led a tranquil life in those days because they used to drink urine. A urine drinker will never get excited, nervous, or upset. Regular drinkers become quite and more relaxed, reabsorption of urine having calming agent, hormones have a calming influence. Melantonin and other hormones are released during sleeping time, so its reuse has a deep relaxation effect, such a valuable hormones should not be wasted, as they are produced with lot of energy and time.

38

Preserved Urine

Human urine is a natural substance that can be preserved without decay. It can be prevented from decaying by treating in a particular way. It can be stored well remarkably in original state in good condition for a week's time. Urine will not change or damage by age or weather.

The stored urine will have a medicinal quality, since preserved or old urine is of higher concentration of ammonia. It acts as a therapeutic medicine against skin diseases and rashes. For external application and massaging stored urine can be used more effectively.

In the process of preservation, it increases the strength of the urine by reducing its volume. It becomes like concentrated orange juice, concentrated solution of salt in water.

A fresh urine can be made as old urine, when it is stored in a dark bottle, closed tightly and kept away from light and the sun up to seven days.

A little quantity of urine can be applied directly on the skin all over the body. Like scent spray, urine can also be sprayed on the skin, mixed or added to skin locations, creams or moisturisers.

39

Urine the Mysterious Liquid

God created the physical body. It is something that is difficult to understand or to explain. Though the modern science found something about its anatomy, compositions of the body. But still there are many more secrets and so the body is one of the great unsolved mysteries of science. The motive of creation itself remains a mystery.

A physical body that is strange and interesting because we do not know much about it. Life itself is a mystery because its existence is a mystery tour, as we do not know where from we have come, where we are going, what is the fate of this decaying body, soul's journey.

The quality of health, quality of being difficult to understand or to explain especially when this makes something seem interesting and exciting. Mystery surrounds body's appearance, disappearance and reappearance. We know much about it.

A real story, or fictitious story, a film, movie or a play in which a theme, crimes, social event and strange events can be explained at the end. The secret knowledge of the functioning of the body, health, decay are not known. Secrets from religious postulates, a religious belief cannot be explained or proved in a scientific way.

We know nothing about the truth of urine. Do you think you know truth? I do not think you know the whole truth about the nature. But it is true that there is no truth in rumours about urine. The fact is believed by most people to be true is not really true. It is half truth, but health truth, medicinal secret. Truth is stranger than fiction and rumour.

Therapists used to say these things that actually true, are often surprising than the rumours that are invented. The truth will out, if you practice urine therapy, you find out the true fact about it even if you try to keep it secret.

The secret truth if you discover, you will come to know how little you really know. All through these ages, inspite of all philosophies, religions, sciences, spiritual texts, urine remains mystery, and very often upsets all our pet theories.

We are born with urine tight bodies. We are thus born like this, it affects all the organs, that is mysterious; because it matches as a drug to innumerable diseases.

People who have practiced the urine therapy lived the longest and suffered the least. The inference that is to be drawn from this is that in recent years most people suffered from new, degenerative diseases, some of them died of modern medicine and not of disease which is based on basic principle of many drugs, many diseases. The mystery of urine therapy is that one drugless drug for many diseases. It is not a specific medicine for a particular ailment, but to whole health.

There is nothing equal to urine. It is based on long experience, why it is mysterious, as well as is that it seems to be an 'unpleasant' idea self-discipline. But life itself is a discipline. We consider it as dirty rude practice because it is connected with genital.

Urine therapy has become a mystery because, it is strange and interesting because we do not know much its natural contents of healing properties. People bathe, drink, gargle, massage, sniff with it. No wonder, it is not just faith, religious, the healing liquid possesses many chemicals and medicinal substances, that is the mystery, this book piercing this secret.

Give a chance to urine to treat, it will work in its own natural way, though we not understand its mysteries.

Truly, nature's way is not our way, it superseds all our disgust beliefs, barbarous superstitions, orthodox tenets, it has its own way. 'Urine the unknown' is the super-medical panacea to public health.

40
Mystic Power

A person who believes and tries to drink urine becomes disease-free and maintains, good health and normal living through devotion and regular practice. He understands the important curing things that are beyond normal human understanding.

We consider human excretion urine as wasteful, but practitioners, believers understand that it has spiritual power of qualities in prevention and curing which is difficult to understand or to explain. Partly human urine has mystical force and power. Many people who have benefited from auto-urine therapy have felt an almost mystical experience, unbelievable being waste, showing wonderful results.

Shivambu, a therapy formulated and advocated by Lord Shiva, the belief that knowledge of God, the Creator of the body, who knows the internal secrets of the body functioning.

So, the real truth of the treatment results can be found through trust, and belief in God's words rather than through reason, the senses and scientific supports. Simply people are made confused because they do not understand this mystified by barbarous superstitions and disguest beliefs.

The fabulous medicinal and curing quality of the urine being mysterious or secretive it makes auto-urine therapy interesting or attractive. Because of this reason uropathy has become famous.

As a traditional medicinal practice it has been in existence from ancient times. We cannot say that this therapy does not have historical documentary evidence. It is not fictitious, but real.

The therapy is connected with ancient mythological subjects. It is an ancient practice of Indian culture. The idea of urine therapy as a treatment modality is a fact.

41
Animals' Urine

It is a customary practice in India to drink cow's urine in large quantity. It is done even today for the cure of many human ailments and other afflictions.

Some pharmaceutical manufacturing companies in advanced countries are breeding horses to collect their urine to produce drugs and injections for curing human ailments.

In 'Sunni Islam', the 'Sahih Bukhari' collections quote that prophet Mohammad advocating drinking camel's urine as a medicine, when a group of people from Uraina tribe came to Madina became ill.

It is a household medicinal practice in many families to give infant babies donkey's, goats' urine and milk as a preventive medicine like vaccine against polio and other degenerative diseases. Thus, the health giving properties of urine have been known in India for centuries. Some people drink one's own urine regularly, they never fall ill and live long, healthy.

But one's own urine is superior as a preventive and curative agent to animal's urine. Patient's own urine contains medicinal properties according to one's body's requirements. The wiser of the ancient *yogis* used nothing but urine for the treatment and longevity. Country side people even to this day use urine as the same measures.

In rural areas the drinking of one's own urine has been widely practised.

In rural side, the use the cow's urine is recommended by many people for boils and many chronic internal ailments. Patient's own urine is superior as a curative agent to cow's urine.

42

What Conditions Can Urinopathic Medicine Treat ?

Urinopathy is sometimes called panacea, something a drugless drug, isopathy that will solve all the problems, ailments of human body. It is the medicine of holistic approach to life, that cures the whole person rather than just the symptoms of a disease. It eradicates the cause of the malady rather than suppressing the symptom of the ailment.

The treatment does apply universally, cure is universally availabe, universally known and universally accepted. A universal medicine does concern all the people in the world, true or right, at all time, and in all places, and the drug is always with you and in you.

The intrinsic value of medicine has been recognised. It belongs to you, on the part of the real nature of the body. There is nothing intrinsically wrong with this self-therapy. It is good in itself. There may be a misconception that it is a waste product, and hence not drinkable.

As a matter of fact the list of diseases for which urine therapy is said to be effective is around 175 known diseases, really abnormal number of ailments for any type of medical practice.

'Ease' and 'Dis-ease'

The immunity system, hormonal, nervous, detoxification, elimination are the basic risk factors which should always be in a balance-state to restore optimal health. When they are in a state of balance, the body is said to be at 'ease'. Otherwise it is said to be at 'dis-ease'. Human urine is a vital force which promotes self detoxification, builds immunity system, self repair and auto-pathogen. So, human body has the innate ability for self–healing and it makes you feel at 'ease'.

The philosophy of urinopathy ensures optimal wellness, wellness enhancement and 'ease' management but not 'disease' management.

Classification

The therapy will be invaluable for the present youth, and for the future generation. It is the only the last resort or first choice. Further and future research should prove the valuable things of urine that prevent and cure emerging innumerable and incurable human ailments. Urine possesses curative properties. So, all illnesses can be cured. Even incurables as we consider today like cancer and AIDS also become curable with urine. What that cannot be cured need not be endured, if urine therapy is properly practised.

Disease

The disease of a body is an illness affecting a person often caused by infection or virus or chemical imbalance and other means. There may be many more reasons which cause a disease. It is a suffering from bodily disorder, not feeling well, or in an unpleasant way. It is a state of getting affected very badly by a disease causing pain, sadness, inconvenience, trouble and discomfort. The sufferer of an illness is said to be suffering from a disease.

Disorders

The body of a person is said to be in order when it works in a normal way and logical way as nature designed establishing a calm, orderly life, good health and normal living. Body is said to be functioning in a disorderly way when it has an illness that makes a part or organ of the body stop functioning well. It is a state of suffering due to mental, physical, emotional or psychological disorders which require correlation and proper planning of life.

For instance, a blood disorder, bowel disorder, eating disorder, psychiatric disorder, respiratory disorder, behavioural disorder, emotional disorder, cardio–vascular disorder, hair, nose, eye disorders, mental or physical disorders are the result of lack of correlation and planning.

Common Diseases

All common ailments can effectively be cured by applying your own urine without often visiting a doctor and eating dangerous drugs like pain killers, antibiotics and others which will have side-effects, ill-effects and after-effects. These are a group of illnesses which are more frequent, happening often in large numbers or in many places. Some kinds of complaints which are common in day-today life like allergies, cough, skin infection which are quite commonly faced by or belonging to two or more people or by the people in a group in all places and the diseases have the same characteristics by the same cause.

Some Common Curable Human Ailments

Fever	Indigestion	Hepatitis	Cold
Gas/acidity	Dry skin	Flew	Nueasy
Eczema	Cough	Allergies	Troatache
Malaria	Infection	Weight loss	Chickenpox
Insect-bite	Measles	Scorpion poison	Miscarraiage

Menstrual problem	Dysentery	Itches	Wrinkles
Piles	Fistula	Fissure	Urticaria
Nephritis	Bed wetting	Mucus colitis	Rheumatic fever
Rash/Wart/Hump	Cataract	Glycoma	Hair loss
Hypertension	Chronic ear	Viral infection	Fatigue
Rabies	Fungal infection	Polio	Candida
Anemia	Urinary diseases	Hives	Tinea
Wounds, Injuries	Epilepsy	Burns	Cuts

Acute Diseases

A group of diseases which are very serious or severe are classified as acute ailments. They have those features which quickly become severe and dangerous. For instance, acute pain, acute illness, acute appendicitis, acute allergy, or body's acute general health problem are very sensitive and fast developed.

Auto-urine, or urinopathic medicine can treat either alone or in combination of other complementary therapies like massaging and water therapy. Some of them are : headaches, sore throats, ear infections, intestinal disorders, cold, flu, etc.

Chronic Diseases

Especially, a class of ailments lasting for a long time, they are of the nature which are difficult to be cured or got rid of easily. A person may have had a disease for a longtime: for example, chronic bronchitis, chronic arthritis, chronic asthma, chronic sinus, chronic blocked nose or congestion or chronic fatigue syndrome.

Some acute and chronic complaints curable with urine are :

T.B.	Psoriasis	Eczema
Pemphigus	Gall stone	Lyme
Cholera	Acne	Migraine
Pelvic information	Ulceractive Coatings	Fatigue syndrome
Hasnimoto	Chronic cystitis	Prurigois
Uslicaria	Ulcers	Digestive disorders
Whooping cough	Hives	Tooth abscess
Prostate Enlargement	Parasites/viruses	Epilepsy
Lumpe	Ring worm	Sores
Enteritis	Diarrhoea	Gastroenteritis
Pneumonia	Gout	Blood urine
Immunological disorders	Infertility	Insomnia

Urticaria	Obesity	Papilloma
Lumbago	Infections	Abrasion
Gangrene	Sinus	Bronchitis
Breathing congestion	Nasal blockings	Typhus
Tetanus	Cosmetic disorders	Mouth and Dental ailments
Stomatitis	Gingivitis	Pyorrboea
Dandruff	Constipation	Conjunctivitis
Orchitis	Respiratory problems	Laxative disorders
Tendon	Jaundice	Asthma
Heart complaints	Musculoskeletal pain,	Gynaecological problems
Gastro intestional		

Degenerative Diseases

It is a type of disease of a human body where a part or organ whose characteristic feature is that it cannot make a part or organ to develop and grow strong again. Once destroyed, torn out, or dead or exhausted, they cannot be regenerated. The regenerative power of the body made by God is lost forever. The affected part or organ becomes worse by becoming lower in quality, strength and energy. It becomes weaker and weaker finally becomes weakest which cannot be rebuilt. The body loses its orderly status and normal standards which fall to a very low level which is not optimal for good health and normal living. Body lacks in originality that is usually present and required. This type of illness gets or likely to get worse as time passes and the body cannot be repaired, restored to its natural position due to these diseases.

The degenerative diseases are :

Arthritis	Diabetes
CAD	Kidney disorders
Cancer	Paralysis
Angina	Tumor, etc.

Opportunistic Infections

This infection is an illness that is caused by bacteria or a virus which affects one or other part of the body. An opportunistic infection is a serious illness harmful to the people whose immune system is weak either because of disease or due to use of drugs. Some types of diseases may be waiting for an appropriate opportunity, a time when a particualr situation makes it possible to attack. These types of infections or diseases can be passed easily from one person to another by any means. These are the infections that can easily spread to others. They have a character of spreading the disease through touching or contact as they are highly contagious.

These infections are extremely dangerous, harmful and of fast spreading nature. Diseases caused by viruses which are living things and too small to be seen without a microscope, cause infections diseases, some of which are deadly. For instance, venereal diseases (VD) which are passed on to others by having sex with an infected person.

Instances are :

1. AIDS (Acquired Immune Deficiency Syndrome),
2. HIV Positive (Human Immuno-deficiency Virus),
3. Syphilis,
4. Ganorrhoea,
5. Skin,
6. Urine, etc.

Inherent Tendencies

They become serious illnesses or degenerative diseases??

Mental and Emotional Imbalances

The effects of recent stresses, long term pattern of anger, depression, anxiety??

Physical Injuries

Wounds, injury, infections, trauma, skin-burns, cuts.

A separate volume is required to write the list of human ailments that can be cured by urine therapy.

There are thousands and thousands of ailments which positively responded to urine therapy. Even incurable ailments are successfully treated all through the years. I do not want to increase the pages of this volume by including all such variant diseases. It is a long and big history.

Many of the patients who were previously ignorant of the existence of urine-therapy, tried other therapies and pathies, both modern, traditional and natural, but failed and finally resorted to urine drinking.

43

When Can You Expect Result ?

How long will it take to work on a patient's body ? The recovery time varies greatly depending on the individual body response and the type of condition. Acute conditions can respond to treatment within a few days. Chronic conditions require more time for recovery due to their complexity, stage and can take one–two months, even, three-four months to treat cancer like conditions to notice improvement. Even degenerative, opportunistic conditions ultimately respond very successfully to urinopathic treatment.

Treatment aims at supporting and helping the body to heal itself with the use of inherent life forces. It treats the underlying cause within the body to achieve optimal health.

Nature-cure-treatment agent like urine is to treat the cause or root of the disease but not to suppress the symptom of a disease which is the function of allopathic medicine. It will take time to remove the obstacles on the way of health. Allopathy suppresses the symptoms and gives quick and temporary relief but urine gives permanent cure as it cures the cause.

Urinopathic medicine does not offer a magic cure. Each individual has his or her own unique set of symptoms and reaction. It is a customised treatment protocol.

Urine theraphy works in two ways such as :

1. Preventive maintenance,
2. Specific disease cure.

If a person is taking urine regularly even without any illness, it works as a preventive medicine. It stops any illness that is going to happen rather than curing the disease after it has happened. Prevention is better than cure, preventable from complaints. An ounce of urine which acts as a preventable medicine is better than a pound of curing medicine. Prevention is the best cure.

Truly, great results come from removing obstacles, maintaining balance between risk factors and building immunity system. Prevention requires to maintain balance between immunity, hormone, nervous, detoxification, elimination and demands regular proactive for the body to respond to prevention.

Wonderful results within a short period of therapy are reported in cases of many acute, common, chronic, skin, sinus, bronchitis diseases.

When can you expect results from urinopathic medicine is a matter that depends on each type of illness, body nature, etc. The respone time varies between quick, immediate, short, medium and long term.

A Magic Liquid

There is no any magic secret power of treating a disease and curing it by saying words, or doing special things.

Do you believe that there is magic in urine therapy?

But the results seems too wonderful to believe. But urine has a special and distinct medicinal property that makes curing seem wonderful.

There is no magic power supported by evil spirit.

A urine drinker is not a sorcerer, having magic power.

It has a mesmerising effect on the illness that you cannot find in allopathic therapy or anything else.

There is no black magic to use the power of the devil in order to perform evil.

Urinopathy is a natural approach to health and healing with the emphasis on integrity of the whole individual.

It is vitalistic household medicinal tradition in India. It prevents, cures and maintains through stimulation, enhances, supports, refills immunity and promotes inherent healing-capacity through self-healing. It works with patient's life force.

Urinopathy is attempting to stimulate and support one's own system to address the cause that has been responsible for the ailment. Often long-term underlying disturbances must be corrected in order to allow the body to realign to its natural state of optimal health and remove the deep rooted cause of the disease from the body. However, preventive maintenance of the body requires regular drinking of urine.

44
Success Stories

For centuries, many people who have come forward with miraculous stories of having been healed with self-therapy by drinking urine. As a last resort in survival situations, people used and were surprised. All advocates have offered for evidence of the efficacy of urine therapy, information of case studies are held back, to the public for some reason, for centuries. This is only hardcore public experience in support of this therapy. Otherwise there is no much hardcore scientific and medical evidence. Of course, the medicinal value of urine therapy is difficult to establish, because most people would probably do not want to come to public, or to conduct research studies.

This is the reason why the people continue to wonder how urine can cure. The idea of using it for treatment, the successful stories of power may seem shocking. For centuries, urine therapy has long played a crucial role in the holistic medical traditions of households of societies all over the world. People have been getting benefited with urine's incredible curative powers for diseases ranging from common to serious ailments.

Urine thus has been the best penicillin, tonic, natural vaccine for your body. It has to its credit many case histories of people, fills volumes to write, who have been successfully cured. Today this surprises even scientifically advanced countries like USA, Germany and Japan. It works to treat a wide array of ailments.

Use of urine as a medicine for all bodily problems is a common medical tradition of rural people, *yogis, kapalis* who lived close to the nature. Besides, there are numerous medical, scientific, clinical studies, investigations on urine application and effects.

There are many testimonials from authoritative sources about abilities of urine healing qualities and medicinal character.

The success stories, shocking news, survivors' reports, provide a good resource for understanding the uses, and supporting evidence and contemporary users are the most compelling argument for trying urine therapy. Inspite of this, still it is very difficult to convince a layman, majority of people that one liquid can cure a number of diseases.

More and more people are recovering, regaining their health, new and new variety of diseases are cured. Extensive and specific research studies are undertaken adding it to their healthcare options, became as an individual and family health care system.

45

Urine – A "Doctor of Divinity"

Your Personal Doctor

Human urine, as a medicine has its roots of divination. It means the act of believing, saying and practising urine therapy that will effectively work, acts as preventive in the future and cures present human ailments. The origin and source are in religious texts. Urine is a nature's elixir, means a magic liquid, that is having capability of curing illnesses, and make people live forever. Heavenly nectar of life or youthfulness.

Natural urine is a divine nectar. A nectar is a sweet liquid that is produced by flowers and collected by bees for making honey. Likewise human urine is a watery solution of the body that is produced by the complicated and intricate process of blood filtration, extracted by kidneys and nephrons process.

It is a serum, the thin liquid that remains from blood when the rest has clotted. Derived from blood can be taken as medicine to protect from diseases, poison, etc.

So, it is a liquid-like water in blood tissue, mixed process of God's power, biologically coming from connected with God. A divine intervention in the production process, deposited, an intrinsic medicine, a help from God to change or improve a health disorder. It contains the qualities of God or like God. The study of auto-urine therapy is partly a study of divinity, the study of nature of God and religious belief. Urinopathy is this called as a "Doctor of Divinity".

There is no particular reason, how it works and cures. It is just wonderful and people are very much surprised by its nature of working. People using it have a feeling of surprise and admiration they have when they see the unexpected results. Something intrinsic force or quality in urine that fills us with surprise. Prevention and curing quality is one of the natural wonders of the world, God has created. That is the wonder of divine body, one can always discover in physical body.

A neglected, but still a new wonder drugless drug, has a very good effect on the health.

It is not surprising, it is little wonder that it impressed. It is strange that what we have considered as wasteful body excrete, it is wonder that it has become life saving medicine. I have no words, or phrases to be used to express surprise and pleasure at this naturopathy.

Wonders, divine gifts will never cease, work wonders to achieve very good health results. Dietary styles and exercise programme coupled with drinking one's own urine has worked wonders for many people all these centuries. It is remarkable what you can do when you have to. Regular practitioners in way that exhibited unusually surprising results, feeling tremendously exciting challenge, keeps the body remarkably in good condition for its age, without disease, decay and figure change.

46

Urine–Your Personal Doctor

1. Respiratory System Problem

Drinking urine helps a person who experiences difficulty in breathing and makes one breath again in normal way. Urine liquid makes it possible for a sufferer to breath over a long period when he is unable to do so normally. Respiratory problem is connected with breathing, i.e., inhaling and exhaling. It repairs, and removes disorders in respiratory tract, breathing system, and heals the respiratory ailments.

Urine therapy alleviates the ailments of asthma, hay fever, T.B. and whooping cough. Hay fever is chronic illness that affects the nose, eyes and throat, it is caused by pollen from plants that is breathed in from the air.

Whooping cough is an infectious disease and urine is an anti-bacterial. It is especially of children that makes them cough and have difficulty in breathing. Similar is T.B. a serious infectious disease in which swelling appears on the lungs and other parts of the body.

2. Ulcers

One's own urine has a therapeutic property purported to have healing benefit in case of various ulcer complaints. The urogastrone component of urine cures on the outside of the body, or on the surface of an organ inside the body which is affected and bleeds or produces poisonous substance.

Urine therapy helps in preventing peptic ulcer and also correct and promote the healing of existing peptic ulcers. It is an ulcer in the digestive system, especially in the stomach. Similar benefits can be obtained for duodenal ulcers and gastric ulcers. Duodenal ulcer originates at the first part of the small intestine, and then spreads to the stomach. Gastric ulcer connected with gastric juice, i.e., the acid in the stomach that helps to digest food. Mouth ulcer affects small area in the mouth.

3. Eye Drops for Complaints

A drinker of urine will have a good ability to see. Eye-sore and uncomfortable looking problems can be solved. If you are a regular washer of your eyes with urine, there is no need of a surgeon, or physician.

It is good against all eye problems. Wash your eyes with urine; it cleans, strengthens the sight. You never lose your eye-sight throughout your life. You will have a very good eye-sight. No disease will affect your eye-sight. You can use fresh or boiled urine for eye-application. Urine can be used as eye drops.

Urine is a liquid medicine that you can put one or two drops at a time into your eyes, so that the problems like eye pain, burning, tired eyes can be solved. It reduces or removes an unpleasant feeling, makes the problems less serious and prevents future occurrence. You will be relieved to feel your sight, job and work safe and comfortable.

Urine mixed with a bit of water in order to dilute is also very useful. Conjunctivitis, an infectious eye disease that causes pain and swelling in the parts of the eyes can effectively be cured with your own urine. In case of those who are wearing contact lenses continuously, the skin part of the eye area near nose top sore, painful or irritative, urine external application will give relief. Any scare or mark left over will disappear soon. Clearing, sore eyes, weak sight, pain, burning, tired eyes, conjunctivitis, irritation, etc. are solved.

4. Throat Disorders

The tube in the neck that takes food and air into the body is always inflicted with common ailments, disorders and infections: for instance a sore throat, a sob cough or wound. A throat sore is painful, and often red especially because of infection, injury or because of muscle has been used too much, either by water, air, food etc. One's own urine is a specific medicine to reduce soreness, swelling or tightness. Different types of throat inflammation can be cured by gargling with one's own urine.

Usually, soaked stockings in urine and wrapped them around the neck in order to cure sore throat.

Urine gargling is useful to cure sore-throat. Taking urine into your lungs as you breath in through your mouth gives wonderful results. The method of inhaling of urine is adopted by people who have problems with breathing. It relieves blocked sinusitis, a problem of painful swelling of the sinuses. Any of the hallow spaces in the bones of the head that are connected to the inside of the nose is a sinus ailment.

Respiratory diseases relating to respiratory track, blocked with blood or mucus known as congestion problems are also cured.

5. Teeth Problems

Teeth must be strong for biting, chewing food, drinking. White teeth are good for appearance. Whoever else cleans the teeth with urine will have white teeth. What you piss, you can use to brush, teeth, red gum, so that your teeth look polished. Urine is a medical substance you can use to rub surface to make it smooth and shiny. The shiny appearance of the teeth after polish is really fabulous wonder of urine. Gargling and polishing teeth regularly protects the teeth.

In Roman times, there was a tradition among the gauls to use urine to whiten teeth. There is historical evidence for this.

Dentists are removing wisdom teeth unnecessarily, which is actually not necessary. Most of the pain or illness of surrounding wisdom teeth is not caused by the teeth themselves as we think. A report by dentist Jay Friedman in *American Journal of Public Health* reveals that 67 per cent or more of preventive wisdom teeth removal is unnecessary. 6.7 million wisdom teeth are removed unnecessarily every year.

6. Mouth Diseases and Disorders

Mouth disorders, diseases, infections or any other health problems are an untidy state, an illness that causes the mouth to stop functioning healthily and smoothly. Uropathy is recommended for prevention of medication. The usual method of gargling with urine is an effective way to fight gum problem, tongue disorders or other mouth infections. Besides, toothaches disappear quickly and teeth stay, healthy. It can also cure paths speedily.

You can spit out urine again after sometime. Gum problem, foul smell, toothaches, tooth decay, tooth stay healthy mouth and tongue disorders, voice problems are cured.

7. Insects Bites

Insects are small creatures with legs, body, sting and wings. For example, ants, bees, flies and other crawling creatures, spiders, scorpion stick, etc. A bee has a sting. Scorpion has a sting in its tail. An insect may touch your skin, or make small hole so that you feel a sharp pain. The sharp pointed part of an insect that can go into the skin leaving small, painful and sometimes poisonous wound. A wasp or bee sting is painful not necessarily serious. An insect bite can be painful and itchy. Urine can effectively work when it is put on them to relieve the discomfort.

External urine application is a natural treatment and home remedy which relieves insect stings bites. A bee or wasp sting can be painful and traumatic for a child. Sometimes delicate even adults are surprised at just how painful an insect sting, such as wasp sting, can be. Weals and itching caused by bites and stings heal naturally within a few days. So, how simply home remedy can relieve !

8. Tuberculosis (T.B.)

It is a serious infectious disease in which swelling appears on the lungs and other parts of the body.

The world has 100 million active cases of tuberculosis, a disease that claims two millions lives every year, according to the Medical Research Council,

Cambridge. The disease is known for many complexities. It was significant that it took one billion to develop new drugs.

One must know the structural biologists and pharmaceutical companies alone cannot solve the problem of drug resistance.

There are many bacteria in our body which should be removed to be free form disease. The urine alone can do that work. Human bodies have some 10 million human cells, but the body has 10 times the number of bacterial cells; means 100 trillion to be precise.

9. Bone Marrow

In human urine there is one hormone substance by name Erythropoietine, minutely deposited in urine. The scientific research in it resulted in isolating and extracting this hormone. It is very useful to make bone marrow to develop or become more active. Bone marrow is soft substance that fills the hollow parts of bones. Urine stimulates the bone marrow to increase the rate of production of erythrocytes, i.e., red blood cells.

10. Anaemia

The valuable substances deposited in human urine are useful which have capabilities to increase the rate of production of red blood cells. A patient suffering from the ailment of anaemia, is a medical condition in which he has too few red blood cells in his blood. Such a medical condition makes the people look pale and feel weak. Patients of a anaemia will derive a substantial benefit, by drinking his own urine.

11. Numbness

In these days of modern life style, sitting life, no work or leisurely work, idleness, numbness has become a common ailment people experience. More sitting without physical work and exercise makes you unable to feel anything. The body, leads to numbing effect on mind, hands, legs, etc., a condition of body that you lose the ability to feel through your sense of touch, lose of sensation.

Washing, rubbing the hands, legs or any other affected area with your own water it cures numbness, chap and sores, makes the joints limber. Massaging with urine at joints is necessary in order to stretch and prepare your muscles to be active to do work without strain, pain, and take part in race, walking, sporting activity, etc.

12. Trembling

The common ailment of body shaking that cannot be controlled can be solved. Generally, a person especially because he is nervous, excited, frightened, he feels trembling. For instance, trembling of legs with fear or voice, trembling because excitement, trembling hands, shaking slightly or trembling at the thought of having to make a speech, trembling knees, such disorders can be solved by washing and rubbing one's own warm urine into the skin directly after urination.

13. Digestive Tract

If a person drinks urine as a medicine, it makes digestive part, bowels empty easily. It has laxative effect, as it cleans digestive part clean. Urine is a substance sum total that causes and increases in the flow of urine. So, it has diuretic effect also.

14. Eases Ear Ailments

Human urine has strengthening and curative characteristics concerning many ear deficiencies. Ears can be washed with urine as ear drops. A person who is unable to hear anything or unable to hear very well is a problem of deafness can be solved and improved.

Pain, burning and itching ears can be relieved by applying a few drops of fresh urine. With or without diluting the urine can be used as ear drops. For pain inside the ear, urine is a liquid medicine that can be put into the ears. The ear drum which makes you able to hear can be cleaned with urine. It is a piece of thin tightly stretched skin inside the ear which moves by sound waves. Ear aches, infections and for other ear ailments dropping urine is the most effective treatment. Self-urine may be used as ear drops.

Ear pains, infections, deafness, noise problems can be alleviated.

15. Leprosy

This disease is one of the most dangerous and dreaded ones. The urine therapy is the best remedy prevents and also accelerates the healing of existing leprosy. It is an infectious disease that causes painful white areas on the skin and can destroy nerves and flesh. Leper is a person suffering from leprosy ailment, other people avoid because they have done something that these people do not approve. If urine therapy is practised for nine months, one is freed form leprosy.

16. Alleviating Migraine

It is a very severe type of headache which often makes a person fall sick and have difficulty in seeing. Auto-urine therapy is recommended to alleviate migraine ailment.

Human urine has analgesic effects useful for treatment of migraines and migraine related depression. Migraine headaches are a neurological condition; sufferers often experience missing time for hours or days.

17. Nose Ailments

Self-urine may be used as nose drops. It loosens mucus and cleans up blocked nasal passages. All disorders connected with the nose can be cured.

Treatment of stuffed nose, sinus, nasal disorders, respiratory canal, breathing problems, clears upper part of the bronchial tubes.

18. Tonsillitis

Tonsillitis is an inflammation of the tonsils. It generally happens due to viral or bacterial infection. It is a common illness, causing discomfort to children.

In allopathic treatment, there are only two methods that the physician recommends. They are:

1. Prescription of antibiotic drugs to treat the condition.
2. Recommend to remove tonsils to cure recurring bouts of tonsillitis.

As household medicine one can use herbal urine, and urinopathic medicine for effective treatment of tonsillitis.

19. Light Body

Makes the body lightsome and cheerful, keeps you always in less than average or usual weight, gentle, delicate, easy to do usual works, would not make you tired, free form worry, happy, full energy, cheerful, smile, fine voice, tone, giving you a feeling of joyfulness, comfortable.

20. Other curable Diseases

- Cures sickness
- Enhances beauty
- Fights flu
- Common cold
- Broken bone
- Kaposis scrcoma
- Asthma
- Morning sickness
- Hangover
- Chemical intoxication
- Enteritis
- Edema
- Congestion
- Lumbago
- Fatigue
- Fever
- Gonorrhea
- Small pox
- T.B.
- Immunological disorders
- Infection
- Insomnia
- Jaundice
- Hepatitis
- Lymphatic disorders
- Urticaria
- Hypertension
- Obesity
- Papilloma virus
- Rheumatism
- Stroke
- Eczema
- Typhus
- Gastritis
- Depression
- Gout
- Cold sore
- Migraine

- Tetanus
- polio
- Rabies
- Anamia
- Ebola
- Lungs
- Weight loss
- Cataract
- Malaria
- Dropsy
- Parkinson's diseases
- Diabetes
- Throat inflammation
- Sexual energier
- Piles, anus
- Thyroid
- Uterus of women, sists
- Venereal Diseases
- Bed-wetting

It has wonderful properties – divine qualities, incarnation and treats endocrine related diseases.

21. From Spiritual Angle

Divine sight

Ego

Cosmic intelligence

Divine manipulations

Kundalini unleash

Intuition power

Moral superiority

Spiritual effects, mental intellectual level

Distemper, egoism in ward out ward

Lightsome, cheerful

Strengthening aura

Spiritual energy

Progress to Samadhi is smoother

Sidhies

Godly Qualities

Self-realisation

Conclusion

So, what can we conclude after reading all these fabulous medicinal qualities of urine? As a matter of fact, the list of diseases for which urine is said to be effective is around 175 known diseases, the list is inclusive. There are many substances in urine which are not yet isolated and extracted from urine by intensive research, which have the beneficial effects of treating many incurable, innumerable modern diseases like cancer, AIDS, arthritis, etc.

Many pharmaceutical companies have already ventured and exploited urine ingredients for medical purpose. Many drugs are made from urine constituents. Today, research is going on large scale non-stop in labs attempting to isolate specific elements of urine in order to make new drugs from urine. Many companies in western countries have grossed billions of dollars from sale of medicine made from urine compounds. Miraculous stories of research finding on urine are found in medical literature.

Dr Armstrong suggested that clinics in which urine therapy could be practised and where it could be supervised by doctors would be a great convience to those who could afford to attend such institutions. And with this extremely unusual and surprising facts in which everything is explained, controversies settled, is exciting.

47
Curable Diseases

Cosmetic Purposes

Face Beauty

Use of human urine for cosmetic purposes means that it is intended to be rubbed, poured, sprinkled or sprayed on the face or other parts of the body appreances or introduced into the skin or otherwise applied.

The purpose of using one's own urine is for cleansing, beautifying, promoting attractiveness. It alters appearances, and looking.

The external application involves massaging too. Urine contains urea which is a valuable moisturiser. It is intended for curing, mitigation, treatment or prevention of diseases, disorders, eruptions which affect the beauty, attraction, etc. or affects the structure or any function of the cosmetics.

Other instances of urine for cosmetic purposes may include deodorants, antiperspirants, moisturizer, sun-protection and treats dandruffs.

The whole affair of a urine for cosmetic purpose is still shrouded in secrecy. It is a fact that nothing is known about magic fluid. Sex workers, beauty queens and a few other know about this hidden secret. Put your own urine on your face or body to make it more attractive. It improves the outside appearance of the skin. Today many people, particularly young men, women are greatly concerned about their appearance, worried the way the face looks on the outside. A pleasant look of a face is an interesting and enjoyable, attracts the attention of the people.

Regular use of urine makes the skin completely smooth and soft, and even without any lumps, holes or rough surface. It is a natural medicinal lotion, that makes your skin feel soft, and smooth, pleasant to see and touch, skin even and regular.

Any flaw, crack or fault on face is something that makes it less attractive. Urine touch makes a flawless complexion. The natural colour, and condition of the skin on a person's face will completely change. A pale or bad complexion disappears. It changes the way that a situation of skin appears.

If you value your face to be smooth, flawless skin and appearance, use your own fresh urine daily and massage, you find miracles happening on your face.

There is no need to use costly, modern chemical-based cosmetics like powder, face cream, costly lotions, going to beauty parlors, which have emerged in recent years even on corporate level, with variant names as natural beauty parlour herbal beauty parlour, etc.

A person especially a woman whose Job today it has become to give beauty treatment to the face and body, involved and spending more to make herself more beautiful, to bring the quality of being pleasing to the senses and to the mind. Many beauty products are made and available in the market.

Put urine on the face, massage and keep wet for 20-30 minutes and wash with hot water. Daily two times also can be practised. It can also be used as aftershave lotion. One can take bath with urine by diluting the urine with water.

The urine urea, is one of the primary ingredients in many face and skin creams. It is one of the best moisturisers, very scarce product. It is the most customised face medicine you will ever find available. Please try urine application to the face, and you can experience miraculous wonders almost immediately.

A woman can easily be judged to be the most beautiful in a beauty contest, it is the secret of beauty queen. Those who are interested to participate in a competition for young women in which their beauty, personal qualities and skills are judged, urine is a cosmetic secret. Modern beauty products are all expensive but urine is a cheap natural material.

Self-urine is an excellent cosmetic for moisturising and healing skin blemishes. Urine is absorbed when massaged through the skin. The hormonal and protein based contents are slowly reabsorbed into the face skin.

In Thaiwan, nearly more than two lakhs people are drinking their own urine like bed coffee, tea. It appears a wonder, but it is true. They are giving public statements on open dais, propagating in women's organisations. Urine is the secret of their face-beauty.

Prevention of Heart Attack - Natural Home Remedy

Cardio Vascular Diseases

Heart is a part of the body, an organ on the left side of the chest that pumps the blood to all parts of the body. Heart pounding in chest. The heart trouble or failure is due to a weak heart. If a person's heart stops beating for a few minutes, seconds sometimes he will die.

Heart attack occurs due to a sudden serious medical condition in which heart stops working normally, sometimes causing death. He is said to be suffering from coronary disease, connected with heart.

The arteries take blood to the heart. An illness relating to coronary is called Coronary Heart Disease. Either of the two arteries that supply blood to the heart.

A blocking of the flow of blood by a blood clot in an artery supplying blood to the heart leads to heart attack. It is known as coronary Thrombosis, blood or cream clots, it forms thickness, lumps or clots. It is a lump that is formed when blood dries or becomes thicker due to cholesterol.

Tubes that carry blood from all parts of the body to the heart are called veins.

A person suffering form coronary heart disease, may have to undergo a open heart surgery or stunt depending upon the magnitude of clot formation. A heart attack takes life, operation is a costly, because medical operation on the heart during which the patient's blood is kept flowing by a machine to operate.

Angina is a common complaints of the people suffering from heart disease. Angina is a severe pain in the chest caused by a low supply of blood to the heart during exercise because the arteries are partly blocked.

Human urine potential stops blood from clotting and prevents heart attack. So, natural urine has a medicinal hormones, that acts as a blood clotting dissolving agent or factor. It may be heartening to note that cardiovascular (C.V.) disease related deaths can be prevented effectively with regular auto-urine practice.

One Home – One Heart – One World

The term of "One world, one home, one heart" can be achieved with this therapy. The theme is observed every year on "World Heart Day".

Urine therapy practice is to be underscored, it is the need to take immediate steps to curtail heart ailments which are on the rise to day.

Be Alert

'One Home' theme means all the members of the family necessarily have to adhere to healthy life style. It means banning smoking, planning healthy food options, checking blood pressure and cholesterol levels regularly.

The theme 'One Heart' stands for educating public on warning symptoms and signs of heart attack and stroke and to call for medical help at the earliest.

The 'One World' signifies the campaign taken up globally to adapt a few household behaviour.

You are required to watch for warning symptoms like chest discomforts in the form of squeezing, pain spreading to other areas of the body arms, neck, jaw or stomach and shortness of breath with or without chest discomfort.

Every one must be careful about weakness or fatigue, anxiety, or unusual nervousness, indigestion or gas-like pain, breathing out in cold sweat, nausea, vomiting, light headedness and collapse, etc.

It may be pointed out that change in life style on account of modern civilisation industrialisation, urbanisation, dietary style, life style are the chief enemies of health.

Lack of physical exercise, excessive consumption of fatty food, stress factors are also the contributing risk factors to the malfunctioning of heart and ailments.

In recent years heart ailments have increased by ten times and about 40 years ago, there was no need for cardiac care.

Diabetes, hypertension and B.P. are also contributing to the heart problem.

In fact C.V. diseases alone account for 29 per cent of deaths globally each year. Average age of a heart attack in India is 35 as against 65 in the west.

Your Urine Saves Life

Your heart is a water pump, because it works like a pump. It makes blood flow in a particular direction. When the pump becomes weak, it is not able to pump enough blood and provide nutrition to various organs of the body. This situation of the body is referred to as heart failure.

The incidence of heart failure is increasing day by day throughout the globe despite advances in healthcare.

The reasons are:

- Increased life expectancy,
- Increase in the size of aged population,
- Better awareness about the condition of the ailment.

The deadly ailment heart failure is the final pathway to cardiac diseases such as :

- Heart attack
- Valvular heart diseases
- Hypertension
- Higher blood pressure
- Use of certain drugs
- Lack of physical exercise
- Diabetes
- And many unknown causes.

The incidence is one per 1,000 population per year. About the age of 80 years the incidence becomes 10 per 1,000 population per year. The risk of death in untreated cases is five-ten per cent annually.

The common symptoms in the early stages are :

- Breathlessness
- Swelling in legs and face
- Extreme breathlessness
- fatigue

A majority of studies have shown that high blood pressure, when remains undetected and untreated can result in the gradual enlargement of the heart accompanied by the weakening of heart muscles, resulting in heart failure.

Modern medical treatment is oriented towards relieving the symptoms in proving the quality of life and reduced mortality and instances of repeated hospitalisation. Studies have shown that readmission rate within one year is up to 30 per cent in such cases. This resulted in increased demand for corporate supers speciality beds. The patient's financial conditions may not permit such a costly treatment.

Besides, the number of cases of heart failure is bound to rise exponentially in the years to come due to changed life styles and occupational styles, stress, tension and depression.

Therefore, everyone of us should not wait till such a surge happens. There is a need to prevent, and be prepared in order to tackle the situation before heart failure poses a threat.

Here is a divine nectar urinopathy which saves your heart, prevents heart attacks and cures all types of cardio vascular ailments.

The disease management methods are either by means of drug therapy, devices such as pacemakers of special type to improve the pumping capacity of the heart, or finally cardiac transplantation.

Pacemakers are very expensive and are limited battery life, cardiac transplantation method has its own limitations in terms of availability of suitable donors. So, early detection and prompt medical treatment are key to managing the rising number of cardiac cases.

If we observe the trends in developed countries, there are special heart failure clinics, for such patients. Many of them may need domicilliary care. These aspects of care are yet to come to India.

Pacemaker devices and cardiac assist devices such as artificial heart, which is a bridge to actually cardiac transplantation are expensive. The cost may come down as more and more patients seek to undergo such a therapy.

Many of these patients suffer a psychological impact also and develop depression due to chronic illness, recurring hospitalisation and financial burden.

Here is Preventive Medicine in Urine

Enzyme, is one of the substances that is contained in urine. There are many enzymes, among them, one is called urokinase. In a special research study on this, scientists found that urokinase vasodilatation resembles nitroglycerine. It has the ability to strengthen the bloodstream from coronary artery to cardiac muscle. Today it is used as blood clot dissolver for unblocking coronary arteries. The enzyme urokinase is used in drug form and sold in market which is showing miracle results. So, the effectiveness of urokinase in urine will explain why the urine therapy is said life effective against arteriosclerosis, heart attack, pulmonary embolism, etc.

It prevents the formation of blood clots in the blood vessels, and dissolves clots already formed. Thus with urine therapy heart attacks may be prevented and cured.

Dr Mezel, Edgewater Hospital, Chicogo, injects urokinase into the bodies of the victims of the heart attacks. Therefore, human urine has powerful medicinal properties aborting the attack and saving the lives of the patients. It is a life saver.

Normal human urine has been found to contain a powerful artery dilating often to resembling Nitro Glycerin in the ability to increase coronary blood flow to the cardiac muscle used for the relief of Angina Pectoris (*Science Digest*, July, 1958).

"An extract from human urine shows great promise for treatment of certain deadly diseases caused by formation of blood clots".

Research Physicians disclosed at the scientific sessions of the American Heart Association. The extract is called Urokinase, activates substances in the blood stream that dissolve the clots. Experience has been obtained with about 200 patients with pulmonary embolism the most common of serious Lung diseases. Dr Sherry Pointed out. (Press Report, San Francisco, USA).

Similarly, in India Dr Salaria, a renowned surgeon,-Ahamedabad used to give an injection of the patient's own urine before taking up surgery.

Infertility Problem Made Curable

Infertility is a major problem in recent years because of changed life styles and occupational styles as well as environmental changes. Infertility is a biological problem of a woman, wife or husband. Such people are said to be infertile couple who need a fertility treatment.

Today, many women experience impregnancy because of fertility problems. The chronic problem is that hormonal deficiency, or changes occurring in the body on-production of chemical substances which influences the growth of fertility hormones are cases of fertility hormonal imbalance.

Natural human urine contains fertility hormones, as well as a female sex hormone called oestrogen. The disorder of humans not able to produce children can be treated with urine only.

All sorts of infertility problems are remedied by its use. It works fabulously against infertility also. To our surprise, human urine also works wonderfully well on impotency and sexual debility. The condition of impotency is an apparently insoluble problem male impotency.

Fertility Hormones in Urine

The hormones which are responsible for causing fertility or pregnancy are deposited in plenty in the couple's urine. They are called with following names:

1. Testosterone, 2. Progesterone, 3. Oestrogen.

Urine is the main drug for infertility problem.

A regular drinking of one's own urine improves and converts impotency situation into potency. Women's urine contains fertility hormones. Even immunological analysis of urine is the basis of most pregnancy tests.

It was reported in 1938, that an extract from urine of pregnant women has prophylactic and therapeutic effect on ulcer in dogs.

Shortly, thereafter the study group noted that an extract from urine of normal urine has similar effects.

The urine of pregnant women when injected into a frog, the frog within 24 hours releases eggs. It is because of the fact women urine contains fertility hormones. The research found out this.

During the period of pregnancy the urine possesses full of oestrogen hormones. It is a hormone produced in women's ovaries that causes them to develop the physical and sexual features that are characteristic of female and that cause them to prepare their body to have babies.

Sometimes, men may also be responsible for infertility due to non-production of male hormone. Men's hormone is called Testosterone. It is a hormone produced in men's testicles that causes them to develop the physical and sexual features that are characteristic of the male body.

Similarly, progesterone is a hormone produced in the bodies of women which prepares the body to become pregnant and is also used contraception.

After recognition of the importance of the hormones which are hidden in urine, having medicinal value many pharmaceutical companies extracted by isolating them to make fertile drugs.

With a view to solve the problem of infertility, fertility hormones have been extracted and drugs and injections are developed.

For instance, Profassi Injections made with urine, a drug which is useful, now available in the market converts infertility condition into fertility that gives birth to babies.

In advanced countries, many multi-national pharmaceutical companies are actively involved in this industry and spinning millions of rupees.

It is reported that one of the marketing companies in Hyderabad, India is exporting such urine in large quantities to Japan (Dr C. Chordia, *Uropathy*, 2007, p. 22).

Dehydroepiandrosternoe is one of the substances found in urine, isolated and extracted, a hormone related to testosterone.

Urine is said to deter ageing.

Successful Case Study

Before concluding this topic, I would like to refer to the real story of fertility that actually happened by drinking urine in case of a infertility couple.

Dr Arthur Lincoln Poul, a Canadian doctor and author of a book titled "*Shivambu kalpa*" has referred in his book about a case of urine therapy of a infertility couple. This interesting case inspired me to quote here to prove the fabulous medicinal character of urine.

A young man aged 27 years old, an Anglo-Indian, got married to a young girl aged 18 years. But no babies. To verify their fertility position medically, a few years after their marriage, they consulted a doctor, revealed that the male spouse was not verile and his semen lacked active sperm. Hence, his wife did not conceive. He did not possess strong and full sexual energy. It is a sexual power in men, considered typical in case of men which he lacked.

In order to conceive, men's semen should contain sperms. A sperm is a cell that is produced by the sex organs of a male and that can combine with female to become pregnant, produce babies.

He has a low sperm count, i.e., very few live male cells in semen.

As a therapy the couple drank each other's urine everyday, and also on alternate days drank their own urine.

They put each others urine on parts connected with outer sexual organs called genital organs.

The practice for sometime resulted that he became mark potent and his sperm count in semen increased satisfactorily. Within a couples of months his wife conceived and became pregnant, delivered and they had sons.

Urinopathic medicine produces amazing results in reversing infertility condition. Today, of all available treatments for infertility, urinopathy is one that people usually think first .

But as you will see in this section, urine is actually one of the safest, priceless and most effective treatments for infertility known to modern science.

Why does it work so well?

Because urine possesses fertility hormones.

What exactly means inversing infertility?

Here is an answer:

Ease Menstrual Disorders Naturally

Urinopathy is effective to ease women's menstrual problems. They are connected with the time when a woman menstruates each month. The average length of woman's menstrual cycle is 28 days. During this period, there is a flow of blood from her womb, usually once in month.

Menstrual pain, sudden pain that they feel during the period, something almost every women has experienced, while some may only experience them in the form of mild discomfort, other may experience severe and often debilitating pain during their menstrual cycle.

The good news is that there are several urinopathic remedies which can be used.

Menstrual sudden pains actually result in change in women's brains, similar to those produced by chronic pain. She may experience extreme tiredness, severe stomach pain, discomforts for several hours and even longer. The discomfort, pains and other menstrual disorders can be avoided naturally with urine treatment as home remedy.

Urine-use is a natural remedy for endometiosis which is in the form of pain, scarring, menstrual problem.

Urinopathic medicine is effective in reducing and relieving period-pain, experienced by women who are going through their cycle.

Other Problems

Especially, women are prone to some special type of disorders or diseases by virtue of their body composition and reproduction system. Urine therapy proved to work wonderfully to correct disorders. Some of them are as follows:

1. ***Leucorrhoea (Leukaemia)*** : It is a serious disease causing weakness and sometimes death.
2. ***Irregular Menstruation*** : They are connected with the time where women menstruates each month. In an irregular cycle, there is a flow of unusual blood from her womb. An irregular menstruation at irregular intervals is a disorder.
3. ***Pre-menstrual Tension*** : It is case of causing heat and inflammation the women menstruate before menstrual cycle. It causes a feeling of fear and excitement that is created by premature cyclel giving a feeling of muscular tension, a state of stretched tight causing pain.
4. ***Fibrosis, Swelling of Fibres, Firous Tissues.***
5. ***Tumor :*** It is a situation of a mass cells growing in or on a part of the body where they should not usually cause medical problems.

Relieves Arthritis

The word arthritis complaints is wide that encompasses over 100 different health conditions. It is a degenerative disease characterised by inflammation of joints, surrounding tendons, ligaments and cartilage. The illness causes swelling of the joints, stiffness and pain that can range from slight to crippling.

Urine helps to reduce back pain, grow bone, prevents osteoporosis and even prevents bone cancer, reduces the arthritis pain. The patients have to bear with the limited and slow movements due to the disease, but they actually have to suffer through the pain, there are no pain relieving options except painkiller drugs in allopathy. Urine is a healthy diet and drug supplement, relieves arthritis pain naturally.

It is a condition to describe joint pain or inflammatory condition such as osteoarthritis, rheumatoid arthritis nothing but an auto immune disease and gout.

Joints are natural shock absorbers for the body. They are cushioned by cartilage and supported by muscles, tendons and ligaments. The wear and tear of daily activity, injury, ageing, obesity, repetitive motion place stress on joints and cause them to wear down. Urine is a natural solution with vitamins, proteins that relieve and eliminate joint pains.

In recent years, a great variety of joint health supplements are available in the market for treating gout joint pain and others.

The products as well as painkillers have possible side effects, please despise them before using.

Urine is rich in potassium which reduces rheumatoid arthritis, symptoms preventing painful gout attacks.

Urinopathic treatment has a long history in treating and curing gout. Its variant remedies are useful to reduce the swelling and inflammation and as well as aid in the healing of the joints. Gout is caused by the build up of uric acid in the joints.

Gout is a disease that causes painful swelling in the joints, especially of the toes, knees and fingers which is one of over many forms of arthritis. Luckily, it is highly treatable, try with this natural drug, and remedy for gout has been very popular.

The primarily reason for this is that modern gout medicines have severe side effects and are not safe for long term. Your own urine is a natural drug very safe to take and depend on.

Please learn how urinetherapy relieves arthritis and joint pains. It is a nature's answer to joint pains, that the therapeutic value brings together a variety of nutrients hidden in urine. Which can support healthy joints and relieve pain, associated with arthritis patients suffering form chronic joint pain, they can find effective natural remedy from his own body-made medicine.

In arthritis health market, human urine is virtual nectar, has joints-health promoting properties.

A cup of your own bladder tea relieves pain with no harmful side effects at all. The watery solution is a powerful pain reliever that works just as well.

Allergies from Urinopathic Angle

In simple terms, an allergy is a response of the body to certain substances which are foreign to our bodies. These substances are called 'Allergens' , like food, perfume, cats, pollen, drugs and dust. A contact with one or more is enough to become sensitive or allergic to.

Some people are more susceptible and some acquire throughout life. The immune system of the body becomes sensitive and reacts hyperactively, when it touches the allergen.

The allopathic medicine is suppressive drug, does not treat the underlying cause of the problem. It gives numerous side effects, worsens our health by regularly suppressing the immunity system. Depending on drug medication throughout the life is harmful.

An allergy is a bodily disorder caused by an allergy, an allergic reaction, rash, etc. It is a medical condition that causes you to react badly or feel ill, when you eat or touch a particular substance. Urinetherapy has been recommended to completely alleviate, eliminate allergies. A person faces allergic situation because of renegade white blood cells which attack substances. White blood cells are called antigen receptors, which is a nerve ending in the blood that reacts to changes such as heat, cold and makes the body react in particular way.

To cure the allergy, the disorder is to be corrected which the urine therapy can take care of. You may be shocked to know how urine liquid cures. The medical research findings showed in 1982, when the urine is reintroduced into the body, the body develops antibodies which work against these antigen receptors. The antibodies stop the allergic condition (Dr William Linscott, in *Basic and Clinical Immunology*).

The remedy for this disorder is to eliminate the allergy causing antigen receptors. And that is what the urine is exactly doing. Allergies can completely be eliminated with this simple self-urine therapy.

To conclude, the body producing allergy causing antigen receptors, the excreted urine when reintroduced into the body, the body manufactures antibody to fight against allergy causing antigen. So your own urine is a powerful healer inside.

Hair and Head Disorders

Head and hair are the two important parts of the body commonly associated with several types of disorders, and health problems. Head is the part of the body on the top of the neck containing the eyes, nose, mouth and brain.

Hair is a substance that looks like a mass of fine threads growing especially on the head.

Make a point, drink your own water, and apply to the head, take your head bath and it cures all the disorders. Loss of hair, white and looks extremely clean and neat with urine application now and then. It washes and shapes hair, old urine and fresh urine both can be used. The skin that covers the part of the head where hair grows will be nutrious and wet. Otherwise a dry scalp can lead to develop dandruff.

The dandruff symptoms like very small pieces of dead skin seen as a white dust in person's hair is a common head disorder which can effectively be managed with urine.

Understanding the urine therapy and knowing about your hair problem is the first step in this direction.

Hair is one's crowning glory. Any kind of hair loss, whether temporary or permanent has a deep psychological impact, irrespective of age or gender. It is your duty to take some natural therapy in order to protect and prevent hair-fall and preserve or enhance. God blessed your good hair beauty.

The main reason for hair-fall is nutrient deficiency such as iron, calcium, proteins, vitamins. Besides there are external factors such as pollution, using wrong hair care products, excessive blow drying. Urine contains multiple qualities of proteins, nutrients vitamins which when applied to the head are reused and keeps hair healthy, prevent hair fall. Urine is a right drugless, priceless, natural hair care product which otherwise is being washed.

The problem of lack of oily scalp and dry hair ends can be solved by urine application. Dry brittle hair and subsequent hair-fall and breakages can be prevented and cured. Fully nutrients urine will strengthen the hair roots and stops hair shedding.

Use of modern chemical based factory made hair products on the hair either to alter the hair type or smell also leads to hair fall, damages the hair shaft. Similarly excessive blow-drying causes bubbles to form in the hair shaft making it weak and susceptible to breakage. Use of colours also is not good for health of hair , can cause not only hair fall but also allergic irritation, itching ,infection etc.

With sensible use of urine, excessive hair fall, dandruff, dryness etc., are not only manageable but can also be stopped as well.

The itching and redress over the scalp and surrounding skin disorders can also be effectively treated.

Urine is a wonderful remedy for lifeless hair and even baldness and hairloss. Apply urine to the head, keep it wet, massage and keep it for 30-45 minutes, hair roots absorb, enter into the head all proteins, nutrients, vitamins are reabsorbed by the body. Take bath with hot water. No need to use soap, shampoo, lotions and other chemical based hair and head care products. Hair becomes clean, keeps shining quality of surface, no question of losing lustre. The quality of being the hair look special in a way that is existing , thick lustre hair special added lustre, the effect is even more powerful.

For this purpose, both preserved urine as well as old urine can be used. Hair is made beautiful and vital. One does not appear with grey hair, maintains original hair colour throughout life. Regular oral and external application results in growing hair again on bald area.

Dandruff, loss of hair, grey hair, colour baldness, bald spots lustrous, poor growth disorders are cured.

Heal Your Skin

Urine improves the health and quality of the skin. Skin is the layer of the tissue that covers the body. More than any other therapy and paths, urine therapy represents the principle of natural medicine used for all cosmetic purposes. All types of skin infections, disorders, sores, itches are cured by body excretion urine. It makes the skin attractive and keeps it healthy. Pour, rub, pack are the modalities of using urine to skin. Injuries, damages, burns, etc. are cured with the help of urine effectively.

Urine therapy is recommended, as it alleviates hives, a skin disease that causes the skin to become red and painful, tinea. It prevents infection of existing wounds.

Therapy is also effective for healing other skin complaints like skin blemishes, allergies, burns, scars, fungus, rashes, cuts, roughness itches, chap, anus piles, dry skin, wrinkles, infections, skin flaws, insect bites, birth marks, blisters fistules, pimples, acne, stings, pemphigus, leucoderma, psoriasis, lingering, obstinate, etc.

All sorts of uncomfortable feeling on the skin that makes one scratch oneself on the body, disappears with application of urine. A skin allergy gives a feeling to rub your skin with your nails usally because it is itching. Like ear scratch, chin scratch, sometimes certain types of itches are incurable and scratching may cut or damage skin slightly with sharp nails, sometimes, awkward to look. The practice damages the surface of the skin especially accidentally by making thin shallow mark on the body.

Urine not only cures the ailments but also, if any scar, or mark that is left over on the skin after a wound, operation also disappear.

Rub the scratch, infected and itching areas with urine. They effectively disappear with correct treatment for a week time.

Urine is an antiseptic agent, sterile, hygienic, can be used as a remedy for cleansing wounds. Urea in the blood is converted into the highly beneficial agent glutamine, and in urine there is ammonia using for combating the common menace of infection, decay, allergies, etc.

Urine miracle cures skin ailments without drugs. It is a drug-free method of healing wounds that proved revolutionary as the discovery of penicillin. It helps clean up wounds of all known types of toxic bacteria.

It does not get stuck to the wound and heals burns, cuts and any septic and infected wound faster than medicine. The urine pack stops bleeding, ends inflammation, eliminates swellings and stimulates skin regeneration.

It also helps kill pain and remove foul wound odour. The most remarkable thing about urine drug is that it contains no antibiotics and is therefore naturally effective against drug resistant bacteria which is the growing problem of clinical medicine.

The modern medicinal way of treating wounds is to apply antiseptic medicated bandaging to kill pathological microbes, whereas urine therapy heals without administering any chemical drug. It is based on long-known fact that urine is antiseptic and has medicinal qualities. Its is anti-bacterial, too.

The therapy works with all types of pathological micro organism and it does not matter whether they are resistant to antibiotics or not. In the twenty first century when more people suffer from various skin disorders, infections the auto urine drug may prove just a ground breading in helping people and revolutionising health care. It is a traditional domestic medical proactive since ancient times, as the discovery of penicillin was only in the twentieth century. It also guarantees 100 per cent protection from viruses, bacteria, and parasites and does not require any additional disinfection.

A person with skin affection can drink the urine in the morning he passes the night before. Sprinkle the urine on affected wounds, injuries; it will effectively treat.

48
Cancer

Combating the Menace of Cancer with Urine

Cancer is a serious disease in which cells, also called cancers, form in the body and kill the normal body cells. The disease often causes death. A serious illness or dangerous human aliment that spreads quickly.

Tumour, on the other hand, is a mass of cells growing in or on a part of the body where should not normally grow, usually causing a medical and health problem. For instance, a brain tumour.

Its nature is invasive, means cancer cells, spreading very quickly to other parts and difficult to stop. It is known as invasive cancer, demands an invasive surgery.

The cancer is the most dreaded, life disease of the present century, threatened the very existence of mankind. The whole humanrace is terribly frightened by this draconian situation. It is taking lakhs of lives every year. Tobacco claims 50 lakh lives, poses threat to 10 lakhs lives in the twenty first century. Breast cancer is the most common cancer in women world wide. Cancer is a leading cause of death across the world, accounting 7.6 million deaths every year. In India, every year nearly 10 lakh cancer patient cases are being registered on average at any time, 15-20 lakh cancer patients wanting treatment.

The symptoms are pain, no pain, inconvenience, feeling of growth, and we use the word for them as cancer malignancy or even tumor. It may be in the form of growth, lump, nodules and others cancerous growths that form on the human body. All growths are not cancer.

Types of Cancers

Breast cancer, bowel cancer, gullet cancer, rope cancer, armpit cancer, lungs cancer, throat cancer, breast cancer, oesophagus, larynx, mouth, kidney, bladder, pancreas, stomach, blood, bone cervix, colon, sarcoma, lymphomas, skin, uterus, lever, prostate, uvula, neck cancer, etc.

Causes

Malignancy and other growths are due to a diet deficient in natural salts especially in potash [Dr F Forbes Ross].

Long time meat eating with excess spices, oils, fats, salts, etc.

A long time vegetarian starts eating meat.

Women do not have children and mothers denying breast feeding to babies.

Living in a house situated over an underground stream.

Unmarried women suppression of sexual desire.

Excessive use of common salt.

People live on ill balanced or denatured diet.

Deficiency of sodium chloride.

Psychological fear and thoughts.

Tobacco consumptions.

Passive smoking and smoking cigarettes.

Use of poisonous substances such as nicotine, cadmium, polonium, hydrogen cyanide, and radiant isotopes.

Hereditary Cases.

Hookah smoking.

Use of smokeless tobacco products, *paan*, *gutka* consist tobacco or a tobacco blend which are chewed, sucked, or sniffed, chewing tobacco, nicotine, sweetness and chemicals.

Consumption of alcohol.

Lack of internal cleanliness, neatness, tideness, accumulation of toxins, infection of internal parts or organs, using stomach as dustbin, leads to malignant growths.

Immunity deficiency, perpetual constipation and weak resistance mechanism in the body.

Wrongful, bad dietary habits, changed life styles, dietary styles and occupational change.

Long period suppression or masking of symptoms of diseases without eradication, with antibiotics, painkillers and other opiates.

Metabolism malfunction, eating food stuffs made with inorganic manures, pesticides, antibiotics,

Use of freezed foods, bottled foods, fast foods, non-foods, fluorides, adulterated, polluted water, air and living in impure environment.

Non-noticed malignant growths, nodules, lumps, ulcerous growths, damage of glands, dead cells.

Living away from nature.

Presently Available Treatments

1. *Chemotherapy :* The treatment of disease especially cancer, with the use of chemical substances.

2. ***Radiation :*** One of the treatments that uses powerful and very dangerous rays that are sent out from radioactive substances. It is the heat or energy, etc. that is sent to the affected parts in the form of rays. For treatment of cancer and other diseases radiation therapy is used. The rays that damage cancer cells.
3. ***Radium :*** Radium is a white radioactive metal used in the treatment of disease such as cancer.
4. ***Surgery :*** it is a branch of medicine connected with the treatment of cancer. The surgeon is involved in cutting open the body and often removing cancer affected part, lump, growths, nodules, cancerous cells etc.
5. ***Antibiotics :*** Antibiotics are chemical substances that can destroy bacteria or cure infections, or growth of bacteria.

Side Effects

The following are the side effects of chemo, radiation and surgery modalities :

Physical troubles, persistent nagging pain, nausea, copious vomiting, depression, sweats, diarrhea, numb fingers, toes, dry, irritated skin, sleep disruption, fatigue, urinary track infections, constipation, weight loss, wasting, painful death, hair loss, figure change, decay, headache, change of voice, colour spots on the body, loss of sense of taste, scorch, loss of appetite, invading lassitude, weakness, bad taste in mouth, bleeding, inactiveness, intolerable foul and bad smell, burning sensations, skin eruptions, violent reactions, feeling of heaviness in the abdomen, blisters and herpes growth, shooting pain in the body, temperature, motions and watery stools, aversion to food, torturous side effects of injections and drugs, checks sink, body becomes skeleton, sleep disorders.

Hospitals are not prepared to keep the cancer patients. No one is willing to look after such a patient because of this disease is regarded as highly difficult health management.

Cancer disease has created a grave danger for the extinction of the human race. Modern medicine does not have any such sure prevention, cure sure and no harm successful health care remedy for cancer.

As seen there is no any possibility of finding out any remedy. Extensive and intensive long term, elaborate scientific research, studies, clinical investigations are undertaken for the last nearly 75 years, so far no effective remedy has been found for cancer cure. In the days to come, as it has been increasingly realised, urine therapy will be the only cure for horrible cancer.

Abuse, over prescription and indiscriminate doses of drugs, antibiotics, chemotherapy and other harmful treatments in use in controlling cancer are causing reactions, side effects. The impact of irrational use of antibiotics is very harmful to the body.

The cost of treatment is heavy, for periodical visit to cancer hospital located away, diagnose, drugs, tests, etc. it is great financial burden to the patients, relatives, they became bankrupt and mentally depressed.

Prime Minister Manmohan Singh remarked the impact of high medical cost places an unconscionable burden on the poor, we need to accelerate our efforts to achieve our goal of providing universal access to health care at affordable cost for all our citizens.

Dr Rabagliati, a famous doctor who has performed no fewer than 500 major operations for growths, the result is that there is uniform lack of success with the knife. This situation caused him to search for other means of more effectively treating cancer though unfortunately in vain [Dr J.W. Armstrong, *Water of Life*].

"The mortality from cancer in San Francisco exceeds that of any other American city" [*Victory Over Cancer* by Cyriscott].

It is because of the fact the city has few physicians but hundreds of surgeons, it is a surgically ridden city.

'I have operated on some thousands of cases of cancer, and they all returned but six, and they were not cancer' [*The Breast*, Drs Dearer and Macfarland, quoted Dr J.W.Armstrong, *Water of Life*]

People are frightened and nervous of dangerous treatment of costly modern medicine.

Urine First Choice

Urinopathy is the use of urinopathic medicine for therapeutic purposes. Urine has been used as last resort when the rational patients noticed the benefits of the urine. Urine therapy can be used to help a whole range of cancer problems, both emotional, as well as physical including side effect.

Urinopathy has been proven to help cancer patients reduce the severity of their cancer symptoms. There could not be a better and happier news than this repugnant medicine for the entire global mankind.

Time is now ripe to recognise the necessity of urine treatment, health care modality in the present time. Urine therapy gives a definite hope to the patients who are miserably suffering. The ignorance of this suppressed body made substance causing millions of patients to suffer.

Inculcating awareness among the sick and starving poor and making them to use will be of invaluable help to those suffering people, perhaps it is more than all food, shelter, welfare, development and other welfare projects, it immensely benefits the suffering human race.

Urine has no side effects, after effects, ill effects of the dangerous disease, promotes self-confidence, no pains, troubles, struggles, no cost, gives immense happiness and overflowing joy.

Today, mankind has been surrounded by innumerable over the counter drugs, found utterly hopeless and dejected.

The philosophy of urine therapy is that firstly it has no harm to the body, treats whole person as holistic medicine, cures the root cause of the disease, instead of suppressing or masking the symptoms of the diseases which the modern medicine will do without eradicating the cause of the malady.

The deadly disease cancer cannot exclusively be treated by knife, radium, chemotherapy or medication alone.

Body of every individual has innate capability of natural power of self-healing, urine as a biomedicine is far more efficient healer. The system educates the masses on health management, self-responsibility than just giving fatal medicine.

Orthodox and superstitious practising doctor's point of view that the dread cancer as incurable, the dictum is longer true, can effectively be cured with simple remedy. Auto–urine has a therapeutical value, and a curative agent. Urine is a Queen–of–Terror killer of cancer cells, vanishes lump, nodule, tumor, ulcer and other cancerous growths. The therapy achieved victory over cancer.

Urinopathy is an age old household medicinal treatment has been sometimes remained hidden, fallen a bit into obscurity. The entire suffering mankind has deprived of this drugless, priceless self therapy. Really speaking in these days of emerging innumerable, incurable, acute and chronic diseases like cancer, time has now ripen to be recognised, as the only potent universal remedy for prevention and curing.

The cancer curing natural substances and elements that are end up in urine, which cannot be duplicated, procured nor produced from any other source other than the multimillion dollar manufacturing human body factory. An intrinsic medicine. Incredible cure.

For this paper, the most compelling argument for trying urine therapy is its benefit in the treatment of cancer which has enormous source of curing potential.

Benefits to Cancer Patient

Human urine, and urinopathic medicine support patients undergoing cancer treatments, it is a natural approach to health and healing. For patients with cancer, this form of medicine helps to create a healthy environment both inside and outside the body. The goal of urinopathy for patients of cancer undergoing treatment includes :

1. To Support normal metabolism;
2. To build immunity system;
3. Wellness, detoxification and health maintenance;
4. As a long-term strategy prevention of cancer;
5. To promote health management and self responsibility;
6. To support energy, improves body's performance;
7. To strengthen well-being and over all quality of life.

Treatment Modalities

Fast on One's Own Urine

Fasting on urine and drinking plain cold water daily, rubbing with urine on affected areas, cotton packs wrung out in urine and placing on affected areas will cure cancer. The fabulous medicinal characters of urine is astonishing that no trace of abnormalities in the body of the patient will result. Patient can be restored to perfect health. Within a few days, depending upon the stage of the complaint, no trace of the growth of malignancy can be noticed.

Troubles, sufferings, pains would disappear, no need of surgery or other painful treatments. In many cases, though the doctors adviced the patients to die soon, they followed fast on their own urine, as a result completely cured, living long, looking much younger, strong, fearless and glow in figure. The quality of urine is that it activates the lymphatic system which detoxifies the body and works in the true progress of healing and regenerating cells and tissues.

If the patients do this treatment systematically by following proper method of regimentation, fasting, massaging, enema and oral taking, so that expected benefits can be obtained. Within a short period of practice a remarkable reduction in tumor cells, dissolution of accumulated cancer cells and non-formation of cell groups can be observed.

The specific compounds of human urine which are expected to account for the effectiveness of auto-urine therapy in the treatment of cancer includes :

Human Urine Derivative (HUD),

H-11,

Retina Antineoplastons,

Uric Acid.

Dr Novak, a German doctor reported that therapeutic results of the use of auto-urine extract on malignant tumors (Neitschrift Inn ere Medizine, 1961). He employed with much success injections of a natural extract of patient's own urine to treat cancers of the breast, colon, lungs, uterus, lymph nodes and stomach.

One of ingredients of human urine is named as retinene, which is isolated and extracted from human urine. It was tested on mice with artificially inducted skin cancer and was found to inhibit the growth of tumors when applied larger doses proved to cause the regression of tumors (*Science,* 20, 1571-1572, 1963).

Yet another element extracted from human urine called as H-11, applied and experimented on cancer. It was reported that H-11 is an anticancer urine extract. Many doctors and researchers have found that H-11 is clinically effective in inhibiting the growth of malignant cells in human (*British Medical Journal,* 7 : 43, 1943, Thompson, J.H.)

Joseph Eldor, Theoretical Medicine Institute, Jerusalem on *Uropathy for Patients with Cancer* reported that urine is a new treatment modality for cancer patients as it has much therapeutic value, miracle cure power.

Medical field believes that there are being several other beneficial substances in human urine not yet known to science. Likewise lot of scientific evidences are found which testify that human urine has healing modality works in true process of healing.

Urine Urea–Anti-cancer

One of the compounds found in human urine is urea, a colourless substance containing nitrogen. Urea is medically proven to be one of the best moisturisers and scarce substance. The chief constituent of the nitrogenous waste in urine is urea, a product of protein decomposition, a diuretic.

According to studies, 25 per cent of the urea in an adult finds its way into the intestines where it is decomposed into ammonia by the intestinal bacteria. The extra supply created by applying urine therapy increases the glutamine level in the body, as a result it strengthens the immune system and specialised organs.

Urea is converted through ammonia into glutamine. Urea occurs in sufficient quantity in average person's urine, By utilising one's own urine the occurance of cancer cells can be prevented, sure chance of curing cancer cells.

Human urine urea is a main compound of total composition and is a decomposition product converted into proteins. On an average, 25–30 grams of urea per day is extricated by a person. Every one of us are coming into contact with urea at an early age, as a fetus, in the womb. Amniotic fluid of a pregnant woman mainly contains urea, which we drank, breathed in, swimmed. Thus a cancer patient has a healer within the body made life saver. Dr Evagelos Danopoulos, Greece, reported that urea found in urine has anti-cancerous properties. The ability of urea is that it disrupts the character of cancer cells to group together and kills them, by upsetting some of their normal metabolic activities the doctor found in his clinical investigation.

Introduction to Biochemistry by Dr Pharon found that the highest quantity of urea in 100 milliliters of urine is 1,459 grams, highest volume among all other elements like uric acid, sodium, potassium, creatine. Urine contains 95 per cent water, 2.5 per cent urea and the rest 2.5 per cent is a mixture of minerals, salts, hormones, enzymes, vitamins, etc. The multinational companies are using human urine to manufacture hormones diuretics and cancer fighting drugs. Danopoulos has applied urea in the treatment of breast cancer, liver cancer and several other kinds of terminal cancers. Types of cancers responded to urine therapy are sarcoma, lymphomas, uterus, cervix, eyes, stomach, skin, etc.

Creatine hydrate is another compound of urine to fight cancer. Melantonin is a hormone found in urine which has a power of anti-cancer effect.

Urine Injections For Cancer Patients

We are helplessly unaware and ignorant about precious gift of nature. For instance, antineoplastone is an injection made from urine extract meant for cancer treatment. Dr Burzynski of USA as a result of his intensive long research for 20 years on human urine has developed an injection. Medical professionals in different parts of the world aware of this (*Oncology News*, July – August, 1990). So, instead of wasting urine, when reintroduced into the body improves body's immunity capacity and acts as immunotherapy, as a result stimulates self healing modality.

Urine as Antibody Agent Acts Against Antigen

It has been scientifically established that urine acts as a anti cancer agent responding as antibody force against antigens. Urine ingredients contain antibodies which upon reingesting can strengthen the body to react on specific pathological situations. To work against antigen antibodies are produced by the urine. As the urine and blood are mixed together and circulating through the blood stream, the antibodies are transpierced throughout blood flow and attack the tumor and its cells. The weakness of antigens is non self recognition of antibodies.

Cleansing Tumor Cells

Certain substances which enter the body can cause cancer. Cancer cells actually holds antigens ultimately release several antigens. External toxic substances, toxins substances produced by the bacteria internally both are dangerous which form cells. Enema of urine has potential of cleansing bowl, intenstines, alimentary canal and other parts of the body has a tremendous and powerful effect in detoxifing the body, antigens, and in dissolving cancer cells thus cures the roots of the disease.

Cancer disease is set due to imbalance diet, bad substances, mucus, accumulates, non – vegetarian foods, intoxicating, smoking bidis and cigarettes, chewing tobacco, because of these many became victims of this silent killer. Impurities, poisonous, toxins accumulated in the body are being thrown out of the body by urotherapy with a view to clean and keep the body tumor cell free and acts as preventive maintenance.

Urine–An Immunotherapy

Urine substances and elements prepare and improve the immunity system of the body. It improves the body's ability not to be affected by infection, diseases, illnesses. The reaction of the body defensively to the presence of antigens is very powerful. The immune system in the body is improved by the urine ingredients and helps to fight against the formation of tumor cells. Its task is rid the human body of diseases, unsoluble substance developed in the body, then these substances reach healthy tissues, the blood becomes stronger, cleaner. It acts as autoinoculation, self natural vaccine, this phenomenon of self cure is found only in urine.

Multifarious effects

Urotherapy has ten effects on the cancer cells like reuse of nutrients, hormones, enzymes, urea, immunological effects, bactericidal, virucidal effects, salt therapy, diuretic effect, transumulation, recycling and psychological effects on the patient.

Urine Massaging

In addition to oral use, it can be used for external application as massaging simultaneously. Fresh and old urine can be used in order to get rid of incurable disease like cancer. It helps considerably in early recovery. In outward application on the whole body, the urine enters through the pores, detoxifies the toxins in the body.

Painless Death

Chemotherapy, radiation, surgery, radium and drug administration are presently available cancer treatments. They are very horrible, miserable and painful. As a result they have unfavourable side effects, after effects, ill effects, spoiling the body leading to occurance of new degenerative diseases. Uropathy is simple, safe, harmless, no pains and sufferings, patients can die peacefully, a painless death. This is the fabulous medicinal quality of urine therapy.

Healer of Last Resort

When all paths and therapies fail, as a healer within is a last resort, urine therapy will turn around to work. According to the physiological, constitutional, biological, metabolic functions every body, makes its own medicine particular and peculiar to the body having curative power.

Scientific Supports

1. Dr S.R. Burzynski , M.D., U.S.A., who isolated and extracted a hormone from human urine called as Antineoplantons, which is non-toxic, an anti-tumor agent. It has medicinal capability to make malignant cells revert to normal. This was published in July-August, 1990 issue of *Oncology News* (Vol. 16, No. 4). It is a publication of Academy of Professional Information Services. The hormones he found are naturally occuring peptides and aminoacid derivates. They were first isolated from human urine. He carried out research for 20 years on human urine has developed an injection which reduce cancer tumors. It costs about $ 8,000 and for full treatment it costs about two lakh dollars.
2. Thompson, J.H., he found that the specific component of human urine called as H-ll useful for cancer treatment. H-ll is an anti-cancer urine extract. This study claims that more than 300 doctors and researchers have found that H-ll is clinically effective in inhibiting the growth of malignant cells in humans (*Source: British Medical Journal*, 7.43, 1943).

3. Joseph Eldor, MD, Theoretical Medicine Institutte, Jerusalem in his paper on *Uropathy for Patients with Cancer* reported that Sandweiss, Seltzstein and Forbman in their study found that an extract from urine of preganant women has a prophylactic and therapeutic effect on ulcer in dogs. Shortly thereafter, the same group noted that an extract from normal women has a similar beneficial effect.

   Cancer cells release various antigens which appear in the urine. Oral auto-therapy is suggested as a new treatment modality for cancer patients. It will provide the intestinal lymphatic system the many tumor anti-gens against which anti-bodies may be produced. These anti-bodies may be transpierced through the blood stream and attack the tumor and its cells (The paper originally published in *Medical Hypotheses* 48, 4, April 1997, pp. 309-315).

   Urotherapy is suggested as a new kind of immunotherapy. The urine of the cancer patients contain the many tumour antigens which constitute the tumour. Against tumour antigens, anti-bodies may be produced due to non-self recognition.

4. The report presented at the annual meeting of the Federation of American Society For Experimental Biology in Atlantic City, U.S.A., in April, 1966 under the heading, *Bringing Cancer Cells Into Line*, gives the account of research showing the effect of human urine on cancer cells. The two researchers found that unexpectedly in 1965, that urine extract which they call " Directin", when added to the culture medium causes all cancer cells on which it has been so far been tested, to align themselves end to end into straight rows.

5. Hegyeli A., *Preparation of Retinene from Urine Meant for Curing Cancer*, on this subject the study discloses that a fraction of human urine was isolated and named as "Retinene". It was tested on mice with artificially inducted skin cancer. The results found was that it inhibited the growth of tumors. Larger doses application shown to cause the regression of tumours (*Science,* 20:1571-1572,1963).

6. The Noble laureate Albert Sczent Georgyi has carried out a number of experiments testing the effect of mythyle glyoxal, a constituent of urine on cancer patients, and has considerable success in several cases (Source : http;// www.hpscleansing.com).

7. Dr Evagelos Danopoulos, Greece, reported that urea found in urine has anticancerous properties. The urea seems to disrupt the ability of cancer cells to group together and kills them by upsetting of their normal metabolic activities. Urine therapy has been used to treat cancers of the skin, cervix, lungs, eyes, breast and liver (*Water of Life Foundation*, Mumbai, India).

8. Another study is a by Novaka, Dr on *Therapeutic Results of the Use of auto-urine Extract on Malignant Tumors*. This is reported from German doctor who employed with much success injections of a natural extracts of patient's own urine to treat cancers of the breast, colon, lungs, uterus, lymph nodes and stomoach (Source: Neitschrift Inner Medizine,196l).
9. As per the press report, San Francisco (USA), dated October 24th, 1967, published in a medical journal. Human urine has been found to contain marvellows healing property promising to cure deadly diseases such as cancer, TB, pulmonary and cardiac diseases, etc.
10. Mr Ken Hashibara, President of Hashibara Laboratories, Japan in his letter dated 22.11.1991 addresssed to the former Prime Minister of India, Morarji Desai, wrote as under :

    "On research I discovered that cancer and other incurable disease can be treated with "Leucocytes", a hormone found in human urine. AIDS, hepatitis can also successfully be treated with urokinase and enzyme found in urine, while thromobosis can completely be cured by it".
11. Dr Alexander N. Glazer and Dr Stocker from the University of California, had discovered : The yellowing dye responsible for Jaundice present in urine which was previously considered as valueless bodily waste till now is very much useful to reduce tissue damage in cancer, aging, inflamation and heart diseases (Source: *Uropathy* by Dr Chanchal mal Chordia, K. Chanchal Chordia Trust, Jodhpur, India, p.9).
12. Rabagliati of Bradford, a renowned surgeon of England. He admitted that the surgical treatment of cancer was complete failure. He had performed over 500 major operations for cancer and rarely had any patient survived after operation. Regarding the success of auto-urine treatment in diagnosed cases he testified as under:

    "I have examined a number of women, according to orthodox treatment would have been operated and got one or both of their breasts removed..." When they consulted him, I did not find even a scar to suggest the healing of incurable malignant growth. Some of them found lumps disappeared within a fortnight and others even in four days.

    The so called king of terrible disease can be easily cured if tackled promptly by autourine therapy (Source: *Uropathy* by Dr Chanchalmal Chordia, India).
13. Henry Sigerist reported more than 50 years ago that, I personally have the feeling that the problem of cancer is not merely biological and laboratory problem, but it belongs to certain extent to the realm of philosophy...all experiments require certain philosophical preparation. And I have the feeling that the case of cancer many experiments were undertaken without the necessary philosophical background and

therefore proved useless (Source : Referred, in the paper of Joseph Elder, MD, Theoretical Medicine Institute, Isreal).

14. Dr Hamao, a professor at the Medical University of Kyoto, Japan, has succeeded inisolating a substance from human urine which is beneficial in the treatment of cancer (Source *Illustrated Weekly of India*, August, 26th, 1973).
15. Dr J.W. Armstrong, U.K., he himself was a doctor, cured his own illness of T.B. He has written a world wide famous book, *Water of Life*. He cured many varient cases and cancer with auto urine. The cancer cases successfully cured by him presented in his book are very interesting, convincing and eye opening.
16. Two popular doctors of Bombay, India by name Dr Mani Kothari and and Dr Lopa Mehta have written a revolutionary book of research findings and clinical investigation practices titled "*Cancer Myths and Realities about its Causes and Cure*." The book was published in London and later translated into German and Dutch languages.

    A single copy of the same is not available in any book stall in India. After their deep study and research, it is written. They reported in the book that "If any cancer patient takes routine allopathy treatment his/ her life is shortened, and his/her death becomes painful. Whereas those who does not opt for the treatment they survived longer and their death is painless."

    They further remarked that for the diagnosis of the disease, it is not wise to undergo biopsy, too, bacause of doing biopsy can spread speedily to other parts of the body. Dr Kothari had neither done biopsy nor given any treatment to his parents suffering from cancer (Water of Life Foundation, India).
17. Dr Vasant, P. Mehhta, MD., M.S., of Mumbai, Maharashtra, India who was teaching medicine and surgery in the medical college for one and half decades has expressed that auto-urine therapy has played major role in his recover from throat cancer.
18. Dr C.P. Mithal, M.D., House Physician, N.F. Medical College, West Bengal, India. He has written a wonderful book titled *Miracles of Urine Therapy*. In his book, he writes that he used to ask his patients suffering from chronic and deadly diseases to bring their urine for test on each visit. He coloured and flavoured the same and would return the same in another bottle to the same patients as medicine. He got amazing results in several chronic and deadly diseases. He has experienced so many thrilling recovery stories of patients who got recovered from diseases like cancer, terminal arthritis, kidney failure, ulcer, epilepsy, nervous break-down, piles fistula, etc. (Source : *Uropathy* by Dr Chanchal Lmal Chordia, Jodhpur, India).

19. Late Dr Jivraj N. Mehta, M. D, London, former Chief Minister of Gujarat, India, writes in his foreword to the book, *Manav Mootra*, English edition that the belief that Urine is not an excreta, but an elixir of life, gifted by nature for the purpose of healthy living and for the use as a main therapeutic measure for almost the whole range of human, diseases including cancer, TB, Leprosy, etc.
20. Last, W., *Urine and Urea Therapy* : Cancer resource Centre Website available at http:// cancersource centre. com/articles / alt 114.html.

Survivors' True Stories

The following are some of the case histories of the patients recovered from deadly cancer disease by using auto-urine therapy. The recovery stories are incredible, exciting, thrilling and hair raising to hear/read.

1. The amazing recovery story of Shri Himmat Somaiya who suffered from terminal liver cancer at the age of 42 years. He was admitted into prestigeous Tata Memorial Hospital, Mumbai, India. When doctors diagnosed and declared that he was suffering from liver cancer of last stage. The doctors had advised him to go for chemotherapy and thereafter radiation therapy as last resort. Further the doctore warned him that he would not survive for more than 10 days if he did not undergo the proposed treatment. Against their advice, the patient took voluntary discharge form the hospital. He practised auto-urine therapy on one's own urine, improved a lot and after six months he got checked up in the same hospital and to the amazing of patient's physicians he was declared totally normal and healthy, survived for more than one and half decades nearly (Dr G.K. Thakkar, Chairman, Water of Life Foundation, India).
2. The incredible recovery story of Mr Nanubhai Chitalia, Mumbai, India who suffered from terminal liver cancer. His survival true story has been published in many news papers and magazines in India. He had miraculously recovered from liver cancer by urine therapy had healthly survived for more than a decade against the physician's prognosis of few days. It is he who inspired and guided in above case Himmat Somaiya not to go for harmful and dangerous treatment of allopathy (*Auto-Urine Therapy*, Navneet Publication, India).
3. In the month of December 1988 on Sunday of *Gujarat Samachar*, a leading newspaper of Ahmedabad, Gujarat, India reported 33 cases of cancer patients who were cured by urine therapy with their names and addressee of the patients.
4. The incident is relating to the patient by name Shri Chimanlal Tulsidas Patel, office supervisor in the firm Sri Chimanlal Mangaldas and Company, He is a resident of Ahmedabad. He had cancer Uvula in 1954.

On the basis of reports of local civil hospital and advice, he went to Tata Hospital, Mumbai, India. There they insisted upon radium therapy on the offected parts. Drinking urine has resulted in rapid improvement.

When he reported back the doctors at the Tata Hospital were astonished, they did not prescribe any medicine or radiotherapy. He thanked Sri Babubhai Ochchhavlal Soni, his college who actually adviced and and inspired urine therapy (*Ibid.*)

5. This is a recovery story of Smt Bakula, wife of Indravadanam Chandulal Patel, Baroda, India. The lump on Bakula's neck was detected in 1982, another appeared in the armpit after three months. In 1984, another tumors was noticed in the leg joint. The biopsy revealed as cancerous growths. She had taken treatments in Tata Hospital Mumbai, India but death was staring her on the face. As a last resort, courageously embarking on the course of auto-urine on the advice of Nanumbhai Chitalia, she get completely cured and enjoying a happy life. (*Ibid.*)
6. Dr Vasant P. Mehta, M.D., a professor of a Medical College, teaching medicine and surgery. He suffered from throat cancer. He had expressed that urine therapy has played a major role in his recovery from throat cancer (Cited above).
7. Dr Kothari has done neither biopsy nor given any treatment to his parents suffereing from cancer. He and along his friend Dr Lopa Mehta have written a revolutionary book of research findings and clinical investigations on urine theraphy titled "*Cancer Myths and Realities About its Causes and Cure*". This book was published in London and later translated into German and Dutch Languages, too.

The amazing recovery story of Shri Himmat Somaiya from terminal liver cancer is so thrilling, sensational, exciting and inspiring that is reproduced here in his own words for the benefit of the readers. Mr Somaiya, after his miraculous recovery has become a powerful propagator and mighty supporter of U.T.(*Shivambu*). He has joined our Shivambu Mission whole heartedly. He is ever-ready to help and guide the people suffering from incurable diseases.

"Friends, Had I not stumbled upon U.T. eleven years before, my family members and friends would have been mourning my eleventh death anniversary.

In the year 1984, when I was 42 years old the doctors of the prestigious Tata Memorial Hospital, Bombay diagnosed that I was suffering from liver cancer of last stage. Prior to getting admitted in Tata Hospital, I was treated by several well known Allopath, homeopaths and even Ayurvedic physicians for several months, but my health went on deteriorating day by day as I couldn't eat anything, as a result of which my body was reduced to a mere skeleton weighing 40 kg against my original weight of 62kg. Doctors of Tata Hospital had advised me to go for chemotherapy and thereafter radiation therapy as a last resort. I shuddered at the very thought of those dangerous treatments as I had seen with my own eyes the miserable and painful conditions of my few relatives and friends who had undergone those horrible treatments. I prayed God to save me from this dangerous predicament. And as if God heard my prayer and sent his messenger in the form of one Mr Nanubhai Chitalia whose incredible recovery story of terminal liver cancer had been published by numerous newspapers and magazines. He had miraculously recovered from liver cancer by U.T. and had healthily survived for more than ten years against the physicians' prognosis of few days !

He came to meet me in Tata Hospital to inpire and guide me to do U. T. Instead of opting for harmful dangerous treatments. I gathered courage and took voluntary discharge from Tata Hospital against medical advise and doctors warning that I won't survive for more then ten days if I didn't undergo the proposed treatment.

Being a bookseller by profession I had read few books on U.T. But I had never thought of practicing it. I made up my mind to follow U.T. as a last resort. I Started drinking one and half to two glasses of *shivambu* in the morning and within few days my mouth ulcers were cured and the blood that was coming out from my tongue and gums also stopped! This was not a small achievement for me. I felt great relief as I had suffered these afflictions for several months inspite of spending thousands of rupees on its treatment. This gave me added confidence and inspiration to do U.T. treatment more systematically and intensively.

I started drinking whole day's urine around seven glasses and in between I drank ample water, herbal tea of *Tulsi* and *Pudina*, carrot juice, cabbage juice, vegetables soups, fruit juices at an interval of an hour. After one month of treatment, there was considerable improvement in my general health, and at the end of three months a strange incident occurred. Along with the stools, I passed few tumor like substances which I collected and sent for pathological examination. In the report, it was mentioned that those were the malignant tumours that might have got separated from the liver ! Thereafter there was fast improvement in my health. After six months, I went for check up to the Tata Hospital and to the amazement of my physicians I was declared totally normal and healthy ! Today, after eleven years of my recovery from deadly disease, I am having extraordinary health and stamina which I had 20 years before. I have become a legendary personality amongst my friends, relatives and well wishers.

From my own experience I confidently declare that cancer can be certainly cured by urine therapy if done systematically.

I am attending Shivambu Seminars without fail to narrate my incredible story and inspire the audience to follow U.T. before it is too late. Anybody can approach me for guidance. Jai Shivambu [Source : Dr G.K. Thakkar, Water of Life Foundation, Mumbai, India].

49

AIDS/HIV Positive

Introduction

In the present century, this is a deadly disease and a major health problem of humanrace and is considered a pandemic. It is an illness outbreak that is not only present over a large area but is actively spreading. Sometimes, it is feared that the mankind may extinguish with this menace of AIDS. It is a common instant cause of death.

HIV/AIDS related complications is a major world health problem facing humanrace. Most people are unaware that they are infected with HIV. It is a fearful and terrible disease. The ailment has become the biggest challenge to modern society.

It is a dreaded ailment which takes lakhs of innocent lives every year. A big enemy of modern mankind.

In 2009, the World Health Organisation estimated that there are 33.4 million people world wide living with HIV/AIDS, with 2.7 millions new HIV infects per year and 2.0 millions annual deaths due to AIDS.

In 2009, 2.4 millions people were estimated to be infected with HIV in India.

As per UNDP's 2010 report, India had 2.39 millions people living with HIV at the end of 2009. In 1986, HIV started its epidermic in India attacking sex workers in Chennai, Tamilnadu.

Meaning

The abbreviation, AIDS, stands for :

"Acquired Immune Deficiency Syndrome",

or

"Acquired Immuno-Deficiency Syndrome".

It is a name of the disease caused by Virus named HIV.

The letters HIV stand for :

"Human Immunodeficiency Virus"

To be infected with HIV is to be HIV positive.

HIV the virus, a simple living thing that causes infections/illness, that can cause AIDS disease. It is abbreviated for HIV positive. A virus is a living thing too small to be seen without a microscope that causes infections, disease in people. AIDS is caused by a HIV virus. The Illness interferes with the self-immunity system, making people AIDS to get infections, opportunistic infections and tumours. This disease and virus are together often referred to as AIDS/HIV.

Infection with HIV is the ultimate result of setting in AIDS. HIV is a retrovirus that primarily infects vital organs of the human immunity system. It directly and indirectly destroys cells. Once the number of T-cells of blood drops are below normal level, cellular immunity is lost.

Acute infection usually will be rapid overtime that gives early symptomatic HIV infection and later leads to AIDS. It is therefore, identified either on the basis of amount of T-cells remaining in the blood or presence of certain infections.

Features of HIV/AIDS

The following are the salient characters of the disease/illness and the letters stand for:

1. **Acquired**

   A person may voluntarily acquires the signs of the disease. The patient obtains the illness by the causes given below, acquires by one's own act.

2. **Immune**

   Every individual has immunity system in the body, that produces substances to help it fight against infections and disease. It is a nature's self-healing power and the first line of defence. It is the capacity of the body that protects against a particular disease or illness. It responds against a virus or antigen.

3. **Dificiency**

   The deficiency of the immunity system in the body can cause AIDS easily. It is a state of not having enough defence in the body which is highly the deficiency attracts the virus. It is called human immune deficiency virus. The virus bacteria interfere with the immunity system. The disease gets worse as the deficiency progresses. The illness can not affect the people who have strong immunity system.

4. **Syndrome**

   It is a set of physical conditions of the body, that shows you a particular disease or medical problem. The syndrome is associated with frequent and chronic diseases or illnesses.

   Thus, the abbreviation AIDS, Acquired Immune Deficiency Syndrome, is an illness which attracts the body's ability to resist infection and which usually causes death.

Cause

HIV is transmitted in many ways. Some of the common causes are as follows:

- Vaginal contact,
- Oral or anal sex,
- Recipient of infected blood transfusion,
- Breast Feeding of infected mother,
- Sexual transmission,
- Intravenous drug use,
- Homophiliacs,
- Prostitution,
- Homosexual men and drug use,
- Contaminated hypodermic needles,
- Exchange between mother and baby during pregnancy,
- Contact of mucus membrance or blood stream with bodily fluids that has virus in it,
- Virus contained body fluids are blood, semen, vaginal fluid, preseminal fluid or breast milk from an infected person,
- Sharing and reusing of syringes contaminated with HIV virus, infection, contaminated with HIV infected blood,
- There is a close association between AIDS and homosexuality, bisexuality, hetrosexual sex,
- Lack of awareness and gender disparity,
- Unprotected anal intercourse,
- Unsafe healthcare injections,
- Extensive labour migration and low literacy,
- Exposure to infected fluids or tissues,
- Receptive penile-vaginal intercourse,
- Insertive and intercourse,
- Precutaneous needle stick,
- Immunity deficiency, its collapse leads to complications,
- Infected blood donation and blood products,
- Transmission by health workers, etc,

Living Viruses

Most of these HIV/AIDS related conditions are caused by infections especially caused by :

* Bacteria,
* Viruses,
* Fungi,
* Parasites,
* Mycobacteria.

Opportunistic Infections

The illness interferes with the system and makes the people with AIDS much more likely to get infections including opportunistic infections. An infection is an illness that is caused by bacteria or a virus that affects one or other part of the body. An infectious disease can be passed easily from one person to another.

Opportunistic infections are very harmful to people whose immunity system would become weak by disease or drug.

Instances of opportunistic infections are:

1. AIDS – Acquired Immuno-Deficiency Syndrome;
2. Syphilis – A disease that gets worse over a period of time, spreading from the sexual organs to skin, bones, muscles and brain. It is caused by having sex with an infected person;
3. VDs – Venereal disease is any disease caused by having sex with an infected person. Venereal is relating to diseases spread by sexual contact, a venereal infections;
4. Gonorrhoea – It is a disease of the sexual organs, caused by having sex with an infected person.

Most patients die of opportunistic infections.

These infections are very common in people with AIDS, and affects early every organ of the system. Specific opportunistic infections that AIDS patients develop depend in part on the prevalence of these infections in the geographical area in which the patients live.

T.B. is a unique infection associated with HIV because it is transmissible to immune component of the body of the people via the respiratory route. Once affected, it is not easily treatable even after identification.

Poor resistance is a serious problem. Even multi-drugs resist. In early stages of HIV infection TB typically presents as a pulmonary disease. AIDS patients often develop opportunistic infections that present with low grade fever and weight loss. Pencilliosis is now the third common opportunistic infection.

Immunity Deficiency

The dreaded disease HIV/AIDS related complications are mainly caused by deficiency of human immunity system. The virus or bacteria interferes with the immune system. This makes people suffer from AIDS. The illness generally does not affect people with good and strong working immunity system. The disease gets worse as the deficiency progresses.

The signs of AIDS are primarily the results of conditions of the body, that do not normally develop in individuals with strong immunity network. HIV viruses damage the body's defence mechanism. These viruses are normally controlled by the elements of the immunity system like anti-bodies, enzymes and hormones.

A strong immunity is one that cannot catch or be affected by a particular disease or illness. Strong people are often immune to AIDS. They are protected from virus and therefore able to avoid ailments. In them the reaction of the body to the presence of an virus or antigen is quick and strong.

The immune system in the body produces substances like antibodies to help to fight against infection or disease. So, the immunity is the body's ability to avoid to be affected by virus. Most weak people die of malignancies associated with the progressive failure of the immune system and function. It does not generally occur unless the immunity system drastically collapses.

The immune response is essential and without it, the body cannot fight infections or kill cancerous cells. The gradual loss of the ability of the immunity system is a risk factor.

Generally, the immunity deficiency characteristics of AIDS do not appear for years after a person is infected. The quick immune response eventually counteracts the infection, protects depletion through infection, wards off incidence of deaths.

There is direct correlation between HIV gene products and immune response. Breakdown of the immune surveillance system is the cause for rapid progression of infection and AIDS. So, the natural Immunity system, and refilling deficiency timely to remain active always.

Symptoms and Effects

The diagnosis of AIDS in a person infected with HIV is based on the person of certain signs and symptoms.

People with AIDS often have systemic symptoms, infections such as:

- Fever and vomting,
- Sweats particularly at night,
- Swollen glands,
- Chill,
- Weakness,
- Weight loss,
- Affect bone marrow,
- Affect Bones,
- Affected urinary and gastrointestinal tracts,

- Affect liver,
- Affect regional lymph,
- Affect nodes,
- Affect central nervous system,
- Chronic diarrhea,
- Opportunistic infections,
- Several side effects,
- Neurological and psychiatric disorders,
- Infect the brain,
- Encephalitis,
- Diseases in the eyes and lungs,
- Headache, fatigue, nausea,
- Seizures and confusion,
- Impaired the transmission of nerve impulses,
- Severe weakness in the immunity system,
- Infected and affected, killed, degenerated, functionless,
- Behavioural and cognitive disorders,
- Motor abnormalities, irritability,
- AIDS related mania,
- Cancers, tumours, T.B.,
- Colitis,
- Retinitis (can cause blindness),
- Anemia,
- Decreased production of antibodies.

Survival Time

One develops full blown AIDS some years after contacting HIV. The average time of progression from HIV infection to AIDS is nine-ten years and the average survival time after developing AIDS is only 9.2 months. The rate of disease progression varies widely between two weeks to 20 years.

The rate of rapid progression depends on many factors. The main factor that influences the body's ability to defend against HIV. It means the infected person's general immunity function in younger people have strong immunity system and therefore have less risk of rapid diseases progression than older people.

The infected person's genetic inheritance plays an important role. Some people are more resistant to certain strains of HIV. But generally, it is variable.

The average survival time after infection with treatment is estimated to be about nine-ten years.

Leads To Cancer

Those who are affected with AIDS also have an increased risk of developing various cancers such as sarcoma, cervical, and cancer of the immune system. Koposi's Sarcoma is the most common tumor in HIV infected patients.

The appearance of this tumor in young homosexual men is the signal of AIDS. Invasive cervical cancer in HIV infected women is also considered AIDS. Likewise HIV infected patients are at increased rate of risk of certain other tumors like head, neck and lung cancer. Some of these are caused by virus. Generally, the incidence of many common tumors such as breast cancer or colon cancer are found in HIV infected patients.

In cases where treatment is not intensively attended to treat AIDS, the incidence of many AIDS related malignancies would increase. But at the same time, malignant cancers overall have become the most common cause of death of HIV infected patients.

Non-Availability of Sure Cure Drugs

There is no known sure cure or HIV vaccine presently. Although aniretrovial treatment for HIV/AIDS are at present only known medicine prevailing which can only slow the course of the disease, reduces both the death and new infections. But these drugs are expensive and the medications are not available in all countries.

Due lack of medicine, due to difficulty to treat HIV infections, preventing infections, refilling immunity system is the key steps in controlling the AIDS pandemic. These steps attempt to slow the spread of the virus and prevents.

There is no absolute reliable drug so far available that can cure the disease. Controlling, prevention measure is an alternate best solution.

However, even after almost 30 years of intensive research a drug for HIV has become a difficult target. Present research work should think to improve current treatments for decreasing side effects of current drugs. Further to simplify drug regimes to improve adherence and deteriming the best sequence of regimens to manage drug resistance.

It may take several years before a commercial treatment based on this discovery becomes available to all the people in all countries. A small number of activists question the connectivity between HIV and virus therapy as to the validity of treatment method.

Any new powerful new drug developed, will not work because of characteristic feature of HIV continue to evolve resistance to curing. There is no certainity of survival time which is likely to continue to change.

So, the only drug available is antiretroviral therapy. The long use of this drug and treatment may result in side effects and after effects and reactions like neuro-cognitive disorders, neuropathy, osteoporosis, cancers, nephropathy, cardiovascular diseases, TB, etc.

Before the advent of an effective diagnosis and treatment, there was a danger of common immediate cause of death.

Urinopathy–A First choice or Last Resort

It has been postulated that only a human urine can halt, prevent and cure effectively the pandemic, because it is a natural elixir, a manna from heaven, priceless and drugless being most affordable, universal for developing countries and would not require costly diagnosis, tests costly daily treatment.

A measure to prevent opportunistic infections is most beneficial when treating patients with AIDS/HIV infections. Urinopathy is advised for patients who are not infected with these viruses and are under risk of becoming infected.

Patients with substantial immunity deficiency are also advised to go for urine therapy and the patients may benefit from as well.

Plenty of natural substances of urine have potential that stimulate cell growth, avoid cell death, malfunction, integration but helps healthy cells, reactivation of cells, refilling deficient immunity are suggested as possible prevention methods. If infected mothers take urine, babies who are born would be with resistance to infections with some strain of HIV, it cannot be found in the baby's blood.

The topic of urinopathy and treatment for AIDS has become highly controversial in the past few years, primarily because many medical doctors have declared their opposition to the use of urine as mockery. But recently many scientists too are increasingly recognising and the feel is currently the only means of stopping the menace of epidermic virus.

However, there is a growing openness to faith based methods due to failure rates associated with drugs and their treatment. The yogic and religious approach to prevent the spread of AIDS, *Shivambu*, a Hindu ancient text recommended urinopathy. Cultural and religious changes are needed.

In addition to prevention, some yogic teachers have suggested the treatment on AIDS. Some claim that urine therapy will cure AIDS. Several people have stopped taking their medication for many ills of modern days. The urine, is the water of Life, life force, suspicious water which promotes God's healing. The medicinal water, distilled water will eradicate HIV through the mercy of the Creator.

A household with an HIV/AIDS patient has to spend many times as much on medical expenses as other households. Urine is a priceless and drugless natural therapy. A large number of people suffer and die ultimately of AIDS related complications because of malnutrition, under nutrition poor immunity, health care and medicine. Urine is a holistic medicine, nutrious food.

Throughout the globe AIDS/HIV patients use urine therapy. Today, there is a widespread use of it by people suffering with this infection.

The effectiveness of this therapy has not been established by authoritative medical organizations concerned public health. High quality scientific evidence can be built up by intensive research and case studies of who are taking urine.

There is evidence scattered at household level to support the efficacy of urinopathic medicine in HIV infected individuals and AIDS patients.

As urine contains vitamins, nutritions or mineral supplementation has health benefits. Daily drinking of one's own urine can improve protective mechanism of the body which can effectively prevent and suppress HIV viral burden with an associated improvement. The anti-viral and anti-bodies qualities of urine can be used as an adjustment therapy to other anti-viral treatments.

It is sure that itself cure the infections. More evidence is to be recorded at clinical level before it can be established that urine therapy supplementation reduces mortality rate. There is some evidence that it can be used as preventive maintenance to prevent mortality and improve growth.

Immunologically and nutritionally rich urine shows a number of benefits to daily multivitamin supplementation for both mothers as well as children. Regular intake of urine having multiple micronutrients by the HIV infected people is recommended. Supplementation of natural substances, vitamins of urine can produce adverse effects in HIV positive adults.

Besides, there is currently no publicly available HIV vaccine of cure for HIV or AIDS complications. Urine acts as a natural vaccination, inoculation or immunization.

The only known method of preventative medicine is human urine, which protects the body from viral infections. The reaction of the body of the urine drinker to the presence of HIV viral is powerful and immediate. The antibodies property of the urine in the body produces chemicals to help fight against infection and disease is the efficacy of the urine.

The scientific study of urine's claim of protection against infection is to be taken up by the medical community for verification.

Though human urine has been rejected to day the only current treatment for HIV infection consists of first choice of auto-urine therapy. This is highly beneficial of HIV infected individuals, since there is no alternative to protect the ailing humanrace.

Because HIV disease progression is very rapid and chemical drugs are less predictive of risk for disease progression. However, starting of drinking urine earlier as treatment remedy may significantly reduce the risk of incidence of deaths. It cures the patients of HIV not only, but also protects. Morever, it would take less to clear HIV infection by using urine.

Despite all these merits as reported many HIV infected individuals have experienced remarkable improvements in their normal living, good health, quality of life, wellness enhancement, which has led fall or non-affection from HIV associated morbility and mortality. If strictly followed would increase survival time considerably.

Non-public awareness and non-guidance to the public about the therapy are the major reasons why patients do not get benefit from it. The causes why the therapy is not popular are varied, explained somewhere in this book in detail.

Moreever, psychological, social practices, customs, issues including non-availability urinopathic physicians, inadequate social support, non cooperation from medical community are some of the direct reasons. People prefer to swallow large number of pretty pills frequently and thus drinking urine has become hard to follow.

Side effects, reactions are very serious in case of drugs in treatment of HIV infection related diseases like AIDS. Besides drugs are not only costly but also majority are poor in under developed countries.

In the light of these known facts, in the absence of sure cure for HIV, urine therapy is considered a life saving last effective strategy for enhancing well being of AIDS patients and their dependents.

The incidence of deaths would definitely decline, and it is most appropriate remedy in areas where HIV is the most prevalent. In HIV infected individuals, the cause is normally due to fungal, so urine acts as an anti-fungal medicine.

The use of drugs to treat HIV may lead to after effects of diarrhea. It may also be a side effect of antibiotics used to treat bacterial causes of diarrohia. Similarly, HIV infection may lead to a variety of neuropsychiatric disorders by organism or by illness. Single celled parasites can also infect and cause disease in eyes and lungs.

Universal precaution, universal medicine, universal preventative therapies are normally not available in any medical systems except in urine therapy which is an intrinsic and universal remedy. It gives a ray of hope to the patients. There cannot be better band happier news than this to the AIDS/HIV patients.

The problem of HIV is not merely a biological, physiological and laboratory problem but to some extent it belongs to the realm of philosophy. The whole philosophy of our dealing with modern innumerable and incurable diseases in mistaken. The complete failure of our only modern medicinal approach and lack of proper guidance to the public in natural nutrition and other ways of living are as the ways of progressive medicine.

The laudable belief being that there are many roads to treatment and many means of cure, but for AIDS/HIV for which no alternative roads nor means are available except auto-urine, a cure par excellence.

Scientific supports

Urine therapy may improve the condition of Acquired Immune Deficiency Syndrome (AIDS) patients. There are various anecdotal reports of T-Lymphocytes counts improving in AIDS patients using oral urinopathy.

It is clear that the actual HIV virus, that causes AIDS and has been speculated that oral administration of these antibodies to the HIV via urinotherapy may be responsible for the effectiveness of urinopathy in AIDS patients. Antineoplastons may also contribute to the effects of urinopathy.

The urea component of urine dissolves the foreign proteins that form an antigens. Urinopathy inhibits/kills many types of detrimental bacteria due to the urea content of urine including mycobacterium tuberculosis. Urine may inhibit the growth of the malignant cells that occur in cancer. Many types of cancer that have been reported to respond to urinopathy.

Dr Beastrice Barnett of U.S.A. who is a practising urine therapy has written a book, namely, *Miracles of Urine Therapy,* in which the author had written a special section of treatment of AIDS and given details for the successful treatment of many AIDS patients with urine therapy.

Mr Quique Palladino of New York who had been cured from AIDS by following urinopathy. He has been not only recovered from AIDS illness but has also become healthier than before. Later, he became a researcher, propagator and advocate of urinopathy.

Mr Ken Hashibara, President of the Raashibara Laboratories, Japan in his letter addressed to the then Prime Minister of India, Morarji Desai, who was a life time practitioner of urine therapy. He writes, "On research I discovered that cancer and other incurable diseases can be treated with Leucocytes found in urine. AIDS and hepatites can also be successfully treated with urokinase and enzyme found in urine, while thromobosis can be completely cured by it".

Dr G.K. Thakkar, the then president of Water of Life Foundation, India reported that he had visited USA, there he met several AIDS patients who had immensely been benefitted from urine treatment.

So, any illness spreading from different kinds of viruses, urinopathy provides protection against such diseases because it improves immunity system and refills nutritious deficiency. All types of infections, cancer and other opportunistic infections associated with AIDS can be cured. Urine is antibacterial, antifungal and antiviral. It can be used effectively in treating HIV related illnesses.

The President of Life Science Institute of USA, Dr F.O. Quinn, a famous urine therapist and author of a wonderful book on urine therapy (*Self-Healing Through Intrinsic Medicine*) writes as follows:

"I predict urine therapy will be the only cure for horrible AIDS".

Further says that "I think I will die sorrow it I see another Ethiopian child die due to ignorance of this suppressed fountain of sustenance (urine therapy) for the sick and starving poor. Urine therapy will be of incalculable assistance to those dying people perhaps more than all the food being shipped there".

AIDS–No Stigma

There is a social stigma of AIDS disease to the patients. AIDS stigma exists around the world in a variety of ways. It is a feeling of disapproval that people have about AIDS/HIV and their ways of behavior. Because of serious nature of the complaint the patients are facing many social problems.

Some of them are :

1. Expelling from schools or society because of infection.
2. *Social ostracism* : It is an act of deliberately not including the patient in a group or activity.
3. *Rejection* : Patient is one of the society's rejects, who has not been accepted as a member of the team, group or society, etc.
4. *Discrimination* : It is social practice of treating AIDS patient in a society less fairly than others, treating one worse than others.
5. Avoidance of HIV infected patients.
6. Violence against HIV infected individuals or people who are perceived to be infected with HIV.
7. Keeping a way from others in order to prevent the disease from spreading.
8. Stigma related violence or the fear of violence prevents many people from seeking HIV testings.
9. A reflection of fear and oppression that are likely to be associated with any deadly and transmissible illness.
10. Symbolic AIDS stigma, i.e., the use of HIV/AIDS to express attitudes towards the social group or life styles perceived to be associated with the disease.
11. Stigmatisation of people connected to the issue of HIV/AIDS positive people.
12. Other stigmas associated which may include homosexuality, bisexuality, prostitution, hetrosexulality and intravenous drug use.

There is no longer any stigma attached to urine therapy

Take Precautions

- Avoid exposure to virus.
- Have AIDS health education and literacy.
- Be Cautious to safe sex behaviour, sexual contact.
- Infected mothers should avoid breast-feeding to infants.
- Health workers to reduce exposure to HIV body fluid.

- Use gloves, masks, protective eyeware or shield, gowns, aprons.
- To dispose of sharp objects like needles, scalps, glass.
- Avoid needle exchange, contaminated items.
- Avoid intravenous drug abuse.
- Use condoms to reduce the risk.
- Avoid homosexuality, bisexuality, heterosexuality, prostitution.
- Avoid exposure to infected body fluids or tissues.
- Screen thoroughly donor blood and blood products.
- Have HIV test on venous blood.
- Avoid use of disposable syringes.

50
Self–Therapy

My Own Experiences

My Himalayan yoga guru had disclosed to me the secrets of auto–urine therapy and recommended for life long practice for wellness as health management measure. I drink, practise and I receive treatment at home to help myself for good health and normal living and longevity. It is my personal healthcare medicine even today.

I learnt about its importance later by reading ancient texts, and recently its medical relevance scientifically.

Throughout my life till to day, it treated me in a wide variety of conditions in daily life. This ancient Indian therapy works better and has no side effects, no cost, personal convenience and individualised. We are a society succeeded with so many traditional healthcare methods, practices and cultures deeply familiar with them. The only problem is we lack access and awareness about them.

Millions of people have now become familiar with it. Today, mankind is reeling under incurable and innumerable terrible ailments without an effective remedy. Globally, people are suffering, searching and looking for suitable solutions. But neither the modern medicine nor alternative medicine seems to offer a definite remedy to resolve.

But Here is a Divine Nectar–Urine

"The pain is gone – I cannot believe it".

That is what I want to share my experience with you. My pain suddenly disappeared after two months of unrelenting pain from foot, tendon complaint. The urine treatment practice systematically followed for week time that it profoundly interfered with root cause of the diseases and improved the quality of walk and I avoided to an addition of myriad of pharmaceutical drugs. It saved money, got relief from troubles and the body saved from side effects.

I regularly use my own urine as a household medicine both as medicine for preventative and curative purposes as first-aid and as mainstream , in treating day to day minor ailments, skin allergies, fistula, fissure, cuts, bruises, headache , dandruff and as after shave lotion.

The more I use, the simple is urinopathic medicine to cure, the easier it is for me to avoid frequent and repetitive visits to allopathic physicians.

My practical experience has shown that urine retake promotes the health of hair. To the best of my memory goes I do not apply hair oil to my head. Periodically, I cure my head and hair with urine for some time and take bath after half an hour. My experiment with my own urine to my head has shown external application helped to grow hair thick, prevented hair loss, till later in age, no dandruff, no hair fall and conversion.

Human urine possesses rich vitamins good nutrition to the hair, which are reused by the head and by the hair follicles. A follicle is one of the very small holes in the skin from which actually hair grown from or which is where hair begins its growth cycle.

My bronchitis cough has gone, I cannot believe !

That is what I want to say to the readers frankly when my cough suddenly disappeared after many years of an unpleasant situation during which the cough not stopping or becoming less severe, faced an unrelenting suffering.

I was affected by this type of diseases affecting the two main branches of bronchial leading to lungs. It is called as bronchitis, an illness that affects the bronchial tubes. Those who are affected by this suffer from acute, chronic bronchitis.

It was just with urine therapy of 10-15 days treatment the cough gradually declined and continuous practice for some more days the cough completely absent.

Incredible ! No more medicine ! No sign of repeat of bronchial cough so far in my life. I began feeling like old self.

Friends, family members felt that it was a miracle and were surprised. Besides bronchial cough, serious ailments like sinus, asthma are of many common health conditions that can be eliminated by using urine therapy as a household personal medicine.

Urinopathic medicine is like a nature's elixir that sounds too far fetched to exist in today's world.

However, in these disease prone days I personally feel the therapy will be the only future medicine for the coming generations and is poised to become mainstream medical practice. No alternative to it.

This secret and household medicine is revolutionising health care system for a wide variety of ailments of ailing humanrace.

Many of health problems that have so far been notoriously difficult or even impossible to successfully prevent or manage like cancer. HIV, AIDS, arthritis can now benefit from urinopathic medicine. There are several hundreds of successful stories, recovery conditions by using human urine.

I am seventy years old, never faced any problem in my life time relating to dental or mouth related problem. I am not using brush, paste, no medication, never felt gum problem, capping, cementing or root canal treatment.

I brush my teeth with neem tree stick and gargling and pulling with my own urine. That is the secret of my dental health and care. It removes the pain to the dental patients by using regular urine pulling. No anxiety and phobia.

It is a common phobia that many people have the fear of dentistry. Patients fear of pain, cost, time and possible procedure that could cause them anxiety. Many people also afraid of going to the dentist, because it may lead to a great deal of stress and fear.

Urinopathy has proved its quality as to the safest home therapy for virtually all common dental and mouth concern including bad smell and tooth decay.

Try gargling with urine solution it removes mucus, reduce swellings, eliminates foul smells , protects and prevents from decay, early fall, refills immunity system which in turn help in strengthening long teeth stay.

Urine acts as a pain killer and antibiotic, reduces pain, relieve muscle spasm. Historical records testify that this practice has been there in India for centuries to treat mouth and teeth problems.

Likewise in day-to-day life for all small common concerns I drink or apply externally and I experienced favourable results. The cause of my prolonged headache is tight and sore neck but cured with urine massaging. In many instances remedial massage modality of treatment worked miraculously. No steroid injections nor pharmaceutical drugs were necessitated in case of rare muscle discomforts. I just did massaging with urine my muscles were stretched and untangled soon.

I have no less confidence in this therapy and about doing its wonders but it is the only thing having unknown medicine. One can no longer need frequent drug consumption.

I work hard every day 10-12 hours of tight sitting: reading, writing work as hobby and as the profession demands. As a result, I faced health problems like body pains, back, neck and shoulder pains are the natural effects of prolonged sitting, worng postures, bad postures and straight sitting. The other effects are headache, tension, neck shoulders, arms, forearm wrist and back pain. Urine therapy helped me in several ways and got relief from many occupational hazards.

I am not sure how can I make you to believe and put into practice to reap the benefits of my experiences. But I am convinced that there is some divine worthwhile intrinsic therapeutic properties in urine.

I have explained my success stories, recovery cases to many people of various cross sections of the society, but some people shown little interest and some practiced. But the allopathic physicians though well aware of the medicinal qualities of urine scientifically but do not reveal to the public and strict to the practice of prescription drugs.

Nevertheless, I feel that the therapeutic benefits are too large, so I am spreading the hidden medicine to the world wherever I can, particularly by this book. I like to continue this inexpensive treatment for the rest of my life worthwhile.

But yet urine is not a drug, but drugless drug, almost no one in the medical field in India wants to know or hear patiently about it.

Today, it has become a common sight in every family to have small medical store with full of prescriptive drugs for all common, acute diseases for self medication, like pain killers, antibiotic, antacids, pantacids, analgisics, opiates, and narcotics. They are home over the counter shops.

What many people may not realise is that their dangerous effects to our body. It is an opportunity to me to give a detailed picture of experiences with the urine to the readers without further shy and nauceat. I want to put it before you secret that the man and within himself is there a medicinal substance to cure one's own ailments. The principle that an ounce of truth is better than a pound of arguments holds good.

I quote here the evidences relating to many years of my practice and personal experiences to those who want to know the real facts. I believed and still believe in it and am committed to its continuance. I am satisfied with my self-cure. The drinking of my own urine is a well known proved cure with success for my fissure complaint by external application of my urine just for a few days.

I share my knowledge and experiences with others of different cross sections of the society, advice and supervise the practice of others drinking. Many ailments of modern human race which modern medicinal standpoint of view are labelled incurable are proved curable with urine. Incurability question or affecting to disease does not arise. Urinopathy proved itself its capability with evidence and scientifically testified that medical dogma of incurability is not true.

At my personal level, I am creating awareness among the public by way of delivering lectures, publishing papers interviews and discussions through. TV programmes which are regarded more seriously by the public.

51
Leading Personalities

1. Dr J.W. Armstrong

In modern times, Dr J.W. Armstrong is one of the great persons who supports the idea of urine therapy and cource of action. He is a chief proponent of this system of health care. He belongs to the USA. He can rightly be called as the person who is the first to study, practice, experimenting on himself, and develop this particular medical area of knowledge. Later, following him, many physicians continued to develop.

A pioneer in the field of urinopathic medicine, it is he who introduced new idea and method of urine therapeutic method. When Armstrong pioneered urinopathic medicine, he was one of the first person to do so, a new health care system pioneered by him in America in his hospital. Those days were the pioneering days of auto urine therapy in post industrial era.

It means in those days his urinopathic way of practice was a new and interesting in a way that was different from allopathic that had existed before. To say an originator of the auto-urine therapy.

It was he who brought back into use the traditional medicinal practice into light that existed before. He restored the system that was long neglected back sometime. The way in which he restored the credibility and culturally accepted medicinal practice to limelight is unique.

Nearly seven, decades back, Dr J.W. Armstrong has written a book titled "*Water of Life*", with a foreword in 1944 and first published in London. The book was published based on his own personal experiences and practice.

The book is very famous both in India and England and it was later first published in India in Rupa Paper Back in 1978.

When this book was published in London, the entire medical industry was in a state of great anxiety, confusion and uncertainity. His book threw the country into turmoil, as there was a strong opposition. He exhibited to the public with evidence of live cases, recovery stories, successful treatment case studies as to the efficacy, efficiency, safety, treating a whole person of auto-urine therapy. The news and about this unknown medicine spread all over the world like tornado.

In this way, he had done great deal of favour and obligation upon the world particularly by writing this book. Many people followed footsteps and reaped beneficial results of far reaching miraculous cure.

In India, Shri Raojibhai Patel was a close associate of Mahatma Gandhi. At that time, he was suffering from Asthma and had a heart attack and he used auto-urine and obtained good result.

Indian *shivambu*, auto-urine *rishi* (sage), great devotee, a propagator and mighty supporter of urinopathy movement, centenarian former prime Minister of India, respected late Morarji Desai had received the inspiration to drink urine by reading the book of "*Water of Life*", written by Dr J.W. Armstrong. The book was presented to Desai by Shri Raojibhai.

The book is a beginning. An opening door, eye opener, thought provoking, hair raising, on reading the one hopefully change the opinion. Hundreds of cases of various health conditions cured by him with urine are presented in the book. They are not only interesting to read but they are convincing.

Dr Armstrong was suffering from tuberculosis and at that time this disease was a very dangerous, acute and serious, and there was no effective drug in modern medicine at that time to cure it.

For treatment of his T.B., he had a long and agonising journey from door to door, from doctor to doctor but proved unable to cure him of his T.B. Symptoms. His condition worsened.

When he was reaching to a stage of incurability towards death, the knowledge of urine therapy struck his mind, practised and totally got cured. There are some important reasons which inspired him and decided to try urine therapy as last resort. First of all, the quotation from the Bible, which he read stimulated his curiosity to drink. That is :

"Drink water from your own cistern. Flowing water from your own well".

The second reason is he had childhood memories of his mother smearing urine on his face which was swollen from a bee sting. His grandfather treating animals with urine.

Third, reminded him of the case of a young girl whose father gave her own urine to drink when she was suffering from diphtheria, with the result that She was cured in three days.

Fourthly, a jaundice disease was also cured by the same means, which also came to his mind.

Fifthly, he remembered the doctor's answer to his question when some few years previously he asked him how he could tell from my urine that my lungs and pancreas were diseased and wasting.

He even remembered saying to the doctor in his innocence.

His first patient was himself. When he was at the age of 34, he was subjected to medical examination and was rejected by four examined doctors on the ground that he was consumptive, means as he was suffering a disease of the lungs. He was put under the care of a physician. Later, he consulted a specialist.

His opinion was that he was more a catarrhal, means liquid in nose and throat than a consumptive.

Armstrong not satisfied himself, he consulted another specialist who said that both his lungs were affected.

Later, diabetes set in. He was inflicted with insomnia, frayed nerves and great irritability of temper, suffered for sixteen weeks. He also suffered from sciatica, he felt that cure seemed more unpleasant than the disease. After two years of treatments, he lost his faïth in doctors.

"If I am losing vital tissue and sugar through my urine, then why not drink the urine and replace these elements in that way".

To which, the doctor replied that the organs could not assimilate 'dead matter'.

Armstrong considered this view point as a theoretical fallacy.

The Bible verses, his belief, and many others bear reference to that vital force and acted in accordance with that belief. Fortified by his faith he fasted for 45 days on nothing but urine and tap water. He also rubbed urine into his body which is also a very important modality in cure.

At the end of this treatment, he felt and was 'an entirely new man' weighed 140 lbs, full of vim, looked about 11 years younger than actually he was and had skin like a young girl's.

He was 36 years at that time. He looked and felt much younger than most men of his age, and kept free from those major and minor aliments.

The essential details of his diseases and self-cure are described in his book, *Water of Life*. In 1918, when he was convinced the traditional medicinal knowledge of self-therapy that must not be selfishly hidden under a bushel, and with a view to share with one's fellows, he wrote this book.

After witnessing practical result by experimenting his own urine on himself, and totally got cured from T.B., he found that human urine is a panacea. In his practice, he followed the philosophy and principles of urinopathic medicine, he treated thousands of patients suffering from various common, acute, chronic, degenerative diseases, opporthenistic infections, injuries and natural tendencies of various incurable diseases found and proved discarded by the physicians of modern medicine. Based on the result obtained by practice he had written the book, "*Water of Life*." Even today it is very useful to the ailing human race and future generations.

His first patient was himself, and his complaint, he cured nearly 40,000 patients suffering from various diseases and disorders by auto-urine therapy including medically diagnosed cases of cancer, Bright's disease, gangrene, cases of leucocythaemia or leukaemia, heart diseases, fever, malaria, black water fever, orchitis, veneral disease like syphilis, cure of wounds which would not heal, treatment of burns, enuresis nocturna, menstrual troubles, nephritis, mucucolitis, eye injuries, psoriasis, rheumatic fever followed by influenza, pyrrhoea, obesity, prostate troubles, bronchial asthama, rashes on skin, wart, lumps, jaundies, paralysis, premature old age, loss of memory, loss of hair, cataract, glaucoma, arthritis, and many others which from orthodox stand point are labelled incurable.

He writes :

"The universe keeps gifting us with blessings and we often miss them. Our education or culturisation gets in to the way. I really think the best things in life are free".

2. Morarji Desai

He was the former Prime Minister of India, long practised urine therapy. He is popularly called as *shivambu rishi*, sage. *Yogis* were ancient Indian sages, but Desai is a modern urine-therapy sage, both in India and outside. A wise person especially because he had a lot of practical expericene about this therapy.

He was a great devotee, propagator and supporter of urine therapy movement. He had a long and determined effort to achieve good health and happy living that he believed to be right.

A centenarian, a person who lived to be 100 in good health. He boldly and emphatically declared to the world that he drank his own urine regularly, and that was the secret of his longevity and exuberant health, lived with full of energy, excitement and happiness.

As the most secret it remained long in dark, but most valuable and beneficial information disclosed to the world at large.

Only a few people like him dared to declare public useful things, publicly he supported this medicine. A written and a spoken way, he stated in an open manner so that the people know about it. By this honest and frank declaration, he has received world recognition, glory and greatness. He is an example of generosity, set an example, a shining example how he is interested in public health. So, the whole world, the medical industry is indebted to him for his inner feeling of humanitarian service that inspired people.

He is the most proponent of urine therapy and lamented that India would have been better if more people used this extremely inexpensive and effective way of treatment.

Whenever a group of people meet in the context of urine therapy, they refer to urine as 'Morarji Cola' or 'Morarjin'.

In the year 1978, Morarji Desai spoke to Dan Rather on urine therapy for 60 minutes. He opined that this therapy was the perfect medical solution for the millions of Indians who could not afford medical treatment.

3. Martha Christy

A leading personality in urinopathic medicine is Martha Christy, an American lady. She has published a revolutionary book in USA titled "*Your Own Perfect Medicine*".

There is an interesting story around her, as she had a painful history of 30 years sickness as she suffered from several acute, chronic and degenerative diseases. For nearly 30 years right from the age of twelth-year, upto the age of 42 she suffered from various incurable diseases. She consumed many pharmaceutical drugs, undergone surgery for six times on her body.

She is a urine expert and has lot of personal experience. For long, she fell ill, sick; some of the disorders, diseases she faced are pelvic inflammatory disease, ulcerative colitis, chron's disease, chronic fatigue syndrome. Hashimoto's disease, mononucleosis, severe kidney infections, two miscarriages, chronic cystitis, severe candida, endometriosis, adrenal insufficiency, serious chronic ear and sinus infections, food and chemical allergies, weight reduced, hair loss, became weak.

She has given all her attention to all known medical tests, surgery and drug. Besides she used all forms of alternative and natural therapies and pathies like homeopathy, herbal medicine, mega vitamins and live cell treatment in Mexico. Lot of money and time was spent on many things and even traditional medicine failed to work.

Her husband and herself faced lot of problems in their life. They spent over 1,00,000 dollars to her complaints with alternative healthcare modalities too. All failed, nothing worked. Really it had become a financial burden upon her family member. Treatment for nearly 30 years, spending lacks of rupees by trying various physicians, expers, and health care systems, visited Japan and Mexico for treatment.

Frustrated and discouraged in life, fed up with miserable life, pains and troubles, and very much wished that death should relieve her miserabls.

One fine day, her husband came across a book written by Margie Adelman, USA By reading this book, she inspired by this seemingly strange natural therapy. She practised by which she became free from all diseases. Right from the beginning of drinking urine, she experienced lot of relief and general health improvement. Firstly, she felt almost instantaneous relief from her chronic incurable constipation and fluid retention.

Within a short period, her severe abdominal and pelvic pain disappeared. The problem of cystitis and yeast infections soon were gone. Other disorders like food allergies, exhaustion, digestive problems, etc. started to heal. Gradually, cold, flu, sore throat, viral symptoms disappeared. After long period of 30 years of repetitive, non-stop illness, she was safe and healthy again.

Later, she became a strong believer, propagator of auto-urine therapy and became the author of a world famous book.

52

The Urine and Immunity Connection

What Is Immunity System

Immunology is a newly fast emerging branch of health care subject, which is a scientific study of protection against diseases. It is a cellular structure and immune system constitution of the body of an individual. It is the defence mechanism of the body that protects us from diseases and infections, bacterial, parasitic, fungal, viral infections and from the growth of tumor cells.

Every human being has a natural immune system in the body that produces substances to help it fight against infection, or disorder, therefore, an immunity is the body's ability to avoid or not to be affected by infection or disease.

A human body is a system which has a number of sub-systems. They are mental systems, nervous, hormonal, cardio-vascular, reproduction, respiratory, urinary, skelton, muscular system, etc. connected, inter connected and interdependence in their metabolic and physiological function.

Contrary to them, the immunity system of the body is quite distinct, separate and it is an autonomous system that functions independently of many other sub-systems of the body.

It is like a sac with full of multiple variety of powerful cells, it has no fixed anatomy, having mobile character travelling from place to another place within the body and not staying anywhere permanently.

The system operates individually, and its cells kill viruses and bacteria. Whenever, wherever, there is an antigen, that is a substance that can cause disease or infection, the immune responses quickly by way of reaction of the body to the presence of an antigen.

The immune system is a fluid, distributed throught the body by the two circulatory systems like blood and lymph, they put together carry fluids to every cell.

How the immunity system erects influences on health is one of the neglected as well as hottest areas in recent years. Many therapies and pathies exhibit unkind laughter or make remarks that show us to think immunity system and its impack on health as ridiculous and not worth considering seriously.

The exact nature of an immune system's response is unique to each individual due to variance in the constitution of the body.

The naturopathy and other complementary and alternate therapies addresse the root cause of the disease relating to immunity. In a real true sense, the immunity deficiency makes one physically sick. In addition, many of the changes overtime in the body from day to day are driven by fluctuations in one's own immunity system of which we are unaware.

The system preserves and conserves energy. It is the body's rapid first line of defence against risk factors or causes of disorders or diseases. It also activates response by releasing hormones, enzymes and other medicinal qualities to respond.

The deficit makes a person dis-ease from 'ease' conditions. The clinical observations also have proved the role of this natural health keeping mechanism, their direct positive correlation between changes in the immunity system with day to day variability in health condition.

This is really an exciting time that every one should know that changes in life force substances that constitutes the system alters proportionately the health system.

It is not very unsual any more to think of this mechanism as regulating health function. Many of the modern innumerable and incurable degenerative diseases like cancer, arthritis, cardio complaints, allergies and opportunistic infections like AIDS, HIV positive, VDs are due to immune system failure and they are not healed because of this. Such conditions are commonly referred to as immunological disorders whose symptoms are caused by immunity process of the sufferers rather than external causes.

The interaction between illness causing factors and the immunity system is a specialised theme of naturopathy. This is what is known as auto immune disease or disorder or health condition which caused by substances that usually prevent illness. Human body has unique physical, mental, emotional, genetic, environmental, social and spiritual make up, to suit naturopathy has carefully tailored treatment strategy.

The body has self-healing power of nature through the response of the life force, which first does not harm, treat the cause and heal the whole person than suppression of symptoms of disease specific.

So, it is a wonder of very complex puzzle, the puzzle of what creates and maintains hormony and well being. What many of us are unaware of at a common level is how necessary our natural system to maintain to good health and normal living. Our present life style, dietary styles and occupational styles are some how responsible for complete loss of all or some immune functions suddenly. As a result, we are subjected to ravages of invading bacteria, viruses and other pathogens or even subjected to AIDS, cancer and arthritis.

It is everybody's health responsibility to build refill and maintain one's own immunity infact always. So, immune system's constant vigilance and response are absolutely necessary for health and wellbeing. It has a wide reaching effects on the body's state of health.

Urine–A Immunity Booster

Human urine is the only natural substance which has immune boosting potentiality to build and refill the system. All the substances required to form a complete immunity system are fully deposited in multiple quantities in auto-urine. The solution possesses all elements of minerals, proteins, nutrients, hormones, enzymes, vitamins, matabolities and host of others which together contribute to the defence system.

The presence of this system in the body that produces armed services to help fight against infections, parasites, viruses and refills internal chemical imbalances. It also activates response by releasing hormones, enzymes, etc. contained in urine.

Urinopathic medicine is a specialised field of health care system which builds natural healing power of the body. The reintroduction of one's own urine into the body enhances person's immune response and can prevent from diseases usually caused by resistance deficiency disorders.

Urine is a major internal factor or player. Auto-urine contains body generated chemicals which promotes and maintains well being. So, urinopathy typically focusses on self-healing strategy. It is a branch of bio-medical science that explores the correlation between the immunity and health. It is concerned with elucidating the links between our state of defence mechanism and our state of health.

This is the reason why urine is called as healer within, means strong presence of defence, its dysfunction or malfunction is a sign of illness. Urine drinkers will never experience these kinds of health problems because of this.

Why do urine drinkers stay healthy and others do not?

Why do drinker's immune system seems balanced?

Why do some people easily succumbed to cancer, AIDS, HIV, allergies?

Of course, these are complicated questions to answer. But reingesting urine certainly plays a direct role and therefore, health is your state of defence and strength.

How Do It Work ?

The basic premise is at the physical, mental level and express themselves. The connection between the two circulatory and the immunity are bi-directional. The brain transmits to and receives information back from the immunity system. It is the way in which state of the body influence the health.

A number of things will happen to the health when this system's responsiveness is activated. Today, poor defence mechanism has become a serious threat to the health of many people because it has come to be influenced in many events in our daily life. When the immunity is weakened it may lead to many symptoms of allergies, sinus, infections, disorders and even more serious illnesses like cancer, AIDS, arthritis, diabetes, asthama, inflammatory, bowel disease, chronic fatigue syndrome to name but a few.

The relationship between urinopathy and health offers possibility of prevention and maintenance. The nature of the therapy has provided a robust self-repair, self-refilling mechanism inside.

Between land and seed, the question is which is important. Whether land should be fertile, or seed should be qualitative? The answer is that land should be given top priority and preferecene. But modern medicine is putting all its efforts completely on the seeds means the symptoms, risk factors, probabilities, possibilities, which are external to the body rather than to identify the internal cause of the malady. The land is ignored, that is the body whose fertile system is to be strengthened like using organic chemicals.

Naturally, the farmers have to improve the ability of the land by adding organic matters, than chemical fertilisers that naturally destroys the natural potency of the land.

Likewise, human urine has many immune boosting modalities in its armamentarium. It contains rich organic substances which basically strengthen the defence system of the body by way of prevention, curing and refilling immunity.

The protein and nutrient rich urine acts medically and naturally to prepare the one's own immune system. Urine will do what it has to do. When it is taken back it may be the best tonic available for your immunity system. As a herbal and natural tonic, a medicine that makes one feel healthier and happier. Upon reingesting, it will help the body to react on specific pathological situations, reflects the individual body's functions.

It acts as natural vaccines, antibacterial, anti-viral, anti-cancer, anti-fungal, anti-carcinogenic agent as well as hormonal balancer and allergy relievers.

It is difficult to convince a majority of people that drinking ones' own urine can act as immunity booster. The reason is that modern medical science has ignored to do research to show evidence. It is a open secret among the drinkers that our own urine has enormous source of strength and life force.

The blood circulating throughout the body along with others carries critical immune defence elements like hormones, enzymes, anti-bodies plasma, etc. which are made at different locations in the body.

53

Describing About Urinopathic Medicine

It is a natural or traditional medicine(T.M). WHO gives the following definition to TM :

"It is the sum-total of knowledge, skills and practices based on theories, beliefs and experiences indigenous to different cultures, whether explicable or not used in the maintenance of health as well as in prevention, diagnosis, improvement or treatment of physical and mental illnesses".

Urinopathic medicine is generally defined as any form of a urine, the urine mixed with herbs in the form of plant, plant products including leaves, stems, flowers, roots and seeds. Urine medicine may contain a single herb or combination of several different herbs that are believed to have complementary effects. The herbs to be extracted may be in its dried or fresh form.

The use of herbs in urine, their combinations, doses, course, duration, etc., have been documented in *shivambu*. But there remains a lot of more experience, information and knowledge scattered around in some households, communities, families, tribes, drinkers and practitioners, which has potential health benefits .

Use of urine with herbs is very popular in ayurvedic medicine. The rich and long experiences and knowledge held by families, individual drinkers which constitute entire treatment regimes used by them in their daily lives. There are also secrets family held recipes passed on from generation to generation. Given the collective impact of all modern life, much of this practice in this medicine will be lost to the world with the time, unless documented early.

The urinopathic medicine is sound and safe assurance inherent which is therefore naturally of paramount importance. So, the use of urine remedies is often justified by its long history of usage from ancient times too. The age-old wisdom always guarantees the health.

Urine-based medicine is inherently different from modern allopathic drug, pharmalogical treatment.

Urinopathic medicines are defined as urine substances that are administered to patients. It includes the herbal power, liquids leaves and are mixtures of urine and urine substances and other urine constituents. The scientific evaluation of safety and efficacy of urine medicine is now well established. There are proper scientific evaluations in its favour.

It is generally regarded as safe based on their long-standing practices and use in Indian culture. However, there are no case reports of serious adverse effects after drinking urine or urine medicine. As a whole, urine has no risk of adverse effects. It is, however, absolutely safe to drink that is proved based on long human experience of drinking mid-stream urine, which is toxicity-free, contamination–free. No report exists in the literature indicating the urine contains micro organism, microbial toxins, pesticides, fumigation agents radioactivity and the presence of toxic compounds of toxic metals. Apparently, those other contaminations constituents, ingredients have not at all been harmful to the body.

Urine medicines are largely unregulated as drug, as is available at body sourcc, has an important role in primary health care all these centuries. There is a lot of scientific information which provide safety, efficacy, effectiveness and medicinal property, support. There is no inherent prejudice exists against body substance. There is a lot of experience of safety and toxicological studies.

There is any insignificant risk associated with drinking of our own urine substance. It has not resulted so far unfortunately any fatalities, side effects or harm, is considered highly healthy, nutrients, clearly there is no danger to the patients, risks which could arise from the ingestion of one's own urine.

Urinopathic treatment is a 5,000 years old system of medicine that utilises one's-own-body prepared urine doses of medicines contain various medical substances. Urine drinking is preferred, for its capacity to work at the cause of disease, and agument their defense response.

Just as vaccines and allergy treatments are in part based in this same premise, its nutrients cause immune response when regularly taken. Urinopathic medicine is a system of helping the wisdom of the body defend and self heal.

In urinopathy, each ailment is considered specific to individual, each disease has a specific physical and psychological symptoms and each patient has his or his own subtly different medicinal substances in urine specific and peculiar to individual body.

Medicinal substances of each one are slightly or overtly different from each other, is a significant feature for urinopathic treatment. In fact, this treatment tends to be easier as it is a body made patient's own medicine, individualised. This situation actually makes it easier for drinkers to treat themselves successfully.

Other features of urinopathy over conventional drug therapies are no cost, convenient and avoidance of side effects as well as reactions that can be life threatening.

Urionpathic medicine is natural system of healthcare within the scope of complementary and alternative medicine. It is a quite distinct therapy of primary healthcare, an art, science, philosopy and practice of diagnosis, treatment prevention and improving immunity system,

Urinopathic medicine is distinguished by the principle, method upon which its practice is based. Its techniques include traditional modern and scientific, empirical methods. The modalities of practice are tested in the light of scientific studies, researches and clinical investigations.

In this primary healthcare system, it uses natural methods and substances to support and stimulate the body's self-healing process. It provides a complete customotised, individualised natural forms of medicine. It is a medicine and its use is the art and science of diagnosis of aliment, treatment and prevention by using natural therapies including biology, hydrotherapy, clinical Nutrition, *yoga*, meditation, naturopathic manipulation, life style, counselling, prevention and immunity building measures, nutritional therapy.

It is primarily based on the belief that the human body has an innate self healing ability.

Urinopathic medicine in practice considers the fundamental substances of the body's excretion urine, its biochemistry in order to cure an illness, restore the balance that we describe as good health. The principle empowers the individual's body material as being responsible for the level of health he experiences.

The therapy is known for a comprehensive care because it treats the whole person. In allopathic medicine, you may prefer to consult to three or four or more different physicians for cure in a self-therapy, the system assesses the symptoms as a whole, as they are interrelated, when a root cause of the symptoms is treated all of the symptoms improve and cure.

54

Is Urine Therapy Really Essential Today?

Today, we are living on industrial medicine which is called modern medicine system or allopathic medicine for our healthcare. In modern life style, dietary style, way of life, we are totally dependent on synthetic pharmaceuticals. Today, modern medicine and doctors have taken over the health care industry in an organised way.

In starting the case of ancient nature-based system to healing, we must consider whether urinopathy is really essential to the humanity.

In other words, if allopathic medicine is really meeting the human healthcare needs in cost effective, affordable, accessible and treating incurable, innumerable diseases and in sustainable manner then we can say that urine therapy is a redundant and unnecessary.

It is true that the highly specialised techno-centric approach to medicine and treating as has evolved in the west has remarkably failed to meet the needs of growing poor sections of the society. It has become not only costly but also not within the reach of common primary healthcare needs. It is evident that the time, place, person constraints are clear in case of allopathic medicine.

The cost of medicine and healthcare are rising at alarming rates. At the same time, global market is growing steadily, the bulk of the population lack access to modern medicine.

Urine therapy as household traditional healthcare practice many are fared much better in health by relying primarily upon their own culture based knowledge and health practice systems.

Truly, it is evident that allopathic system has failed in respect of treating many modern ailments like arthritis, cancer, asthama, allergies, diabetic, etc. and could not provide preventive maintenance medicine.

In recent past, people are increasingly realised the harmful effects of pharmaceutical drugs, side effects, after effects, ill effects, reactions, mostly drugs are antibiotics, painkillers, opiates, narcotics, antacids, analgesic, destroying natural immunity system.

People of present generation have fully appreciated the potentially grave losses that could occur for future generations if they continue drugs. Patients are more inclined to focus on sustainable health and wellness than drug for disease, curing symptoms than health management.

Urine therapy is really essential even today because it gives scope of " health for all" which is a dream and goal which humanity at large wants and strives for.

Unfortunately, it has now been evident without doubt that modern pharmaceutical drugs are out of reach for a large proportion of poor human population.

Due to poor access to modern health care services, especially in rural areas, many people even today rely on urine, urinopathic medicine for their primary healthcare needs. Nevertheless, the system has not been neglected in rural areas, households, even today and its therapeutic potential have been well established. Moreover, the integration of the practice of urine therapy into the formal health system can seriously be considered. The progress made so far in this direction has proved for a wide recognition as heritage benefiting the majority of the people.

Even in district centers, cities, state capitals where modern medical facilities, services are more accessible and specialised, those who do aware of this therapy continue to drink. This may be due to the cultural acceptability as healer the respect and belief they have.

The treatment process is often carried out in an atmosphere of private and secret, mutual confidence and shared experience and knowledge.

Modern medical practice usually emphasises only on physical well-being. The socio-economic, cultural, psychological, emotional variables are ignored. Only clinical trial methodologies like parameters such as improved morbidity, mortality, reduced pain, reduced discomforts, improved appetite, weight gain, reduction of blood pressure, reduction of tumor size, maintaining reduction of blood glucose, improvement in electro-cardiogram and measurements of radiological, or image devices.

Health is not just a medical laboratory, physical evidence issue but many other issues as well influence on health. Medicine does not necessarily to mean a pure compound, and interventional material medicine.

Moreover, many dangerous and side effects have recently been reported including direct toxic effects, allergic reactions.

Health for all is a dream and goal for which today's human race is striving. Fortunately, it has now been proven without doubt that urinopathy remain within the reach for all today and for the foreseeable future.

This has created an appreciation and a need for the use of alternative traditional source of healthcare which provide and meets primary and common health benefits. So, urine therapy can effectively be utilised for disease prevention and health promotion.

Urine medicine has become a popular form of healthcare on these counts.

The system of modern medicine ignores most often social well-being of an individual. It is not intimately related to its nutritional and psychological aspects, its analysis is judged only by physiological, and biological indicators. Allopathy, on the other hand, is relatively more focussed on particular diseases on specific and etio pathological entities.

The vast majority of population not only in India, but also in many developing countries lives in rural areas where the healthcare coverage is low and the government assistance is being stretched to the limit. One of the greatest challenges facing the health sector is to recognise the essentiality of urinotherapy even today to narrow the gap between 'haves' and the population whose access to them is very limited 'have nots'.

People's reliance on this natural therapy is also reflected by the fact that migrants in different countries continuing using their own urine. Many people do not have easy and cheaper access to modern health services.

The national average physicians to population ratio is less. The physicians specialists working in government health services also poor and found only in big towns, district head quarters and state capitals.

The specialists, private practitioners also prefer to work exclusively in large towns with a aim to earn wealth, the patients could not approach them due to lack of money.

Having recognised and identified the significance of modern medicine, more recently, one can decide whether urine therapy is really essential today or not. Greater attention is to be paid by one and all to promote the awareness and widespread application of the urine therapy in health care sector. In this topic, some of the major reasons have been summarised in an attempt to provide a brief overview of relevance of urinopathy in view of innumerable and incurable diseases that human race is facing.

Moreover, an attempt is made to review the essentiality of the natural therapy today. Other main reasons were explained in different sections in the book.

55

What The Future Holds For Urinopathy?

Since ancient times, there are several hundreds of life-changing stories from the household urinopathic medical practice. In more than 50 years out of my 70 years of yogic life, urinopathic consultation, experience, advice, service no therapy has impacted more than auto-urine therapy.

It is inevitable in the days to come in the light of innumerable and incurable illnesses. This is the only therapeutic medicine that holds good as more healthcare practitioners, patients, drinkers, propagators, believers learn, adapt and promote this power medicine. No doubt about it, urinopathic therapy will become a very popular mainstream therapy.

It will soon become not as the 'last-resort' but the 'first-choice' in managing health and promoting optimal health.

The idea is that body of the patient should not be chemically poisoned the sick with toxic drugs. Indian culture takes the view of recognising the role of the Creator in making the human body who has equally assumed the responsibility to guard, maintain the good health and means to achieve. Hindus believe urine as the sacred gift from the God, the intricacies, complexity of the body functioning. There is a high appreciation of its value. It is the law of nature of the body which reorient our life. So, urine has the power of Creator.

Notwithstanding, urinopathic medicine is a healthcare practice of myriad of generations, centuries gathering knowledge, ancestry's oral transmission and continued practice as household practice guarding of its value by generations. It is a wealth of accumulated medical experiences and knowledge become as a part and parcel of their life. Besides, modern science came to the conclusion that the reexamination of urine in the quest for new therapeutic means for new diseases, has led to the remarkable conclusions. The studies brought to the light a rediscovery of various therapeutic agents deposited in urine. Many of the substances of urine are found valuable in modern health and medical science fields.

As a distinctive medical system, the urinopathy is still alive, and vital and clearly it has its own place and role to play in the days to come in the future to cure human ailments.

It offers many areas, hypotheses for further research and enable to give substantial contribution to the healthcare industry. It posses enormous potential of medical properties.

Many noteworthy examples are there where urine application has richly paid, and attained 100 per cent recovery level for even many fatal conditions.

Today, it is increasingly recognised at different cross-sections of the society the need to curb the growing dependence on synthetic pharmaceutical drugs and prefer to use traditional, natural medicines.

In India, the Water of Life Foundation is playing a vital leadership in encouraging a renewed reliance upon urinopathic medicine in primary health care. Urine is non-toxic, safe, inexpensive and culturally acceptable to the community since time immemorial.

There are many texts, records of urine therapy which is said to be effective against to cure many human ailment and usually without any side effects.

The public education and awareness represent a fundamental strategy in the strengthening community self-reliance in healthcare, by encouraging continued usage.

There has been a long and established history of its efficacy and effectiveness, no apparent adverse side effects.

Urinopathy is based on wellness and holistic, less formal, historically relied on precedencies, oral, with metaphysical base, no uniform standardisation, structure, documentation, evidence.

There is no imminent danger of losing this valuable healthcare practice. The practice of knowledge is passed on from parents to children, generation to generation, it is naturally preserved in the nature, the valuable knowledge will not be lost and is available for the benefit of future generations.

Although in recent years, we see evidences of varying degrees of interest in and support of people's practice of drinking their own urine. But evidently in Indian, to this date there is being no major official strategy, policy, funding, research for this therapy.

In day and age, there is a good reason why urinopathic medicine could not be used more fully when human race is suffering from so many incurable diseases.

Till the recent past, urine therapy was considered, very exotic, private, personal and secret practice, as being a forte of the hermits and *yogis*, monks who practised it in aloofness to attain deaging , longevity and attain spiritual attainment.

But this trend has changed dramatically in recent years with therapy coming to light and catching researchers and science, as well as western countries, gained popularity especially as a primary healthcare system. As a result, a network of urine drinkers' associations have come up. There have been known several cases of ailments being cured by this therapeutic medicine. But to make more popular, a lot of research work needs to be undertaken in this filed of medical system.

Recently, there is an increasingly growing awareness about health among the people. Many health conscious, literates, experienced, senior citizens have started reviewing the rational of allopathic medicine. This is why a system like traditional medicine is brought up and gaining more and more acceptance across the globe.

The existing lot of urine drinkers play a very important role in making the therapy wide popular. This is not surprising since urinopathy is more prevalent and popular in China, Japan, Thaiwan. Besides India, there are many countries where the therapy is being practised regularly for treatment of many disorders.

Since the causes of most of modern diseases from which people suffer, are the result of modern life styles, wrong food habits and living pattern. Here therapy of this type has the potential to set right and cure them. With the changing life style and global scenario, there have been change in almost all the streams of traditional sciences to suit changing requirements.

The fast changing face of our ancient therapy should not be buried, be worked with contempt, or as a threat to our cultural system. It should be made an integral part of today's life style.

Today, the trend has shifted as people and health fanatics have started looking to past, to preserve their health. In ancient period, this therapy was taught by *yogis* to disciples, but this role has been taken over by multinational corporations, who do started making medicine from urine, and has been as a multi billion dollar global industry.

Due to all these ressons, the face of urine therapy has also undergone a dramatic change.

56

Why The Therapy Not Popular?

The Question

If urinopathy can effectively prevent and cure many conditions, then why is it not popular? And then why is it regarded as unworthy of official recognition?

Various reasons have been put forward.

One is that urinopathic medicines are inexpensive, priceless, self-therapy is worthless, is the human psychology.

Also, patient does not require the free services except very rarely, of all or any of the expert assistants towards diagnosis, tests, imaging to whom the allopath now a days resorts.

This means that no money or less money is spent by the patient under urinopathic treatment than under allopathic treatment.

Urinopathy advocates also to use urine as preventive maintenance, preventive assurance against all such diseases which many people are reluctant to practise. Preventative is recommended for almost every imaginable type of ailment.

It is the nature of the public to go for treatment when they are facing health problem, specific disease based cure, but not prevention and maintenance.

They do not believe in prevention themselves, becoming drug addicts.

But so much the lay public have been influenced by prevailing fads and fasions that there is no priceless, natural, self-cure healthcare system. Many ignorant members believe to approach a physician, any path, pay and get their money's worth prescription drugs, pills, drinks of poisonous nature. Certain class of patients believe in swallowing pretty pills, drink liquids given in multi coloured bottles by the doctors with dramatised diagnosis.

Non availability of case-wise, disease-wise, successful recovery stories, treatment evidence based records.

That there is no formal recognition by the government or other competent authorities, which is a common practice, tradition and formal of many other health care professions such as allopathy, homeopathy, naturopathy, etc.

A group of drinkers, practitioners or urinopath or as urinopathic physicians or doctors as may be called are not publicly visible at all places to practise, educate, promote the knowledge of this healthcare system.

It suffers from want of some legal, and or regulatory protection and recognition. There is no regulatory co-ordination authority to regulate this practice.

The entire modern medical industry composed of druggists, doctors, pharmaceutical companies pretty are well aware of therapeutic value of urine for centuries, decades and years. But the unsatisfactory state of affair is that the public have ever been informed and educated about it. May be, because it has become highly controversial. It is not knowing something value that exists and is important, being made interested. An awareness of the importance of drinking a healthy liquid, there is an almost complete lack of awareness of this issue involved.

Special studies, research findings, clinical investigation results all are not evidently available, and the concerned people know about the astounding efficacy of natural healing power of life force.

Auto-urine therapy is so divided and the people are misinformed, that the problem seems to be even worse.

Urine therapy if it becomes popular, it adversely affects the livelihood of doctors who are living on prescribing modern medicine, and suppressing symptoms quickly rather than cure illness.

Drug manufacturing companies have to close down their factories, if there is no demand for medicine. Hence they don't want to popularise urine therapy.

Why? May be due to some known reasons:

1. Many are shocked to listen about a waste as a medicine, and hence disapproved.
2. I think people are really not aware of just how much medicinal value is hidden in it? Every body should be made to realise the therapeutic benefits involved.
3. There is no financial, or the amount of money offered for helping and telling public.
4. People have ample money, have much purchasing power try to avoid unpleasant drinking, is the nature of present thinking.
5. It is a open secret and understanding among the concerned people of modern medicine and other traditional and complementary medicine to do something harmful to this therapy. A conspiracy to over throw this therapy, a conspiracy in silence. People are not taking publicly about this natural drug and want to remain secret.
6. Though the medical industry and its allied branches has been well aware of wonderful efficacy of urine for centuries, but none of us have ever been informed about it.
7. An ailment which cannot be treated by urine no other therapy else can cure.

8. The members of the public or patients are not able to approach a urine clinic, nor demanding urine treatment advice from a urinopath, because they are ignorant, innocent of the existence of such treatment nor such clinics visible in the market.
9. The doctors are virtually conservative and soft pedaling, safe sailing not to take risk by experimenting with urine. Urine therapy is a biochemistry therapy is a newer and better system of medication.
10. Many cancer patients have died while surgeons and physicians are preoccupied with modern medicine only, while urine therapy on the other side saving the life of the patients. "Is the patient for the welfare of the doctors?" They are in favour of dangerous drugs, knifes only like chemotherapy, radium, operation, still no life guarantee.
11. Heal yourself with your urine? Patients are deprived of incredible urine medicine.The modern medical science has been severely criticising that it is useless and poisonous, though they well knew the medicinal properties of urine.
12. Traditional cultures, customs, have deep rooted feelings, idea, thinking for a long time and discouraged it to be used for medical purpose. A kind of disgust towards urine is deposited, hammered in our minds.
13. The medical profession, doctors, journals and books are speaking loudly about medicinal qualities which the public at large do not read. But in practice they are neither recommending, nor creating awareness. They are not disclosing the real facts to the general public. Tight-mouthed, closed lip.
14. They favour allopathy and allopathical practices only, urine therapy they consider unworthy of practice, and regard it as quackery. Modern medical professionals consider themselves and behaving themselves as that they are more important and intelligent than others. They are making pure imaginary, theoretical argument against urine therapy before ignorant people. Again they are not able to provide information, or evidence to prove that the therapy is useless. They do not consider it seriously, and substantiating their theoretical opinion.
15. Besides, there is no monetary returns for recommending people what the science knows about the medicinal secrets of healing properties of the urine.
16. Lack of publicity and awareness, mass practice is the fact that many people think urine is not drinkable, toxic and a waste product, body excrete.
17. Another reason is that urine is excertion from the sexual organ.
18. Though there are hundreds of scientific findings, research discoveries, clinical results on urine therapy which have not been brought to the public notice.

19. As a matter of fact, it is a free service, and financially not rewarding, people do not show much interest.
20. For medical practitioners, urine therapy has been too controversial, as they have not studied much in their education, as it is not included in their syllabus.

In the light of the above issues raised in connection with biomedical research model to assess the whole system of holistic healthcare field of urinopathic medicine, the following inferences may follow:

1. There is lack of wide research on practice in this field.
2. The present medical research institutions carry research widely in allopathic medicine only.
3. The research infrastructure in this field is still poor and new.
4. The sources of funding should be made available.
5. This medicine is not able to secure research moneys as that of allopathic institutions.
6. However, the organisations like WHO, medical councils, yogic institutions, health ministries must take interest in this fields.

Research in this field must attend on urinopathic medicine.

57
Exceptions

This therapy though has many distinct features, advantages and sure-cure of many hundreds of cases of large variety of diseases, even incurable one, it does not mean that it is without exceptions. Like other therapies both of orthodox and unorthodox, which too have exceptions, urine therapy, too. Though it is categorised as holistic medicine, it does not mean it will cure every disease of every patient. The law of exception applies to urine therapy also. With very few exceptions, urine gives the best curing results. In bulk of cases of various complaints, urine has cured well, except in exceptional cases.

Urinoapthy is not a fail safe healthcare system for each and every type of acute, chronic, degenerative, opportunistic infections, injuries, fatal and other diseases affliciting human race. A panacea means all humanly possible like any other systems of therapies, pathies or medicine which also cannot cure all diseases. Even the allopathic medicine, homeopathy or naturopathy or any other health care system which have been worked successfully for a particular disorder, may not prove equally efficacious to all diseases to all patients suffering from the same condition.

Recurring diseases, multi-drug resistant infections no medicine proves equally effective all times, to all patients. It does not mean that it never makes failure. The therapy is not infallible. A therapeutic medicine that never fail, such a statement is very extreme or impressive only but not reasonable or practical. It is like giving or writing a wrong idea or impression and making the public believe the therapy that is not true. It is not even scientific to give such an opinion.

As a matter of fact, there are some misleading statements about it on auto-urine therapy, probably this is the reason why public tend to mistrust or lose of confidence in urinopathy.

If the immunity system or hormonal balance, or resistance power of the body have been totally destroyed and so beyond restoration, rejuvenation, it is not possible that urniopathy would prove useful.

The following are the exceptions to the application of urinopathy:

1. Trauma,
2. Karmic conditions,
3. Last stage diseases,

4. Therapy not followed as strict procedure,
5. Pregnant women half-way through facing discomforts like pains, vomiting, etc.,
6. Death bed patient,
7. Hypertension, stress, depression,
8. High blood pressure,
9. Structural damage of the body in cases like accidents, etc.,
10. Grave kidney disorders,
11. Extreme diabetes,
12. Diseases of impossibilitics.

58

Urine–the Medicine for Physical Immortality

What is Physical Immortality

Human beings are mortal. According to the principle of creation, order of the cosmos, it is the universal law. The word mortal is derived from 'mortem' which means death. Mortal is one who has death. Mortal means that the physical body must die after limited existence, which can not live forever, no permanency and eternity. The principle of mortality of the law of cosmos drives them towards death, Thus man's corporeal existence is subject to mortality.

Within the lifetime destiny, of whatever may be the life period, during the time of existence a person must live without disease, decay, figure change with longevity, without premature death or death by disease. Healthy and happy and physically, mentally and spiritually strong existence with good health and normal living is called physical immortality.

The Creator has introduced a revolutionary concept of physical immortality by way of drinking the nectar of body-made liquid, an elixir, that will guarantee physical immortality to human physical body. The body-made liquid as designed by the creative orgin is auto urine which has capability of destroying senility, diseases, disorders and illness of any kind.

One's own urine is the annihilator of senility and disease, stimulates and energies the senses, one acquires divine vision, and freedom from all diseases, extraordinary strength, purification, detoxifies all the organs of the body, conquers deageing, longevity frees from the cycle of birth and death, realise inner-self, acquires happiness, frees from all disorders, makes one physically, mentally exceptionally strong, acquires divine radiance, escapes from the ravages of time, frees from all ailments.

It conquers unnatural death, acquires a merry life, lightness of the body, eliminates the possibility of senile, degeneration, possesses divine attributes, nourishes the body, far sighting, pleasing, attractive, intuition power, will power, desired attainments, frees from ageing and death, conquers lust, makes master of one's desires, peace, cheerful frame of mind, becomes omniscient, pure memory, one can expound all branches of scriptures as one acquires immesurable mental power, etc.

A urine drinker acquires all these rare qualities that make a personal body as physically immortal.

This gives a new life wave principle in the history of human evolution. The main theme of urine therapy is to give physical immortality, giving a healthy endless physical structure, endless life, destined permanence and finally bliss and eternity. It means not to subject to physical mortality, living healthly during life span during that time that physical is not subject to mortality.

Practice makes a man perfect, is an old axiom. Urine drinking is a faith and practice to become complete and perfect, then only the concept of physical immortality becomes a reality as designed by the Origin Himself.

Direct upkeep is a process and principle by which all the parts, components, organs, centres, joints, particles, tissues, cells, endocrines, hormones, immunity system, elimination of the body system are pervaded and occupied, then the diseases, dirorders, decay of the body are arrested and the physical body is kept physically immortal and eternal.

Multiples of ample quantities of medicinal substances deposited in urine readily available are rich source of vigour, vitality and life force to the body which greatly help to achieve physical immortality. By the order of creation, all the experiences of spirit are realised to conquer mortality. So, the physical system is to be rectified, adjusted, remoulded in such a way as to receive the experiences of pure spirit involved in it.

The new life wave principle, or the new life wave activity as introduced by the subtle life force will create a new physical structure of its own required for physical immortality in the very nature of our nervous system.

With this dedicated long amaroli practice and yogic power, many yogis have attained and enjoyed the fruits of physical immortality, highest wisdom, unparalleled mystic powers, supernatural vision, will power, intuition without physical disease, decay and death. They enquired by practice and revealed to us the secrets of evolutionary order to unearth the hidden reasons for absence of physical immortality to the manform physical.

Many people do not know the need to establish a link and contact with the healer inside the physical system even since the evolution started. The secrets of remedial measures to relieve humanity from the cycle of death, diseases, decay, miseries and cosmic troubles are available well written in ancient texts.

It is everybody's desire to attain the immortal body to lead a happy life which is not possible without a contact with body made substances. This is the creative order of the cosmos, to liberate humanity from diseases, decay, death, miseries, troubles, and to establish the desire of physical immortality.

The underlying theme of *shivambu*, as designed by the God Shiva, is that it has revealed the new life force principle for the first time in the history of human evolution for achieving physical immortalty.

So, the physical body is to be made first fit to receive new life force from urine to form new physical structure for physical immortality.

The speed, pressure, and stress bearing capacity of the present physical system of the man-form body is very weak, and limited and hence prone to illness, disorders, diseases, decay and premature death. Accordingly, the original weak form of physical body is to be made strong by additional body-made life force.

Continuous remoulding of physical body is to be carried on, so that old body made with changing cosmic material will slowly be thrown out of the body and filled with new life forces. This leads to the character of disease-free, deathless state of immortality.

Thus, the making of healer inside, the inner is something like that of the egg stuff growing inside the shell. So also, the inner life force has to make outer physical immortal.

The *shivambu* develops the physical body to such a state to resist decaying and to be giving vital energy to our physical system. So, many cells, tissues, parts, organs, so many valves, so many fittings, centres, joints, glands are to be rectified, adjusted, remoulded, immunity system to be refilled, protected and guarded to achieve this immortality. The work is assumed by the human urine.

It is the aim of the urine drinking to protect our physical frame from decay and disease. Such an important work has been given to the urine by the Creator according to the revelations discoursed to Goddess Parvathi by Lord Shiva about *shivambu*.

For the establishment of physical immortality, new life forces are to be given to the physical. The mortal physical is the most important of all the bodies to turn it to physical immortality.

The present man form physical system has only the limited life force and became mortal. But it should be made to fill with unlimited supply of life force to be immortal physically. The human urine has that unlimited supply of life force, to stand to be without disease, decay and death.

This emphasises the importance of an integration body-mind-spirit medicine, so that the physical state remains immortal and independent of want.

The eternal happiness, i.e., *Brahmanandam* or ecstatic delight can be experienced only with physical immortality. Therefore, the principle of establishment of physical immortality is the core theme of spirit dimension of meditation and *yoga*.

Physical state means not the physical structure composed of flesh, blood, bones, nerves, veins, arteries etc.

The physical body is the etheric matrix, the body of *pranic* energies which helps itself unchanged for a life. This is the real immortal physical body.

Everyone wants to maintain the body intact and live for long, but how and what is the mean to achieve is the critical issue. The goal of evolution is physical immortality and to banish death, disease, decay due to old age.

The reasons for the debility of the physical body is the accumulation of foreign matters, poisonous materials, adulteration in the body, lack of detoxification and weak elimination process which create problems, hurdles and troubles to attain immortality. The urinopathy has designed a mechanism as to how to perfect, and purify human form physical, and to convert to unchanged timelessness and immutability with subtle lifeforce.

The mortal body must be transformed into immortality by the entry of supreme energy of superior, and finer quality of spirit into the human body. This is the secret of physical immortality to be established. Otherwise this great concept would be only an abstract, illusion, fiction, a notion and not a fact.

The conception of this idea cannot be possible without practising our ancient healthcare measures like urine drinking, *yoga,* etc. to convert mortal bodies as immortal bodies.

The *shivambu* practice promised physical immortality and eternity. This should be known by everyone by practice and experience.

When once immortality is established–birth, death, disease, decay will not affect such bodies. This could be attained by sustained belief, strong faith and regular practice.

Your physical immortality denotes a life of changelessness, timelessness, devoid of sorrow, misery, cosmic troubles, diseases, decay that itself is a merry life in reality.

Cleansing process of the body should be done by you to clean yourself.

59

Body Mind Spirit Medicine

Today, it is a new age talk, and the interaction of the body and the mind is the neomedical science. There is direct correlation between mind and body, mental related health problems.

A balance between them is non-controversial. Eventhough doctors have rejected the idea, research points out a circuit linking between mind and health. The behavioural and psychological events can equally influence health.

In true sense, mind makes one physically sick. Besides, many of the changes over time in thinking, understanding, feeling, mood and their impact on body are drastic, of which we are unaware. There is a clear communication path between mind and physical parts of the body.

Body-Mind-spirit-medicine focusses on the interaction among the physical body, mind and spirit. They are powerful ways in which they can together directly affect health. It regards it as fundamental approach that respects and enhances each person's ability for self knowledge, self-responsibility and self-care.

The trinity of this approach emphasises the techniques that are around this approach. These three dimensions focus on human intervention strategies that are considered to promote health and wellness. It includes relaxation, herbal medicine, Yoga, meditation, spirituality, prayers and behaviourial therapies.

This system of healthcare views an illness as an opportunity for personal growth and transformation.

The therapist of body mind spirit medicine are the healthcare providers, acting as catalysts and guides in this process of healthcare.

Health dimension can be analysed, studied and practised in three dimensions Body, Mind and Spirit.

Health as : Physical dimension,
Mental dimension,
Spiritual dimension.

Urine-therapy is only the medicine that offers true synchronisation among body, mind and spirit.

In other practices, often these three elements are kept separately, dealt separately and practised separately.

The modern medicine is mainly concerned with physical body and the other two are left out. These days for complete health, the body-mind-spirit connection is well recognised, as in ancient days the *yogis* and *rishies* did to practise these three elements.

In allopathy, the spirit is still left out and only material things, chemical aspects of the body are considered.

Naturopahy, an ancient traditional healthcare system, considers all these three elements for good health and normal living.

Body : *'Hatha' yoga* system is meant to keep the body healthy and practise physical fitness.

Mind : A meditation practice brings, calm, peace, stillness to be free from ills of stress, strain, tension, irritation, conflicts, mental abennation and frustration.

Spirit : One should not therefore ignore the soul inside the body, which should be realised.

In the modern days, man is mentally tired, physically exhausted, does not find time to think about what he is, who he is, feels frustrated, unable to realise himself.

These are the causes of stress and strain which cause cardio-vascular ailments.

We see that today the whole world is increasingly realising the potentiality of these three dimentions in health care system. Many scientific research studies are undertaken in many countries on the inter-relation of mind-body-spirit in health.

Many countries are looking at India for our traditional medicinal pratices to provide inspiration and enthusiasm. *Yoga* and meditation systems for health are receiving very good response because they provide prevention, cure, promotion and maintenance of health and wellness.

The systems of mental health practices increase intake of oxygen, improve the metabolism and expulsion of carbon-dioxide. Accordingly, the immunity system, nervous system, hormonal system, circulatory system, lymphatic system, brain colonies are tuned up for optimal level of health.

Thus, the body-mind-spirit culturing provides good physical health, mental health, which together help in self-realisation.

These three factors connect the immune system which is the hottest area of special study now a days. It is a complex puzzle, the puzzle of that creates and maintains man's well being.

The word physical refers to the body. It is often used with reference to various bodily features such as physical strength, physical appearance, physical parts, organs, physical development and changes.

As a whole, it constitutes a system which is a set of things working together as parts of a mechanism. It is parts forming a complex whole, has an inter-connecting and inter related network.

The human body is a system made up of different sub-systems to constitute a body. The are :

1. Skeleton : The structure of bones that supports the body of a person. The human skelton consists of 206 bones.
2. Muscular : Connected with muscles, having large strong muscles. Musculature is the system of muscles in the body or parts of the body.
3. Respiratory : The act of breathing, blood pressure and respiration, respiratory track are physical systems subjected to diseases.
4. Circulation : It is relating to the circulation, there also two systems, blood circulation and lympatic system.
5. Digestion : One of the physical systems of the body that changes the consumed food stuffs into substances that body uses.
6. Urinary : A part of the body connected with urine or the parts of the body through which it passes.
7. Genital : Organs of the body connected with reproduction, outer organs of a person.
8. Nervous : The system of all nerves in the body, deals with brain, spinal card and the structure.
9. Endocrines : Connecting with glands and their functions.

All these and others form a part of the whole complex body, which is called physical body.

Accordingly, the modern medicine is primarily based on the principle that all human diseases are caused generally by infections, parasites and internally by chemical imbalance. Based on this philosophy, allopathy makes drugs with physical material and chemicals to suppress the symptoms of the diseases or disordes rather than eradicating the cause of the malady.

Mind

Mind is a part of the body, is invisible, something that cannot be seen, and intangible and exists in everybody but that is difficult to describe, understand or even measure. It exists as a physical thing but is still that we cannot touch or feel, not seen anywhere in the body like any other body organ. There is no separate place or location like any other anatomical part of the body and as a matter of fact it does not require any space for its existence.

The great size and importance of this part of the body, degree to which it is large or important is immesurable with any yard stick. It possesses the great quality of subtlety. It is made up of matter of quality not very noticeable of various grades of density with different rates of vibrations.

It is nothing but a power of spirit over soul. Many people even highly literates do not know the nature of very existence of mind and its functions.

In other words, it is known as '*atma sakthi*' the power of soul realised by *yogis* and *rishies* with rigorous practice of meditation and introspection and its nature, ways, dimensions and subtle workings.

It is a part of the person, a part of the physical body, inside the body that makes him able to be aware of things. To think and to feel are the functions of the body, and all kinds of thoughts are running through the mind.

Drugs are associated in most people's minds with drug abuse. A person's ability to think and reason depends upon the health of mind, It is the work of mind.

A person's ability to remember things is based on mind's maturity. The way a person feels or thinks about something at a particular time indicates this frame of mind.

Mind and Brain

On the other hand, a brain is the organ inside the head that controls movements, thoughts, memory power and feelings. It possesses cells known as brain cells.

Like other physical organs, brain is also subject to diseases or disorders. A temporary or permanent damage to the brain may be caused by illnesse or accident. It is called brain damage, brain tumour. A person may die of brain tumour.

Memory

It is your ability to remember things, the period of time that you are able to remember events, things, etc.

The types of memory:

1. Short memory,
2. Long Memory,
3. Limited Memory,
4. Pure Memory,
5. Trick Memory.

Pure memory is relating to knowledge of your past and future births rather than increasing knowledge or using knowledge.

Intelligence

An advanced level or a mind of a person is termed as intelligence. It indicates the ability to learn, understand and think in a logical way about things. Intelligence quotient is a test that measures how well a person is able to understand and think a logical way about things.

It is of three types :

1. Higher intelligence, 2. Lower intelligence,
3. Average intelligence.

Artificial intelligence is an area of study concerned with making computers copy intelligent human behaviour.

A wrong functioning of the mind may cause much injury to the body. Similarly, a bodily disease can also affect the mind. So, the mind and body are not separate entities. They are one and the same.

During this century, particularly during the last few years, it has been increasingly recognised in understanding their intimate relationship with each other and their influence on our well-being. They are together incorporated into the very structure of our physical.

Modern medicine, based on evidence and science material does not mean to ignore and discard their relations but it is our ultimate natural duty to understand and relate them for better understanding of human health care.

Role of Mind and Health

The mind of the patient should not be ignored in the treatment. It plays a pivotal role in the administration of drugs. Nearly all drug trials are scientifically invalid due to influece of the mind. It is the mind of the patient which actually determines the effectiveness of the pain or the drugs, but not exactly the chemical effect of the drug itself.

"It is phenomenal it is really cool. It is one of the best analgesics we have and the brain's influence can either vastly increase its effect or completely remove it" (Professor Irene Tracey, Oxford University).

The mind is the main determiner of the effectiveness of many drugs, not the chemical profile of the drugs themselves. This has been proven out again and again not just with painkiller drugs, but also with anti depressant drugs which have consistently failed to out perform placebo. It is the mind that makes them real.

The effect of the mind on the drug as well as its working cannot be ignored. The expectations of the patients on the drug and its results are in the minds of the patients. It is the mind that makes the drug work.

The drug effect and mind effect go together and they cannot be separated. The mind of the patient is a necessary variable in the outcoming drug results, The various psychological effects of the patients influence the genuine chemical action of the drug.

Mind definitely plays an active role in the physiology of the body.

It is not a correct opinion that the chemical imbalance of the body alone would decide the health of a person, and mind has nothing to do with it. Any medical system dealing with healthcare, with such an approach is a wrong direction.

The mind has equal role to do with health. In fact, scientific studies have also revealed that the mind can make a placebo 'real' and render a drug useless.

The mind factor as a variable has influence over the results of the substance of the drug. The modern science in the name of science, has almost never taken mind into consideration. If the mind and its control over other variables is ignored, technically speaking it is scientifically invalid.

Truly, there is no way to know exactly the rate of mind as the rate of drug. The cure can never be due to the drug effect alone.

The drug making companies should not ignore the power of the mind of the patients while designing their drugs to work because the expectations of results are in the minds of the patients. The mind has over all control of the body, a great censor and hence drugs cannot work in their own way in the human body, regardless of chemistry of a drug.

Modern medical science believes only in material evidence, chemical characters, chemical imbalance as reason for diseases and use chemical based drugs for treatment ignoring key variables like the mind and spirit.

As a matter of fact allopathy totally ignores the very existence of mind in human body and its influence on physiological functions. Allopathic physicians, having doubts that claim or existence of a mind is true, do not believe that there is such a thing as the mind.

They believe that human bodies are like biological machines that can do some tasks that the humans can do and that works automatically based on the principles of chemistry and physics and while the brain is a mere molecular robotic machine that functions out determining action purely based on above principles.

The mind, they understand, does not exist. There is no mind at all.

There is no wonder that the drugs are made without taking the mind into account. Hence, their drugs are not holistic, real cure, but only suppressive, harmful to the body, and by now are proved as medical self-delusion. It is a false belief or opinion about modern medicine as the only scientific one, with a belief that it is more important than it is in reality.

It is unscientific to think that their drug alone is the mainstream and there is no alternative in the healthcare industry as scientifically accepted and thus they ignored the mind of the people that delivered the results.

It is a false notion that durg is the only remedy scientifically validated. It is the mind which has everything whatsoever to do with drug results.

So, the young allopathy pharmaceuticals are trying to defy the existence of the mind. That is why medical education also does not show interest in the power of the mind. Even medical syllabus also shows partiality in giving priority to body-mind-spirit medicine.

The human mind is so powerful, that it can exercise its powers to examine a drug, and makes the substances ineffective which are considered dangerous to the body, and sometimes renders a drug obsolete.

The allopathic physicians should truly understand the nature of mind, harness the power of the mind and utilise the natural self-healing power of the body, and avoid precribed drugs. They need to act as a teacher and educate the patients that they have the power within themself to heal and the chemical drugs have only the effect of substitute and are suppressive of symptoms rather than curative of the root cause of the disease. This is long by tradition culturally accepted medical knowledge.

The modern medicine proves that the existence of mind is wrong, it is not true. It denies its influence on the body. All diseases are materially generated : bacteria, parasites or chemical imbalances. As a result any healing measure must come from intervention, external application either by chemicals, surgery or radiation. The same is included in syllabus and taught in medical colleges.

It is the duty of the doctor to teach health management, self-responsibility, maintainance of wellness and how to heal themselves without drugs. It is dangerous chemical intervention to the natural body. There must be a revolutionary change in the belief of the people that external drug is harmful to the body. This is the real treatment.

Spirit

The thought of spirit which is quite separate from the body is believed to live on after death. Though a person dies, his spirit lives on. It is the spiritual part of a person believed to exist after death which is also called soul.

Body is mortal, while spirit is immortal. Spiritual, moral, meditation qualities are the other side of the human soul.

The soul lives on and lasts for ever. The soul is immortal. It is the part of a person that includes their mind, feelings, spiritual value and character rather than the body. It is connected with the human spirit, rather than the body or physical things or mind alone.

It is the holy spirit which means God in the form of a spirit in human body. It is the bondage between the Creator and the man. Having gone so deeply into the Trinity of the life, we are now, at the last passage of moving into the re-connection of these three elements. At this time, the neglect of our inner body is spirit. No one understands any more what the landscape, and the language of the spirit is.

Human beings are embedded in the world of spirit. Every physical body carries cosmic element that has come from the eternal bodies. Human bodies are the living expression of spirit, but many do not know this.

Spiriual field and activity is a very slow and orduous practice of attunement of self realisation. This is a practice of whole life time, and many life times. It is to be achieved by spiritual ambition, dedication, belief and practice.

Body Spirit

It is self responsibility of every individual to keep not only bodily health but also soul. You have to keep body and soul together to stay alive with just enough of food, clothing, etc. that you need to survive.

Spirituality

It is the quality of being connected with religion or human spirit, a search for spirit or soul. A spirituality is different from religion in many ways. The former provides an insight-into the nature of consciousness. It is free from religion and prejudices. Spirituality explains the concepts, and laws of metaphysics and offers code of conduct, and practices which mould character and give an ethical base to life.

The principles are universal for entire humanity. The practice of spiritual meditation makes life free from tension, awards peace and tranquility. It has a universal appeal, values, and fully developed and accepted ethical code, covering human love, kindness, purity, non-violence, tolerance, etc.

The spiritual consciousness gives the experience of peace, freedom and eternity. Every person has a spiritual centre which is the real master of one's personalities. The ultimate aim of spiritual life is freedom from this bondage for achieving eternity.

It teaches about the physical world and the spiritual reality. It integrates science, religion and philosophy. The spiritual life gives meaning and purpose to life and solace to the suffering humanity also. It synthesises various branches of human knowledge such as science, ethics, philosophy and social sciences.

Inspiring and uniting mankind to a higher level of consciousness, transcendental reality is greatly emphasised in spiritual approach.

Fortunately, this attitude is changing rapidly and radically with the new understanding of the secrets of creation of the body by God. Besides, some new scientific research studies, findings, investigations that are made in the field of psycho, neuro, hormonal, immune systems, the mapping of the brain and their relationship on study with different parts of the body, and how they affect health.

A body is not just a material chemical structure. It is a interconnected system, not separate from mind, brain, thought process, emotions, sound and all are integral parts of the body.

But the modern medicine is not accepting the role of spirit in the name of science and evidence. A spirit is a vehicle of consciousness, the vital matrix.

The environment of the planet, and the cosmos beyond cannot be ignored, and the role of the Creator cannot be neglected. As a matter of fact, the physical body, and other integral parts of the body like mind, brain, spirit are not made according to science, nor working according to modern scientific principle. The sciene is just studying and understanding the fundamentals of the complicated and complex structure and its functions only.

Therefore, the science cannot separate and ignore the part played by soul in the promotion of health of an individual. The body is the outward manifestation of the soul only.

In this topic and the other related ones, where we will be looking at the physical end of the mind, brain, spirit spectrum. So, try to hold in your awareness the wider spectrum of spirit linking to our body existence.

Also, try to understand the basic structure of the body, mind, spirit organism in a larger dimension and in non-physical, chemical, material dimension, the whole organism of the planet and the web of life or organism of the cosmos.

The physical structure of life has one vast tangible and intangible system of relationship and their close connections and inter connection, links and circuits.

We are not thinking of brain, mind and endocrinal systems as they offer us a new way of under standing to control the whole system and as a way of knowing our healthcare better than we do at present. An understanding of this dimension gives us greater insights into the inter connectedness of spirit, mind and body and of feeling, thinking and sensory experience. This greatly helps us to understand our profound interrelationship with each other as well as with our environment and cosmos.

The *yogis, rishies* of those days of cultures experienced life as an invisible and indivisible web of relationship among mind-body-spirit. They felt that they are equally important parts of the life of web and part of this creation.

The spirit as I believe an inevitable corollary of the other. Today, many people are inreasingly recognising, to recollect and to recover traditions that we lost, to revalue these aspects of life. In self-responsibility of healthcare, one has to reconnect nature, spirit, mind and body and bring together as an integral part of holistic health. Many neo-classical people are today at the forefront of this approach, for good health and normal living.

The heart of medical science is mind. In its essence, modern science has very little to do with it. All the qualities have come to be associated with modern medicine in its material, physical, chemical and evidence form. In synthetic drug world, we live in a culture with too much value on pharmaceutical drugs. The allopathy at its most exalted state is of chemical characters, material and physical endeavour.

It is this inner mind, spirit that the scientists must understand, and also surrender to them finally. I have come to believe that disease or disorder is at their very core, a mental route. To me, it means that we must pay more attention to what mind, brain, spirit and what they connect us to, than we at present are separated from them.

These three different interrelated subsystems of the body effect not only our physical health and well being, but also our mental and emotional health and well being.

We have to go back and look at how the age-old *yogi's* habits, life styles of the older brain, and mental system that influenced their well-being and understanding the interaction between this older mental system and the present mental, brain and immune system one helps us to understand in terms of mental health and physical health. The brain, mind, brain chemistry, hormones are so powerful, that they have positive, negative effects on our lives. One has to take a great deal of insight and attention to become aware of these aspects. It is of great help to bear in mind the interconnectedness of the body, mind and spirit.

Psycho-Neuro-Immunology

Mind-body-spirit medicine is also referred to as psycho-neuro-immunology (PNI) in medical science.

The term consists three areas such as :

P = Psycho, means emotions of a body, thinking process and mood flying of an individual.

It is connected with the mind. A psycho person is one who is mentally ill and who behaves in a very strange violent way. The way in which a person is feeling at a particular time. A person may be in:

Good mood,	Happy and friendly,
Bad mood,	Unhappy, angry, impatient,
Mood swing,	Changes of mood,
No mood,	Politeness.

N–Refers to neurological system, such as reflex system and neuro endocrine system. It is connected to the nerves. Neuron is a nerve cell that carries information between the brain and other parts of the body. Some people suffer from neurosis which is a mental illness where a patient suffers from strong feelings of fear and worry.

I = Immunology : It is a branch of medical science which deals with the scientific study of protection against disease, disorders.

It deals with the immune system.

So, the term PNI emphasises the role of mind over the body effect. The thought process and the mind together greatly influence the individual's immunity system. The attitude of the mind plays a direct positive role in the day today health and normal living.

There is always a clear communication pathways between the brain and the immunity system. Even psyhologist established the existence of a link between the immunity system and the central nervous system.

So, the relationshp is termed as psycho-neuro-immunology or PNI. The term acknowledges psyche or the mind, neuro for the neuro-endocrine system, and immunology for the immunity system.

Anger, anxiety, depression, stress, strain are related to emotions which are responsible for most of today's degenerative diseaes or disordrs like those of cardio-vascular origin, cancer, arthrities, immune system failure and less serious one like spondylitis, acne, psoriasis etc.

Thus today, PNI is a specialised field of research that studies the interactions between :

Behaviour,

Brain, and

Immune system of the body.

Today the Mind-Body-Medicine is referred to as PNI which focusses its attention on the interaction of brain, mind, body and behaviour.

They are powerful ways in which emotional, mental social, spiritual and behavioural factors can directly influence health. PNI regards as fundamental the approach that respects and enhances each person's capacity for self-knowledge and self-care of one's own health.

This new approach of mind-body-medicine typically focusses on the interventional strategies which are designed to promote health. The strategies include relaxation, *yoga*, meditation, spirituality, prayer, ayurveda, urine therapy and other naturopathic and alternative medicine. The principle and philosophy of mind-body-medicine views diseases, disorders as an opportunity for personal growth and transformation.

These therapies influence broad energy fields that cannot be measured.

60

Mental Illness and Physical Disorders

Mind has a processing function of thinking, connected with or happening in the mind. For instance, the mental process of remembering. A person is said to be mentally ill, when he feels difficulty in understanding or remembering and he is in complete mental block.

In medical science, it is connected with the state of health of the mind or with the treatment of illness of the mind. A Mental disorder or illness is a symptom of suffering from physical and mental exhaustion.

A mind has an age dimension called mental age. It is the level of a person's ability to think, understand and remember, judged by comparison with the average ability for children of particular age.

To illustrate, a person of 60 years is with a mental age of 25 years.

Psycho Disorders

Though mind is not physical organ of the body it is subjected to illness, disorders, diseases known as psyche conditions or unpleasantness : the mind and its deepest feeling and attitudes.

The unhealthy condition of the mind is called mental illness, technically referred to as psychiatric disorders. Today, speciality hospitals both at individual, and corporate level have emerged to attend to these special types of mental illnesses and are branded as psychiatric hospitals.

Accordingly, specialists also have come up to capture this dimension of health care industry. They are popularly designated as psychiatrists, doctors who study and give treatment to mental illnesses.

Psychos

A person who is mentally ill and who behaves in a very strange violent way is known psycho.

Psychoanalysis

There is a technique of psychoanalysis, a method of treating psychos who are mentally ill by asking them to talk about past experiences and feelings in order to find solution to their present problem. A specialist who treats patients using psychoanalysis is designated as psychoanalyst.

Psychodrama

It is a method of treating mentally ill people by encouraging them to experience the events of their past in order to help them understand their feelings.

Psychological Disorders

Ills connected with a person's mind and the way in which it works, sometimes may lead to both psychological and emotional problems. Symptoms of disorders are more psychological than physical symptoms.

There are clinical psychologists who treat patients with mental disorders or conditions. The science of psychology deals with a scientific study of mind and how it influences the behavior of a person.

Psychometric

The existing psychometric technique is also used in case of some patients to measure mental abilities and processes called psychometric testing. Psychopath is a serious mental illness, that some people may suffer from, which makes them behave in a violent manner towards others. It is a psychopathic disorder or killer.

Psychosis

A variant form of mental illness is psychosis which is also a serious mental illness that affects the whole personality.

Psychosomatic

On the other hand, a psychotic patient is one who suffers from several mental illness. Psychomatic disorders are connected with the relationship between the mind and the body. It is an illness caused by mental problem such as stress and worry rather than physical problems.

Psychotherapy

It is a method of treatment of mental illness by discussing patient's problem with them rather than by giving them drug.

Mental Illness and Physical Disorders

Mental illness, disorder or imbalance is often a risk factor in the development of many physical and mental diseases, disorders which require mind management to deal with problems rather than administering drugs. They are called mentally related illnesses.

For instance :

1. Depression

Depression is a situation that makes one feel sad, hopeless and deeply distressed and disheartened. It may be a depressing sight, thought or experience of loss, troubl, difficulty or sorrow.

It is a medical condition in which a person feels very sad and anxious and often has physical symptoms such as sleep disorders like half sleep, disturbed sleep or no sleep.

A person may suffer from severe depression after loss of job, death of father, mother, wife, poor economic condition, lack of bright future, etc.

In modern life style, depression is one of the common emotion problems throughout the world.

When a person is depressed, it affects the brain's delicate chemistry. The neuron help to send messages between new cells in the brain and regulate mood. If there is low run, one can become depressed and disappointed.

Every individual has some ups and downs in life. The normal events in life can lead anyone to feel sad and depressed once in a while. An extremely depressed person may need medical emergency. It may be severe, mild, short and long.

Causes of Depression

There are several causes that make people get depressed. It is not a single factor. Some of the common factors are as follows :

1. Genetics: Family characteristics which are passed from generation to generation.
2. Events: Death of family members like father, mother, wife, children, friends, relatives, pets, and divorce, separation, remarriage or change of places.
3. Family Conditions: Poverty, homelessness, domestic violence, relationship and loss of conjugal bliss unhappiness, economic, social, negative stress, family atmosphere, frustration.
4. Medical: Immunity deficiency, hormonal imbalance, nervous breakdown, physical or mental illness.

Symptoms of Depressed Person

Sadness,

Hopelessness, helplessness,

Tiredness, weakness,

Loneliness, separation from friends and relatives and total isolation,

Anxiety, anger, irritation,

Poor concentration,

Weight loss,

Sleep disorders, lack of sleep, half-sleep, falling asleep, staying asleep,

Guilt, worthlessness,

Aches, pains, stomach disorder,

Pessimism, indifference,
Suicidal attempts,
Lack of interest and motivation,
Dietary disorders,
Disappointment, pain, grief,
Discouragement, despair,
Lack of Appetite,
Self-humiliation, worthless and unlovable thoughts.

Treatment

Talk therapy, Positive thinking,
Meditation, Vehement laughing,
Change of mood,
exercise, good nutrition,
Yoga, homework, gardening,
Dance, music, games, fine arts,
Keeping oneself busy,
Association with pet dogs, cats and other animals,
Self-care, self-healthcare, responsibility,
Love, friendship, kindness, support,
Consulting therapists, counsellors,
Keeping busy with different activities,
Watching TV, and listening to radio,
Painting, drawing, doodling, reading and writing.

2. Anxiety

Anxiety is a state of worry or fear about something. It may be a situation of feeling nervous or worried that something bad is going to happen or bad going to be heard. A strong feeling to do something or anxiously awaiting something to happen.

For instance, health anxiety, examinations result anxiety, election winning anxiety, competition, betting, job awaiting, decision making, a resolution, etc. It may be anxious look, face, expression, appearance, etc.

It describes a stronger feeling and is more formal. A mother may be anxious about children's safety. A person who always worries a lot, is said to be in anxious state. you are anxious to do something when you want something very much.

Anxiety disorders is a major health problem costing millions of rupees a year. People are making repreated visits of helathcare services because these anxiety disorders seek relief for symptoms that mimic physical illness.

Many people with anxiety disorders more likely to visit a doctor, like to be hospitalised for psychiatric disorders, children are suffering from separation anxiety disorders.

These are a unique group of illnesses that fill people's lives with anxiety, worry and fear. They are the most common mental health disorders that vast majority of people suffer from today.

Anxiety disorders treatment is also individually tailored, they are to be treated by a wide range of mental health professionals.

It is a natural human reaction that involves mind and body. A person feels a physical sensation when the mind and body reacts to danger. A sense of uneasiness or nervousness is the common feeling. The mental health conditions that involve exessive amounts of anxiety, fear, nervousness, worry or dread are the most common mental health conditions that affect the people of all age-groups, with different symptoms. These disorders affect both body and mind, the body releases the hormone which prepares for reactions.

Anxiety is a part of life of everybody. For instance, anxious to take a test, walking down a dark street, traveling alone, living alone, etc.

Anxiety is of two types :

The anxiety do not go away,

The anxiety gets worse over time.

For instance :

While finding a burglar in bedroom at night, your feelings are :

Heart beats fast, or

Palms get sweating, or

Mind races-it is an anxiety.

Again anxiety is of two types :

1. Generalised Anxiety Disorders

It is perpetual worry or fear, nor relation to a particular event or situation. For instance, continuous worrying about a child who is good at education.

Health Disorders : 1. Muscle Catch, 2. Trembling, 3. Dry mouth, 4. Nauses, 5. Irritability, 6. Sleep disorders, 7. Shortness of breath, 8.Tension, 9. Restlessness, 10. Headache and Twitching, 11. Chronic, 12. Worry, 13. Exaggerated worry.

2. Panic Disorder

A panic disorder is a sudden feeling of great fear that cannot be controlled and it prevents you from thinking clearly. In a situation in which you are made to feel very anxious, causing to act very quickly and without thinking carefully, it causes sometimes your heart to beat faster. It gives panic attack. Its symptoms are :

Pounding heart,

Nausea,

Racing Pulse,

Shaking,

Fear,

Embarrassing,

Dizziness,

Death fear,

Chest pain,

Trembling,

Tingling sensation,

Abdominal discomfort,

Numbness,

Mind block,

Throat tightness,

Shortness of breath,

Choking.

If it is not treated, it leads to phobias. Other types of anxiey disorders are :

1. Obsessive-compulsive disorder,
2. Post-traumatic stress disorder,
3. Social anxiety disorder,
4. Specific phobias.

3. Phobia

The word *phobia* literally means a very strong irrational fear or hatred of a particular thing specific, it is a mental problem that keeps you away from living a normal life. Phobias are unreasonable fears that lead people to altogether avoid specific things, or situations, or events which trigger tension, anxiety created by fear being afraid.

Phobias occur in several forms.

For example :

Agoraphobia

It is a fear in any situation that might trigger panic attack. It is very difficult to escape from such a situation. It is a fear of being in public places where there are many other people. When a person is exposed to such a situation he is said to be a person who suffers from agoraphobia. For instance, shopping malls, airplanes, lines, bridges, public transportation, sports arena, queues, speedy driving, waiting, traffic jam.

Many sensitive people face the problem of panic disorders, of panic attack of agoraphibia. They avoid to go to such places where the need for immediate escape is difficult. When they suffer from severe anxiety panic disorder develops.

A person of agoraphobia doesnot feel safe and doesnot enjoy in public places. It is particularly so where crowds gather. some people are especially trapped always home bound, it is safe place for them. Do not go out to public places. But still there is no sure way to cure.

Claustrophobia

It is a state of an extreme fear of being in a small enclosed place, where it is a unpleasant feeling that a person gets in a situation which restricts them. A person who is exposed to such a situation is said to suffer from fear claustrophobic. For instance, the claustrophobic atmosphere of the classroom, enquiry room, etc.

Specific Phobia

It is a fear connected with or intended for one particular phobia which makes one suffer from intense fear reaction from that particular situation. For example fear of spiders, dogs, flying heights, depths, darkness, speed, blood, queues, water, storm, sound, operations, deathbed, gatherings, etc.

It is an unreasonable fear or fright. The remedy for such a situation is to avoid them. Other common phobias are animals, insects, thunder, lightening, driving, elevators, dental problems.

Social Phobia

It is a fear situation of being extremely embarrassed in front of unknown people. For instance, a situation of fear of public speech; it gives a social anxiety disorder. It is where a person being judged by other or behaving in a way that might make a person feel shy, akward, or ashamed especially in a social situation, an embarrassing situation causing to look stupid, or dishonest, guilty feeling or ridicule.

The physical symptoms associated with this disorder may include:

Heart palpitations,

Faintness,

Blushing,

Profuse sweating,

Shivering,

Tense muscle,

Pale Face,

Freezing,

Fumbling,

Sweating,

Racing heart,

Stomachache,

Dizziness,

Crying,

Tantruma,

It is called social anxiety disorder, it is a social performance situation. For instance :

Initial conversation,

Unstructured peer activities,

Public performance,

Classroom teaching,

Inviting others to dais,

Proposing vote of thanks,

Singing, dancing, swimming, acting,

Other socialisation of skills, etc.

It is a fear that others may scrutinise and negatively evaluate the performance, humilitation.

Since many of the symtoms of phobia mimic those of illnesses such of cardio disorders, many sufferers often make visit to emergency rooms or medical services, some may have life threatening, illnesses. It is difficult to have a correct diagnosis, people feel a great deal of frustration, suffer in silence, isolating themselves from friends, relatives. It leads to mental and bodily disorders.

Phobia disorders cannot be exclusively be treated by pharmaceutical drugs. It needs the assistance of multi-disciplinary professionals like psychiatrists, psychologists, clinical, social, physicians, etc. Prescriptions of right drug is risky. Medication alone cannot be very useful in treating phobic disorders. But phobic disorders affect the people.

The good news is naturopaths today understand phobia disorder better and offer better treatment. Phobia disorders can be treated well by yogic method of healthcare systems and mental health experts like *yogis* and meditators.

Meditation, loneliness, and psychotherapy are helpful for treating. Various medications available have side-effects. Self-care measures, life style changes are the effective methods.

4. Trichotillomania (Hair Pulling)

The word trichotillomania is a Greek word, it means sadness or mania. It is a type of psychological situtation that involves a strong urge to pull our hair. It is a behaviour of a person with hair-pulling compulsions when a patient is emotionally healthy.

According to modern medical science it is a condition caused by a chemical imbalance in the brain. The patient exhibits an extremely strong desire for hair pulling. It indicates a serious mental illness of a particular type.

It is the state of having crazy or stupid behaviour that could be dangerous, in a movement of madness.

It is an urge that leads to hair pulling, when one is stressed out or worried. When something interferes with neurotransitters (chemicals) which are part of the brain's communication centre, it leads to a problem of compulsive urge to pull-hair.

This behaviour affects more girls than boys, during adolescent age. Some pull from places like the scalp, eyebrows, eyelashes, public area, sometimes leaving bald patches. Some do nail biting, skin-picking. It is very hard to understand their urges.

How to solve the hair pulling behaviour ? It is not totally a medical condition requiring medication.

They stop doing when they feel. It is a behavioural habit. By passing of age, the practice will disappear. Psychological, behavioural therapies can help to correct the imbalance.

5. Stress

The word stress means a mental pressure, or worry caused by the problems in a life of an individual. A pressure keeps one thinking about unpleasant things for long. When an individual who is under stressful condition does things or thinks that can easily go wrong. Those who suffer from stresses, generally fails cope and to withstand in personal life and public life activities. The condition of stress causes stress-related illnesses. It is often a risk factor and demands skill of stress management to deal with it.

A Stressful state causes a lot of anxiety and worry and tiredness to be able to relax. When a lot of physical or mental pressure is put, one feels highly stressed and tired. Even a heavy physical pressure many cause stress.

It is a disparity between personal expectations and capacity to cope with stress, if resoureses are not sufficient to meet the need or to meet them is a stimulus to stress. Pressures, strains, demands, time for which the body must have coping capacity to respond, otherwise stress sets in.

When all the energetic resources are depleted and exhausted, body fails to perform its normal functions. The body reacts to stressors, by releasing hormones.

The imbalance between hormonal quality and stressors is a sign of stressful situation.

Stress creates an imbalance between demand and resources. Pressure exceeds one's ability to cope.

Causes (Stressors)

Divorce, pressure, unemployment, financial problem, ill health, conflict, deceptions, drinking, child abuse, social, environmental suffering, over work, quality of work, life, exploitation, superiority and inferiority complex, job related factors, lack of children, hostility, lack of relaxation, unrealistic expectations, time urgency, over schedule of work, high expectations, loneliness, difficult tasks, persistent tiredness, restlessness, hyperactivity, future anxiety, negative attitude, worries, fear, apprehensions, threat, feeling of insecurity, boredom and fatigue, death of spouse, jail term, marital separations, retirement, death of pets, personal habits disturbance, domestic violence, marriage maladjustments, readjustment, family separations, failure in personal achievement, living and working conditions, clashes with boss, job related home stress, children's education and health, poor coping ability, etc.

When one faces stress for a long period it leads to diminising health or illhealth. If stress is not managed first health disorder is to face heart attack, angena and other cardio-related problems. The health effect is the disruption of nomeostasis through physical or psychological stimuli. The stressful risk factors can be mental, physiological, anatomical and physical.

If a persistent stress is not resolved it may lead to anxiety and behaviour. An alarming experience may trigger a stress response. Sweatings raise heart rate, chest pain, sleep disorders set in, capacity of the glands deplete, the immunity system is exhausted and the body's functions are impaired.

The impact can manifest itself in clear illnesses like ulcers, depression, mental illness and even cardiovascular problems. It significantly affects the body's capacity and will have negative implications.

There are a number of psychotherapies against stress. These can be used individually or in group format. The therapies are being delivered by a variety of mental health professionals, including psychiatrists, psychologists, clinical and social workers. The biology, physiology, psychology, behavioral manifestations of fight or flight.

Types of Stressors

1. Psychological
2. Physical
3. Role
4. Sociological
5. Physical illness

6. Biochemical
7. Stage of human development.

Physical effects of stressors

1. C.V.Ds
2. Strain
3. Mental illness
4. Numbness
5. Stomach Knot
6. Digestive disorders
7. Heart rate
8. Hypertension
9. Itching
10. Dysponesis
11. Diarrhoea
12. Constipation
13. Nausea
14. Vomiting
15. Chronic pains.

Behavioural Effects of stressors

1. Conduct disorders
2. Change in eating habits
3. Increased smoking
4. Increased alcoholism
5. Carelessness, Rashness
6. Aggressive behaviour
7. Nervous laughter
8. Change in friendship
9. Speed-talking, walking, eating
10. Drug abuse increases
11. Decrease of Energy levels
12. Shifting responsibilities
13. Restlessness
14. Hostility
15. Hypochondrism.

Emotional Effects of Stressors

1. Anxiety, anxiousness
2. Change in emotional traits
3. Depression
4. Anger
5. Annoyance
6. Outburst
7. Impatience
8. Short temper
9. Hostility
10 Jealousy
11. Tendency to cry
12. Self-depreciation
13. Restlessness
14. Narrowed focus
15. Lack of interest.

Cognitive Effects of stressors

1. Poor concentration
2. Low attention
3. Weak recollection of thoughts
4. Disorganised thoughts
5. Break of thread of thoughts
6. Memory loss, absent mindedness
7. Irrational behaviour
8. Error prone
9. Increased distractibility
10. Lack of sense of meaning
11. Mumbling-repeating
12. Confusion-lack of creativity
13. Negative self-esteem
14. Attention deficiency, blurring vision
15. Diminishing or exaggerated fantasy.

6. Trauma

Yet another important cause of mental illness causing physical disorders and diseases is trauma. It is a state of mental condition caused by severe shock, especially when the harmful effects last for a longtime. Every one of us normally comes across rare situation of an unpleasant experience in life that makes us feel upset or anxious.

It occurs in an upsetting situation that makes you feel annoyed or unhappy, on the happening of an unexpected event, gives us a feeling of unhappiness and disappointment.

It creates a medical problem in which a person suffers mental and emotional problems resulting from an experience of life-threatening event or death. He will then suffer from stress disorders mentally and physically.

Types of Trauma

1. Physical Trauma : Physical injury.
2. Blunt Force Trauma : Precursory type.
3. Penetrating Trauma : Skin or tissues are pierced by an object.
4. Psychological Trauma : Caused by stress or life-threatening events.
5. Past-cult Trauma : Caused by disaffection and disaffliction.
6. Situational Trauma : War, genocide, crime, catastrophic mishap.

Causes

Vehicular Accidents, collisions

Intruders, terrorists attacks

Earthquake

Floods, violent crime

Shocks, deaths

horrible events

Tragedy

Gas leakage events

Electrical shocks

Collapses

Hurricanes

Tornadoes

Tsunami

Fire

Hazardous material spills

Injury, impact

Sporting accidents

Assault

Attack by animals

Medical complications, procedures

Rape

Warforce, genocide

Physical or psychological torture

Attack of cancer, AIDS and other dreadly diseases upsetting events

Shyness, introvert attitude

Loss of loved ones including relatives, friends, family, pets, neighbours, loss of home

Property, furniture and favourite belongings

Sexual abuse

Childhood neglect.

Consequences of Traumatic Event

A traumatic event may lead to strong emotions, stress and physical reactions, proactive, realistic, and passive responses. An affected person may face many traumatic symptoms and responses, normal and abnormal, sometimes life or death issues of survival. An event may produce consequences or impact of serious nature. Sometimes it is very difficult to identify the impact of a serious trauma. It affects in many ways, shocks may be immediate, or after traumatic event.

1. Upsetting memories
2. Flashbacks
3. Nightmares, recurring thoughts
4. Insomia, disbelief
5. Fear and insecurity
6. Emotional exhaustion, detachment, dissociation
7. Confused state, agitated resentfulness
8. Mental Block, anger, suspicion
9. Feelings of despair, loss of self-esteem.
10. Depressions, helplessness, hopelessness, loneliness
11. Domestic violence, crying, frustration
12. Pedophilia and incest
13. Life style change, irritation
14. Emotional numbness
15. Mental illness, hysteria
16. Upheaval and long lastig effects
17. Shocks, apathy

18. Stress disorders
19. Avoidance of situations
20. Hyper activeness, anxiety
21. Demoralisation
22. Addition to drugs, rejection of outside help
23. Loss of memory
24. Relationship change with others
25. Philosophical, spiritual and religious change
26. Betrayal, fear
27. Horror, intolerance
28. Impairment
29. Permanent physical damage, Disfigurement
30. Fatigue, irritability, moodiness.

The common signs and signals of traumatic stress disorders may be classed as hereunder

1. Physical signs
2. Cognitive signs
3. Emotional signs
4. Behavioural signs.

7. Emotions

Emotion is a state of strong feeling such as love, fear, or anger. It is a part of an individual's character that shows a feeling, and as a result he loses control over his emotions.

Emotion is expressed when a person is feeling excited, sometimes loses rational thought, entertains emotional thoughts. It is a reason for emotional stress, exhibits an emotional outburst, emotional reactions, loses balance of temper, uses emotive language sometimes.

Emotional health disorders are relating to psychology, sociology, neuro-science, ethics and metaphysics. Emotions are of various types. It may be positive or negative. It affects an organism's ability.

A person who is in emotional state exhibits feelings through facial expressions, body postures, bodily changes, vioce quality, anxiety, sadness, love, pride, depression, euphoric, irritable mood, other body languages. These are the cognitive processing system. Some people suffer increased heart beat, perspiration and fear, tense muscle, experiences like happiness, envy, sadness, angry face.

Emotions mind states affect emotions. They can have a powerful impact on physical disorder, illnesse, memory, forgetting.

They are primary, universal in all human beings, but varies in degree. Changed emotions may create a changed bodily state and expressions like pain, hunger, fear, rage, joy, stress. There is a close relationship between emotions and physical behaviour.

For instance, a sudden sight of a tiger, hormonal production changes, heart starts beating fast, fear arises, increasing muscle tense increased flinch. it may be pleasant or unpleasant clearly visible in baby movements, gestures, postures. Human feelings are displayed as emotion cues listed below.

Emotions are thoughts to be related to activity in mind and that direct one's attention. Meta emotions are second order emotions, may be short-lived or long-lived.

Emotional Cues

Fear	Agitation
Anger	Apathy
Aggression	Arrogance
Violence	Anxiety
Envy	Border
Sadness	Disgust, Delight
Joy	Disappointment
Frustration	Curiosity
Surprise	Embarrassment
Grief	Happiness
Shame	Horror, hope, humanity
Desire	Impatience, irritability
Jealousy, kindness	Loneliness, Melancholy
Aroman	Nervousness, Negatiity
Hate, zest	Phobia, pity, pride
Guilty	Shyness, sorrow, shock
Love, worry	Regret, resentment
Uncertainty	Surprise, Thrill
Confusion	Unhappiness
Calm	Boredom
Pity	Envy, enmity
Mourning, vexation	Compassion
Fright, timidity, wrath	Aggressiveness, love.

8. Neurosis

Mindset changes the chemical level in the brain. Brain of each individual contains about 1,000 crores of neurons and each neuron has capability of having chemical interaction with about 10,000 neurons in the process of finding a solution to our problems.

A neuron is a cell that carries information between the brain and other parts of the body, a nerve cell. A person may suffer from neurosis, which is a mental illness in which he suffers from a strong feelings of fear and worry.

He feels with some degree of depression or anxiety, depressed feelings, lack of emotions, low self-confidence. It is a state of disorder of sense and motion caused by a general affliction of the nervous system, physiologically cannot be explained. It shows a variety of psychiatric situations by which emotional distress, or unconscious conflict is expressed through various physical, physiological and mental disturbance.

9. Nervousness

Nerve is a long thin thread that carries messages between the brain and parts of the body which enable one to move, feel pain. It always affects one mentally or emotionally. A nervous break-down is a situation of mental illness in which a person becomes highly depressed, anxious and tired, and unable to do, cannot live with normal life.

A human body has two types or nervous systems, namely:

1. Central nervous system,
2. Peripheral nervous system.

A central nervous system is a part of the system of nerves in the body that consists of the brain and spinal cord.

When you are in nervous situation it suggests that you are also frightened. It describes how you feel before you do something very important act.

For instance your feelings at the time of interview, concert performance, dancing, singing, playing or something unpleasant. when you are worried or frighened in such a performance, you are said be nervous.

10. Excitement

it is a state of feeling excited, a situation to make somebody feel very pleased, interested or enthusiastic. One feels exited when something that is going to happen. For instance, the job prospects during a year in the country greatly affected, unemployed, or any situation which exetes interest in public. A favourable event certainly exctes one, that makes a part of the body or any part of the physical system more active, a feeling of happiness or enthusiasm The result of examinations or counting of votes causes great excitement. It may be a surge, thrill, shiver.

The word excited is usually used to describe a positive feeling of pleasant news, or event but not negative feeling. For instance, one get excited to hear of promotion but not of demotion.

11. Worry

You are said to be in a worried situation, when you are thinking about unpleasant things that have happened or that might happen and therefore you are feeling unhappy and afraid. So, you look worried. You are worried about your son who has gone to school, or worried about the results, or job. You are always worried over a thing that you cannot change. What worries me is how I am going to become a minister.

So, it is a state of worrying about something, it creates anxiety and makes one sick, family worries, financial worries, job worries, examination worries, etc.

It is a very common feeling that describes how one feels when he is thinking about a problem artificially created, that cannot be solved or something bad that might happen.

12. Tensions

Tension is a feeling of anxiety and stress that makes it impossible to relax. Its character is the feeling of fear and excitement that is created by an unpleasant situation, whose progress builds tension. A state of being stretched light. It may be mental tension, nervous tension, traumatic tension, muscular tension.

At the time of tension, the outer appearance of a person, the feelings, qualities and behaviour of a person that you see or notice are normal, unusual.

13. Strain

A strain is a situation in an individual who exhibits the effects of worry or pressure. More worried and less calm, becoming tight, lack of relaxation to muscles. Lack of way of resting and enjoying oneself, something unpleasant a time to you, no rest, he cannot afford to relax for a movement. His face looks strained and weary, speaks in a strained voice.

It may be a mental strain and physical strain. Trying to do something more than physical ability leads to a strained condition.

61

Pranic Healing

Pranic Energy and Subtle Prana Yogic Dimensions of Healthcare

Today, *yoga* as a discipline has emerged as a new dimension of helathcare system. whereas, over the centuries, and '*yugas*', it is an Indian born traditional health measure which has been in practice based on ancient theories and doctrines. Today, there emerged a revolutionary *yoga* philosophy in health management, which bought a tremendous transformation in theory, thinking, practice and objectives meant for universal healthcare for the ailing human race.

As a result, the need to maintain and promote health by *yoga* practice now seems to pervade us.

By the end of twenteeth century, it was clear, as realised, that the old concept of health by drug was out dated and is not a medicine for self-cure and that the time demanded to have a relook at our traditional health practice methods. And as a result, *yoga* system has brought a revolutionary change as a new model, remodelled healthcare practice.

Today, there is once again an increasing trend, and the mood of the people which is towards truth seeking of health; the pharmaceutical drugs alone were found unfit and unsuitable for today's innumerable and incurable ailments. As a result, the emerging new diseases, disorders led to an increasig confidence in traditional household health practice methods like urinopathy, *yoga* practice, etc. Time is now ripe.

Accordingly, today the trend as visible is that practice of *yoga* has been now widespread throughout the world. The thinkers, believers, practitioners, crusaders, devotees have been increasingly exponential. Accordingly, it reiterates the inherent true limitations of modern healthcare drugs.

Continuous subtle changes in the working of the present cosmos, environment are leading to a paradigm shift in the new millennium. The traditional, natural, alternative and ancient household culturally accepted medicinal practices today have been revolutionarily tansforming people reeling under healing crisis. Today, many people are enjoying by treating themselves and reaping the fruits of new efforts.

Never before, has it been so easy and possible to the people and the truth seekers of secrets of creation of human body, to know about so much about new order of working cosmos, as today.

The Concept

Yoga means unification, a synthesis of factors that are otherwise disconnected into a whole, which can function as a unit. Now, since man remains as a sort of ununited being not only within himself as one divided against himself but also in his relations with the external world, he requires to make himself one and united.

'*Yoga*' in its most general significance means a 'combination' of two or more factors into an harmonious whole of unity to function as one agency to a definite purpose-whether material, psychic, and spiritual.

'*Yoga*' is not and cannot be a 'gift from others'. It is a self-achievement. One should strive hard to play the actor and not to remain as a passive product in one's endeavour to be such a self. Individuality and universality must be unified as one.

The essence of *yoga* practice is a state of mind, practice towards unification. It is a way of life, a part and parcel of life, a life long activity that keeps one in good health and normal living. *Yoga* theory is a part of the social and spiritual domain. As such, a key focus of its analysis is human behaviour which is mutable, unpredictable and reactive.

It is also heavenly content and dependent. *Yoga* is far from exact science and allows wide room for different interpretations, several fundamental bases from the uderstanding of all *yoga* thinking.

The enjoyment of eternal bliss of '*Brahmananda*' is possible only through *yoga* which acts as an impulse to become perfect man-form. The practitioners through contemplation alone cannot experience *Brahmananda* state with the physical alone, unless the existing and long hidden primary atom or *kundalini* within us is kindled to become active.

The flow is to be received to make the body fit and perfect. The fundamental goal of *yoga* is to make every physical body fit to realise the enegy to receive from supreme fountain source within the physical, with this physical, in this life, with full physical consciousness and conscience.

The eternity cannot be achieved by diversity, but by unity. The *yoga* practice paves way to wisdom during the life time itself, before discarding it, to be without disease, decay, figure change, old age and physical immortality.

It is designed for universal physical uplift and to attain eternity with this body, in this birth in physical and in full conscious state.

Without full mental concentration and thought process, one cannot experience the inner kingdom. It is an effort to realise all the secrets of eternal hidden in spirit which otherwise not possible to feel by physical alone. It is based on the principle of etheric matrix, and the aim is to establish the eternity for the entire humanity, for the benefit of entire mankind.

The spirit part of life gives you all branches of knowledge. It cannot be grasped by the brain only but step by step by mental practice.

The finer forces working will act as rectification of all inner deposited bad energy which will be thrown out.

Yogis and Rishies

The *yogis* of India by practice of urine drinking, *asanas*, not only arrived at a perfect state of health but also attained deageing, longevity, contrive to extend life far beyond the normal expectancy.

They believe in human urine as a medicine of body-mind-spirit strategy. The *Shivambu* text speaks that the sagacious practitioners should get up when three quarters of the night has elapsed. After cleansing the mouth and performing the other essential morning functions, one should drink one's own urine which is the annihilater of senility and diseases.

Yoga Teaches - Prana Treats

The mind and spirit part of medicine comes under the broad name of *yoga* practice. It has two distinct parts :

The theory of *yoga*.

The practice of *yoga*.

The short form of it is termed as '*Yoga* Teaches *Prana* Treats.'

Theory – Yoga Teaches

Every *yoga* practitioner must have full knowledge of theory of *yoga* and practice regularly to get one treated by the '*prana*.'

The theory of *yoga* is concerned with the ideas and principles on which *yoga* subject is based rather than with the practice and experiment.

Ancient *yogis* developed the ideas and principles of *yoga* in order to explain why this *yoga* works as a medicine. This formed a theory or theories about it designed to help treat an illness in addition to spiritual progress.

Yoga theory says that a particular idea of practice is supposed to be true in maintenance of good health and normal living.

The subject matter and philosophical aspects of yogic relate to the theory of *yoga*.

Yoga teaches is the theory of *yoga*. It is the theoretical side of the subjects.

Prana Treats

It is the activation of *pranic* energy and distribution of '*prana*' that actually treats the body, but not just the theoretical aspects which cannot treat.

The practical part of the *yoga* consists of regular practice.

Prana treats is the practical side of the *yoga*.

Prana treats is the generation and distribution of *prana*, i.e., supply-and-use side of the '*prana*' to the body.

Our present life is called cosmic life. The entire humanity is under the mercy of planets without independence. As the planets are responsible for the creation of the present human form they are living under the control, supervision and mercy of the planetary system. Even the '*prana*' is being distributed to the human being of limited quality by the planets. Hence, it is called cosmic life.

Prana Distribution and Diseases

For each individual, man-form the *prana* comes from a particular planet. After entering the physical system through nose it :

Passes through paranirvanic centre,

Later goes through the *sushumna* to the *kundalini*, which absorbs it,

The *kundalini* in turn distributes it to the astral system,

The astral system in turn gives the same to the etheric system,

Lastly, the etheric system distributes it to the physical body.

The *prana* received by the *kundalini* at a particular time will be enough for distribution for 49 days. As long as a person does physical work, there will be spending of energy. If you are in a '*samadhi*' state, the entry of *prana* into the physical system will be stopped and the *prana* received by it will be distributed internally.

The *prana* is distributed through the sympathetic nervous system (SNS) to the different parts of the body.

When the *prana* distribution is not adequate, full and proper then there will be disorders and diseases to the body.

Prana is going up for distribution and then coming down through '*sushumna*' *nadi*, meet at a place and it will be retorted horizontally at 64 centres in the physical system. So, there are 64 groups of physical complaints. In yogic science, it is called as 64 breathing principles. If the '*prana*' is equally distributed through 100 centres in the physical body, then the human body will be free from all illnesses. At present, in human body 64 centres are only working instead of 100 centres. It is the defect of physical formation of the body.

The body-mind-spirit medicine emphasises through *yoga* and meditation to rectify the body, adjust and remould to make the body work at 100 centres.

Plenty of Prana

Life force, vital energy or '*prana*' is essential for every human being to live. *Prana* is a non-material substane or divine force and pranic energy which is vital for survival and to keep in good health and maintains disease-free body.

There are two issues to be analysed here, namely :

Limited supply of *prana,*

Plenty of *prana.*

At present, according to the creative order of the cosmos, the supply of '*prana*' is very limited to the human physical figure system.

It is because of this limited supply of *prana*, limited availability in the body the human-form body is subjected to illness, diseases, disorders, decay, premature death, figure change, ageing and less longevity.

The planets supply limited *prana* to the *kundalini*, which is in turn re-distributed throughout the body, through various nerves and nerve centres of the system.

Hence, the present human form of life is called chief life.

Plenty of Prana in cosmos

There is plenty of *prana* deposit somewhere in cosmos in subtle form, invisible and unknown to ordinary people. Getting unlimied supply of *prana* and its distribution gives human beings a quality of merry life, good health, no disease, no decay, no premature death.

There were expert *yogis* who endeavoured to explore the cosmos to find the respository of this plenty *prana*, obtained and reaped the benefit given life to the dead person, recalling, prolongation of life.

If it is made available plenty to the planet earth, the ailing human race can live without disease and decay.

The main task of the *yogi* is to locate limitless *prana* place and get unlimited supply to live healthily. Presently we are receiving this *prana* in limited quantity that, too, at the mercy of the planets.

So, a person will attain eternity and will enjoy merry life, as soon as he receives plenty of '*prana*'.

By spiritual practice, one has to realise *prana* from the supreme fountain source of plenty prana located in cosmos.

To get plenty *prana* one has to go beyond the triple cosmos evolutions. The practitioner by trance practice in etheric body has to go to the higher planes to explore the source of plenty *prana* and supply.

So, the concept of plenty *prana* which is so far beyond the imagination, comprehension, and capability of ordinary human beings, but still remained as eternal mystic.

For the first time in the history of human evolution, the great *kundalini yogi* C.V.V. explored and obtained it. By his Direct Line Yoga Practice, he made it possible to get it supplied to this planet by independent astral routes and channles.

As soon as the physical body is rectified, adjusted and moulded, new structure of physical form is made by purification, it will be capable of receiving new life-wave-flow in plenty. As a result, human form of physical body enjoys the status of merry life, phyical immortality, disease-free, without decay, figure change with longevity without cosmic influence and without depending on the mercy of planets for plenty of prana supply.

The astral body receives plenty of *prana.*

The astral in turn distributes to the etheric.

The etheric body in turn distributes to the physical body.

There is a plenty of *prana* somewhere in the cosmos which is very useful for long life, treatment, longevity and survival.

But the *prana* has no connection to any of the sides, *prana-less* limit. The energy is kindled in less *prana* level.

Nadis

There is a lot of confusion and misunderstanding in the minds of many people about the word '*nadi* ' and '*nerve*'. But these are used synonymously. But in recent times the word '*nadi*' has been translated as '*nerve*'.

The word *yoga nadi* literally means 'flow' or 'current'. *Nadis* are subtle channels through which the *pranic* force flows.

The *yoga* texts write that there are 72,000 *nadis* in the physical body. These are visible as current of light to a person who has developed psychic vision.

Nadis are composed of astral matter like *chakras*. They are not actually part of the physical body.

As against 72,000 nadis in the physical body, ten are major, and of them three are most significant.

These are : Ida, Pinagala, Sushumna.

So, these *nadis* are the astral tubes made up of astral matter that carries psychic current. '*Nad*', which means motion. It is through these pipes vital force, *pranic* currents move or flow.

These *nadis* are intangible, cannot be touched, sensed, physically cannot be seen, made with subtle matter, defy measurement, cannot be made any test experiments in the physical plane.

They are not like other physical nerves, arteries, veins, which are known in medical science, out side the scope of anatomy and physiology.

Though subtle, non-physical, they exert great influence on the physical body. They have gross manifestation in the operation of the physical body. The physical nerves and plexuses have intimate relationship with subtle *nadis*.

They are respectively called and work in physical centres and astral centres.

The physical centres produce vibrations of various types which have desired effects in the astral centres.

The word plexus means, an interlacing of several nerves, asteries and veins and a centre is formed called plexus.

Kanda

All the nadis originate from a central plane called '*kanda*'. It is the junction where *sushumna nadi* is connected with *mooladhara chakra*. This *kanda* is located between the anus and the root of the reproductory organ.

It looks like the shape of an egg and is covered with membrance. It is just about the *mooladhara chakra*. All the *nadis* in the body spring from this *Kanda*.

The *mooladhara chakra* has four petals which are on the sides of this *kanda* and this junction is known as '*gradhisthana*'. It is here the influence of *maya* (trick) is very powerful.

This centre is the fountain of vital force, or *prana*. It is the centre of the astral body, from where *yoganadis*, subtle channels, spring and circulate vital energy, *sukshma prana* to different parts of the body.

In the physical body there is a centre known a 'Canda Equina', which is the astral centre. This is the '*Kanda*'.

In this paragraph, we will dissuss how the nerves have been formed in different planes. At the time of creation of the physical body, the three nerves *ida, pinagala and sushumna* have been created from the seed portion as basic nerves, supporting nerves. These three nerves entered from the seed portion.

The triple nerves, namely, *ida, pinagala and sushumna* start like root from the bottom of *kundalini*. A separate bone called trait coming from *kundalini* starts spreading as nodes about *kundalini* and extends upto *sahasrara* level.

Nadis-Triple Nerve Centres

In addition to the seven stations in the body, there are also three more pivotal stations called :

1. Ida, 2. Pingala, 3. Sushumna.

1. Ida

The ida is a nerve bone link. It is the place of beginning point of physical or *mooladhara* from the left side of the human body. It is a place where the *kundalini* power coils in the root of *beejam* (seed). The seed, intuition, gives a *kamam* to have an intercourse with other sex. An experienced practitioner with finer sight can see it as seven petalled lotus.

Ida nadi emanates from the left side of the *mooladhara* and spirals up the spinal cord. It passes through each *chakra*, in turn forming a criss-cross pathway and finally it terminates at the left side of *ajna chakra*.

Ida is passive, introvert and feminine. It is also known as the *chandra* or moon *nadi*.

Ida starts from the right testicle, *ida* flows through the left nostril. Ida is cooling in nature. Ida is of pale, *saktirupa*. It is the great nourisher of the world.

Pingala

Pingala nadi emanates from right side of *mooladhara* and passes in an opposite manner to that of *ida nadi*, and finally terminates at the right side of *ajna chakra*.

Contrary to *ida, Pingala* is active, extrovert and masculine and is also called '*surya*' or sun *nadi*. The *pingala* starts from the left testicle. The *pingala* flows through the right nostril. *Pingala* is heating in nature. It digests the food. It is of fiery, *rudra rupa*.

Ida and *Pingala nadis* meet with the *sushumna nadi* at *mooladhara chakra* and form a knot there. The point where three *nadis* meet at the *mooladhara chakra* is known as *mukta triveni*. This meeting place is also called '*Bramha Granthi*'. Again these meet at the *anahata* and *ajna chakras*.

The *Ida* and *Pingala* nerves both end in the same place, the place is called Thousand Petalled Lotus, a place of Supreme Being, '*Sri Gurumurthy*'.

Ida and *Pingala* are the two basic supporting nerves which have connections directly with the brain system.

Sushumna

It is the spiritual channel located at the centre of the spinal cord. It originates from '*mooladhara*', or physical plane *chakra*, at the perineum and terminates at *sahasrara*, top of the head. This *nadi* itself a gross spinal cord, in *yoga* literature called *Brahma nadi*, which is within the *sushumna*'.

The central *nadi* extends from the *mooladhara chakra*. It is from the second vertebra of coccygeal region to *Brahmarandhra*. Acording to medical science also there is a central canal in the spinal cord called 'Canalis Centralis'. The cord is made up of grey and white matter. It is dropped in the hollow of the spinal column.

Accordingly, *sushumna nadi* is dropped with in the spinal canal and has subtle section.

It is red in colour like '*agni*'.

This canal is known as *brahma nadi* through which *kundalini* passes from *mooladhara chakra* to the *sahasrara chakra*.

A breath is to be made to pass through the *sushumna nadi*, the mind becomes steady, it is the highest state of yoga. The steadiness of the mind is called: '*Umani Avastha*'. A *yogi* can experience a wonderful state of meditation if he sits when *sushumna* is operating.

There is a *vajra nadi* located within the *sushumna*. It is known for lustrous nature as sun with *rajasic* qualities.

There is another nadi known as '*chitra*' within the *vajra nadi*. It is in pale colour, and of sattvic nature.

Within the *chitra nadi* there is a fine and minute canal, known a *brahma nadi*. In anatomy, it is called 'canalis centralis'.

It is through *brahma nadi* the *kundalini* passes, when kindled, from *mooladhara* to the *sahasrara chakra*.

The door of *brahman* is called *Brahmadwara*, which is the lower eternity of *chitra nadi*. The *kundalini* has to pass through this door to *brahmarandra*. Finally *chitra nadi* terminates in the carebellum. This *nadi* plays a pivotal role in *kundalini* practice. When it is kindled and activated it passes through the *sushumna nadi*.

Psychic Centres–Chakras

***Pranic* Energy :**

In the *yogic* context and psychic dimension, *chakra* means connected with strange *pranic* energy, vital force and not able to be explained by natural laws.

A person seems to have strange mental powers, to be able to do things in the body.

So, it is called by varient names as psychic energy, psychic force, psychic power.

The word '*chakra*' literally means '*wheel*' or '*circle*'. But in *yogic* context a better understanding is 'vortex', or 'whirlpool'. Literally, it means a very powerful feeling, force or situation from which one cannot escape vortex technically means a mass of air, water that spins around vey fast and pulls things into its centre.

Therefore, a *chakra* is a vortice of *pranic* energy at a specific area of the body. It controls, manitors, the circulation of *prana* permeating the entire physical body of an individual.

Each psychic centre or *chakra* is a specific switch which turns on or opens up a specific area of the brain. In case of non-*yogic* people, these *pranic* centres lie dormant and inactive. when we are not concentrating on these centres these *chakras* lie dormant, but able to become active when we work on them.

while performing meditation, the concentration is on the *chakras*, the practice stimulates the flow of energy through *pranic* centres and assists to activate them. The *yogic* practice makes you feel more energetic, active and healthy.

These centres normally are in sleepy state, but the practice in turn awakens the dormant areas in the brain, faculties in the psychic and mental bodies. This also makes one experience higher planes of consciousness which are normally not possible to all.

These psychic centres are in the astral body, the astral body is also called *linga* '*sarira*'.

Linga sarira is a constitution of 17 *tatvas*.

They are :

Gyanendrias	:	05	skin, ears, eyes, tongue, nose.

Karmendriyas	:	05	speech, hands, legs, genitals, anus.
Pranas	:	05	Prana, apana, vyana, udana, samana.
Manas	:	02	mind and Budhi (intellect).
Total	:	17	

Pranic Energy Centres

At present, in human form physical body the major *chakras* are seven in number.

These seven centres are located along with the path way of *sushumna nadi*. It moves through the centre of the spinal cord.

Each *chakra* has a prescribed number of petals, colour and location, and is depleted symbolically as lotus which signifies the three stages. The three stages the *yogi* has to pass through in his spiritual life, namely, ignorance, aspiration and illumination. The names and order are as follows;

	From Bottom to Top	*From Top to Bottom*
1.	Physical (*mooladhara*)	Mahaparanirvanic
2.	Astral (*Swadhi Sthana*)	Parantravanic
3.	Mental (*Manipuraka*)	Nirvanic
4.	Budhic (*Anahata*)	Budhic
5.	Nirvanic (*vishudha*)	Mental
6.	Paranirvanic (*Agna*)	Astral
7.	Mahaparanirvanic (*Sahasrara*)	Physical

Their location, characteristics and petals are as follows :

Chakra	*Location*	*Petals*
Mooladhara	End of Vertebral column	4
Swadhistana	navel	6
Manipuraka	Stomach	10
Ananata	Heart	12
Visudha	Throat pit-neck	16
Agna	Middle of eye brows	2
Sahasrara	Top pit, Top head	1,000

Kindling Kundalini Power

The word '*kundalini*' has Sanskrit origin. It indicates the root of the nature and its reaction. The name *kundalini* suggests that it originates from 'Origin', 'Creator' or 'Brahman'. It is most ancient and as old as human evolution. It is the mother of all creations.

It is well known to the seekers of truth and *yoga* practitioners contemplating on it. Even then most of them are not fully aware of its nature, functions, three kingdoms of evolutions deposited in it, present work and future plans of future evolution of human Kingdom.

Primary Atom

The very creation in the beginning has commenced with the introduction of the primary atom, which in *yoga* literature is called '*kundalini*'.

In other words it is the '*moola prakriti*', the '*Kundalini*', after undergoing three early evolutions is now working through the fourth field of human kingdom. It has completed its three evolutions, experienced three cultures at different phases of time.

Permanent Atom

Thus, the *kundalini* may be described as force of condensed energy or atomised form of life. This in *yoga* literature is called permanent atom.

Condensation Process

In the first field itself, the pure original atoms were condensed. Later on, it realisd that there was no place for further work in that field, and created a second field for further work, in a similar way the third and fourth fields came into existence. The present working field is the fourth field where physical figure structure building work has reached the man-form state.

Form of Energy

Kundalini is a form of energy. The atom is in primary *kundalini* form. What kind of energy is it? It is concentrated energy manifested all activities. It is the conserved energy or stored up energy.

The concentrated states of three kinds of energies are called triple energies. *Briktha* is the field or a plane, it is devoid of all activities. This activity is thus is the starting activity which begins to manufacture '*kundalini*'.

Anu

Anu which is called *kundalini,* has to perform its natural functions in the course of evolution. It is with the help of this energy, a human being can realise the 'Origin' in the present physical form, in conscious state and in this birth only. This realisation of the Lord is possible through the wisdom revealed by the *kundalini*.

Kundalini is the vital force of creation, in which the present, past and future evolutions, right from its first evolutions upto the present and future manform are concealed or deeply deposited.

Kundalini is the limit at which 'unit of life' or '*prana*' now stands. It originates from the 'primary origin of Life'. The unit of life is being evolved by the '*Brahma*' the Omnipotent of the cosmos and has reached the present human stage.

A Blossom of Bud

Kundalini is the cage, where it has been covered in compartments as a blossom of bud, for protruding from the same cage, to show as a reptile or say as a snake form for culturing the developments in the occult powers.

The controlling action of *kundalini* requires the 'will of action', to empower himself with some 'will power', its graduation to go up and to give a feeling or sensation.

It is at Perenium

The place of the *kundalini* is at the middle of the portion called perenium.

This place is the centre of '*mooladhara*' or the lowerst physical plane.

It is being in super energy form, it cannot be seen, touched, sensed physically, as it is intangible and invisible one.

It can be experienced and felt only, by those who are empowered with higher sight as a brilliant spark.

Types of Kundalinis

There are three types of *kundalinis*. They are :

1. *Cosmic Kundalini :* The cosmic *kundalini* is ruling the whole cosmos.
2. *Earth kundalini* It is ruling and controlling the earth.
3. *Physical Kundalini:* It is ruling the 'jeeva' of man-form.

Triple Coated Kundalini

The word 'coating' means a strong cover round holding '*kundalini*'. It indicates a binding given to it by the 'Origin' Himself, in such a way not to reveal its secrets, history of higher fields to whomsoever except to '*Brahma*', that, too, after must descend in physical form on the earth.

The word triple means three or having three parts in *kundalini*. They represent three evolutions, each part is sealed and the whole *kundalini* is in a sealed box. Hence, *kundalini* is called triple coated *kundalini*, because it underwent three evolutions and is presently undergoing the fourth part of it, which is in half way through, in the present form of human evolution. The evolutions are :

1.	Mineral Kingdom	:	first evolution	first coating
2.	Vegetable Kingdom	:	second evolution	second coating
3.	Animal Kingdom	:	third evolution	third coating
4.	Human kingdom	:	fourth evolution	fourth ongoing.

Each field of past experience or kingdom is covered or screen is put over it. Hence, it is called triple coated *kundalini*.

The *anu* or primary atom is termed as triple coated *kundalini*, when it is covered with coating over it, indicating their fields of evolution.

Thus, the triple is the mysteries to the cosmos as is looked on as unity. The life principle is called triple.

The spirit which comes out after concurring matter is called triple, that which has three qualities is triple or the '*Thrimoorthies*', the Trinity of Hindu Gods.

The fourth field is lower one, a man form cover, the present evolution of man form is going in the fourth division of the fourth field. It is still going on half-way through.

The etheric structutre of man-form in this field is to be made perfect man-form in the ongoing course of present evolution. When the work of the fourth field is full and complete, the state of physical immortality is established.

Thus, now the *kundalini* has three and a half coatings, the fourth is half way through of human evolution going on.

Male and Female Kundalini

Female *kundalini* is from stem.

Male *kundalini* is from seed.

Kundalini in human form is triple energy. It is hermetically sealed in a box, with three strong adamantine walls unbreakable so that the energy of *kundalini* is in the field will not be shown and cannot be opened by anyone by any attempt.

Kindling of Kundalini

When it is kindled, it will reveal its past three kingdoms. It is to be activated, or fired, penetrated into it to know the secrets of human evolution and its past. At present, it is in inactive and dormant state.

Its activation requires its kindling to do its activity which is a process that reveals *kundalini* past and present experience.

The three sealed covers, or coatings around it are to be removed, the covers are known as trick covers.

According to the creation, laws of the cosmos, the *kundalini* cannot be kindled by anyone so easily.

Kundlaini Activity–A Mercury Activity

As mercury works in thermometer and barometers, the working principle of mercury activity is applied to the rising of human physical system of *kundalini* activity.

When the pressure is given to *kundalini*, or kindled its activity, it begins to rise.

When the *kundalini* in the course of its rise reaches the major triple level at the bottom of *sahasrara*, then the three coatings of would have to be removed one by one. When the three coatings are removed, the '*antaratma*', inner soul, the *paramatmic* principle works. This is the *jeevanmukti* and the only *mukti* state the man is destined to attain.

The following are the basic defects in the physical system of present human body, because of them one is not able to go to higher levels.

1. Weak physical figure,
2. *Sushumna* is not yet formed,
3. *Pingala Nadi* not working,
4. Incomplete *sahasrara,*
5. Inability to kindle *kundalini,*
6. Spinal column is not complete,
7. Hithu obstruction,
8. Inner levels not yet formed,
9. Bulb not arranged,
10. *Sahasrara* has not yet bloossomed.

Physico-Etheric Functions of Kundalini

Kundalini has got the capability to mould the figure in the womb of the mother, and also to mould the etheric body by its own retort. The giddiness of various states is produced by the *kundalini* only.

The *kundalini* is always in active state in the physical figure of human-form. It is the physico-etheric body does no other work than receiving *prana* mainly from planet and distributes it to the whole body through various nerve centres.

It has no role to play when the *prana* flow supply stops and it remains quiet and the body dies because every organ ceases its function for want of '*prana*'.

So, *kundalini* is now performing its routine work of merely maintaining the body in its normal state for the duration of life.

The cosmic knowledge, and secret powers of the cosmos can be experienced by arousing it.

The adjustments, transformation and rectification of physical body is arranged through this arrangement in the physical structure of human body.

The radiant beam and light enables one to attain excellent power. Its experience is an indication of progress which gives happiness, and joy and permits the practitioner to achieve physical immmortality.

All wisdom, universal wisdom can be obtained. Repeated flashes give self-confidence. Astral vision helps to gather knowledge and power. Stopping the heart beat, going to higher level and returning again is a wonderful and rare experience. It will help you to get more powers, realise everything.

It strengthens all weaker portions and purifies the body. The physical body receives star power which can be used for its developmet. This enables to rectify, adjust and mould the body. Nerves are rectified, and developed and kept always in stable and usable state.

A stage of '*samadhi*' is reached by kundalini rising. It has the capacity to mould the physical cage, continuous rising and working leads to touch pituitary.

Life energy or breathing rests with the origin and *kundalini*, which gives vibrations to the heart in the *budhic* portion and retorts the breathing.

The *kundalini* alters knowing that the body is not fit for further growth, it causes sudden heart failure. Other physical and astral benefits of kindling *kundalini* are as follows:

1. No *karma*, *maya* (trick) in any way affect the people,
2. The body will lead to salvation, independent living,
3. No influence of planets on human beings,
4. Physical consciousness,
5. Free from vicious circle of birth and death,
6. Dissolution of *karmic* bondages,
7. Full consciousness,
8. Endless joy,
9. Free from bonds of fate,
10. No figure change,
11. No disease, decay and death,
12. Deageing and longevity of life, mental, physical and spiritual development,
13. Word power, will power, intuition, divine sight,
14. End of trick working,
15. Pure memory without giddiness,
16. Plenty of life in conscious state in the present life,
17. The present life body without decay,
18. Plenty of *prana* supply,
19. With all conscience reaching to 'Origin'.

Merry life

There are two kinds of life wave principle working in human form physical figure. They are :

1. Chief life, 2.Merry life.

In physical conscience work, chief wave is associated with minor worries, difficulties, troubles, and health disorders. The activity given to us by the planets to live on the earth is the chief life. This life is mixure of pains, pleasures and troubles. This chief life is the present cosmic activity. It is top vertical portion of *kundalini*, where the present activity is going on.

The lower, deep portion of *kundalini* activity is full of merry life. Merry life is characterised without least pain, troubles, worries, with out health disorders and diseases. With *kundalini* activity at lowest part, one can experience full of pleasure, happiness, physical immortality. Hence, it is called merry life.

The Agenda

In the *yoga* for external life, *kundalini* is the only power which gives fruits of all *yoga* practices and experiences.

It is the *kundalini yoga* practice, which is revealing the secrets of evolution of creation of man-form, and universe, cosmic rectification activity and to remove the defects in the existing physical body.

Many practitioners have experienced plenty of miracles physical, mental, domestic and spiritual during their life time and have attained higher levels.

Kundalini, as absolute brahma and its practice is a Herculian task of moulding man-from physical body which is made of continuous changing cosmic material.

All human beings can practise this *yoga* without any discrimination of caste, creed, sex, religion, country and status.

Many of the secret benefits of kindling *kundalini* on physical, mental and spiritual advancements are not yet fully known to the vast majority of the people.

The new life wave works by creating a new structure of its own, in the very centre of our nervous system, remoulding the cosmic nervous system, standing as its outer sheathing making possibile our outer activities go on in their own way, opposing cosmic process.

At present, our life consciousness is not working in higher plane and is naturally cut off contact with the lower portion. As a result, we are living in a state leading to unconsciousness and lack of conscience state leading to disease and decay.

Kundalini practice activates energies of one's own, which set the construction, whether the practitioner is aware or not, intended or not, in the inner most part of the human body.

The primary object of this practice is to realise spirit or soul, within every body's physical body, through the wisdom revealed by the *kundalini* in conscious stae, self-realisation of the Supreme Super Personality of God Head, Creative Origin.

It provides the promise of an improved quality of life, a better life and society, more peaceful world, merry life and physical immortality to the entire mankind.

The structure of human life and its health is enormously complex. It contains many organs, parts, visible, invisible centres which are inter-connected in a vast network through several junctions. The whole system can be divided into sub-sections and sub-networks, which communicate to each other. All these results in intricate patterns of intertwined web network.

Emotional attachment of each other develop through different kinds of sounds, linked through brain and mind. The nerves work like a telephone system with trillions of miles of criss crossing wiring. The cell language communicates across the endocrine, neurological, gastrointestinal and immune system.

So, mind, spirit cannot be esparated from the body. The trinity constitute the life. They are separate systems. 'Body Mind Spirit' let be one word, no hyphen, or comma–but a single organism whole.

62
Dangers of Drugs

1. The Dark Side of Drugs

The shadowy aspects of medical science cannot be ignored, the tendency of omnipotence, its attitude of arrogance of belief in the conquest of human body and health. It demands a free hand .to do whatever it wants to do in the name of scientific progress, evidence, material and physical. Today as a result, nothing is coming on its way, and as a matter of fact must not be allowed to impede that progress.

It ignored many aspects of human experience, human values and culturally and traditionally accepted aspirations. They are considered irrelevant and mockery. In the name of science, many traditional, natural therapies long serving public healthcare are not recognised. The paranormal medicinal practices, i.e., that cannot be explained by science or reason that seems to involve mysterious forces, or supernatural are not recognised.

Challenging scientific ideas are seriously attacked as heretical. My drug, my theory, my right, my copyright, my patent attitudes have emerged. The commercial rivalry between countries, nations, academic, scientific theories, scientist are the common sights and medical industry has become globally competitive.

In today's world of health, the shadow is becoming more and more easy to see as identified under the following paragraphs.

It is reflected in the drive for supremacy, dominance of industrial medicine, even as mainstream health care system. It is also reflected in the serious damage to the natural self-healing power of the body, and the vast amount of money that is consistently being wasted by the people.

2. The Curtain Raiser

Sir William Osler (1905) said, one of the first duties of the physician is to educate the masses not to take medicines.

While Napoleon Bonaparte went one step further and said, "Medicine is a collection of uncertain prescriptions the results of which, taken collectively, are more fatal than useful to mankind".

Voltaire : The art of medicine consists in amusing the patients while nature cures the disease.

3. Violation of Medical Code

The Father of the Medicine, Hippocrates, profounded the ethical imperatives in medical profession which says, choosing the least costly route the least troublesome investigations, always keeping patient welfare in mind, seems not strictly followed today.

Hippocrates, the great priest of medicine, advised the physicians to accept the help of the laity in the treatment of disease, but his advice has seldom been followed.

Like the Kingdom of heaven, the kingdom of health has to be taken by storm, said J.W.K.

While practising, in discharging their basic duties, the medical doctors both of physicians, surgeons and others should make a promise that they keep the principles of medical profession. It is called hippocratice oath.

One of the oath principles is 'do not harm, a person's body'. In most cases, and many professionals are not abided by this fundamental duty.

Modern medicine has become so wide, and global there is a powerful commercial and profitable exploitation as an earning industry, extending its area and benefiting a few. There is a detailed and systematically formulated medical etiquette which the profession is required to wear in their practice. It is a set of moral principles or rules of profession of behavior that are generally accepted by the society to follow.

The system of law or written rules state how physicians, pharma companies strictly have to follow. The medical industry is violating to obey medical code of conduct, and violating the fundamental ethics towards of the patients.

The innocent public are exploited and in India there is no effective legal mechanism and awareness of medical field to get redressal as to the right to legal remedy, right to information, right to compensation and right to redressal in health sector. As a result, the patients are being cheated and grabbing their natural power of self heal of the body.

The allopathic physicians have formed as ring behaving in an autocratic manner. As a mainstream healthcare system, they are acting as rulers exercising complete power, and not caring about other opinions or therapies. Thus, modern medicine has become a system of dominating drug industry and ruling with absolute powers.

So, unless the patients are aware, in view of all this, in ascertaining their position and health rights, they may be facing an ever worse form primary healthcare system in the days to come which is going under the name of modern medical science.

The science too should understand the laws and power of nature, role of the Creator, because human body is not created by the medical science or allopathic physicians. The Creator knows better about the secrets and complexity of the body. Unless medical science understands these basic principles of nature, Creator and the body relations, it is not a true medical science.

Unnecessary human intervention is not warranted, physicians and surgeons have declared that certain organs of the body like tonsils, appendix, gall bladder, pineal gland, etc. are useless for the body and they have no special functions to perform. But from the Creator's point of view they are useful organs of the human body. They have their own secret functions for the existence of human beings. That is the true principle of health.

It is not at all wise to the nature of the body to fill the blood, stomach, immunity system with pills, drinks of synthetic drugs, poisonous medicine throughout the life.

I have every reason to emphasise that what a doctor has to do and what he is doing? Is he dictator of the treatment? They are not doing in educating the patient, side effects of the drugs nutritional value, friendly-interaction, need of instructing the patients how to be well, health management, wellness maintenance, keep well as well the art of living naturally and many reforming measures. Yet let us not forget the present patient is an example and model to his children and next generation. The physicians never explain and encourage our culturally accepted ancient therapy at all.

4. Drug Reactions

The commonly known side effects, after effects, ill affects, reactions, unwanted side effects of using pharmaceutical medicines are pains, nausea, vomiting, burning, depression, sweats, diarrhoea, numbness, dry, irritated skin, skin decolour, sleep disorders, fatigue, urine track infections, gas, constipation, weight loss, rash, irritating, eruptions, loss of hair, dehydration, headache, discomforts, debilitation, swellings, short lives, affecting longevity, loss of immunity, loss of body's self-healing power, general degenerative diseases, chronic-acute diseases, loss of the quality of life, addiction to a myriad of prescriptive drugs, pain killers (may cause patients to commit suicide), post surgical operative pains, emotions and effects, anxiety, interventions (impair ability), disrupts proper hormonal functions disabilities, changes in skin, muscles-internal organs, damage to peripheral nervous system, emission of blood, inside twisting, irritable bowel, lingering, long term pain, psychiatric disorders, mood disorders in young people, infertility problem, lower resistancy, drug related deaths, disability to innate body's natural power, stress, weakness, liver damage, accumulation of toxicity in the body and joints, immobility, tiredness, other detrimental health effects, dangers and limitations.

5. Suppressive Drugs

The modern medicine, called allopathic or industrial drugs, are mainly concerned with the identifying diseases, diagnosis, ascertaining symptoms of feelings from the patients and applying treatment with chemical substances which suppress the symptoms temporarily rather than eradicate the cause of the malady. The drug just works as a substitute.

Using drugs that they only weakening physically but also affecting mental, emotional, behavioural, equilibrium, weight loss, illness, very poor general health, debilitation of the body. These are some of the common distressing features of using synthetic substances. The final result is a complete curing but not real cure of cause, but the cause of the disease will remain intact.

Whether we want a real cure or masking the cause of the disease?

In most cases, the ailments may be the condition of the body but not a disease to be attended by a bio-chemic practitioners. It focusses solely only symptomatic treatment.

6. Non-physical Factors

Allopoathic medicine considers only physical, material aspects and ignores to support the body's natural ability to heal physically, mentally, emotionally and spiritually. The physicians do not consider the organic vision of health and wellness.

Natural body has inherent ability to establish self healing, self-repairing and here the role of physicians is to facilitate and improve the process by removing the obstacles on the way to optimal health.

Ignoring the mental, genetic, emotional, psychological and behavioural aspects in treatment and considering only the physical factors is not a real treatment.

Drug should not cause damage to the body, treating the cause and whole person and the physician to act as a teacher, prevention is better than cure are also equally important in any health care system.

7. New Era of Health Destruction

Today, we live not only in an age of materialism with fast changing life styles, dietary styles and occupational styles associated with occupational diseases and hazards, but also live in an age of synthetic medicine despite the warnings of physicians, and pharmacist about their dangerous limitations. We depend more on serum, vaccines, prescription drugs, over-the-counter pharmacy for all common complaints like antibiotics, painkillers and opiates. Already much harm and damage have been caused by extensive use of these chemicals.

The fast spread of industrial medicines, over abuse of drugs and increased dependence on physicians, specialists, multi-specialists all have combined impact to narrow the innate natural capacity of self-cure. I regard this as being dangerous sign to the public health.

Many doctors are ignoring health management, educational, counselling, nutrition and progressive naturopathic way of wellness as well as unnecessary intervention. We are not understanding what goes on the mainstream medicine and in which direction the pharmaceutical industry is moving? And where will it all end?

For instance, "The history of the art of medicine so teems with delusive, inefficient and capricious practices, fallacious and sophistical reasonings as to render it little more than chaos of error, a tissue of deceit unworthy of admission among the useful arts and liberal pursuits of man [Dr Blhne].

In recent past, we witness the fast emerging specialism, where in an area of study that doctors specialise in. It means they have degrees with a specialism in relation to the special or particular organ or part of the body in which they are specialists, for instance cancer specialist, urology, neurosurgery, artho, cardio, nephrology, gynochology, kidneys.

Now a days many graduate doctors prefer to specialise in a specific areas of health. They have formed as a class or ring.

The orthodox medical system called Allopathy has become the main stream of healthcare and it is even recognised by the government, institutions, where as the other healthcare systems like osteopathy, herbalism, naturopathy, urinopahy, ayurveda, biochemic system of medicine are considered as quackery.

There are a number of traditional, alternative, complementary and culturally accepted healthcare practices prevailing even today which are curing preventing, maintaining public health that have ability to cure many conditions declared incurable at the hands of the allopaths.

8. Vested Interest

Disease becomes a vested interest, and consciously or unconsciously, the doctors foster it as. It is quite common observation that doctors produce disease. Moreover, the whole system and philosophy of our dealing with disease is mistaken [Dr W.H. White].

Knowing well that there is no cure for arthritis or some other disorder, and the results of their prescription drugs are so well known, then why do the doctors continue to abuse and would not recommend other healthcare systems available. Today, we rarely come across enlightened and broad minded physicians, but exploiting innocent patient, or are patients meant for doctors? Modern medicine is thriving at the cost of public health and national health. Today, people are frightened and nervous of healing drugs, entirely created by the medical profession. Quack medicines are prescribed by quack professionals more harmful when the medicine enters into blood stream, lymp, as swallowed.

9. What is Evidence What is Not Evidence

Opinions are also there that urine therapy is not based on science and there is no scientific base, proof or evidence. Our evidence based science has been built on loose sand. There is a lot of difference between life and death. On similar lines, there is a lot of difference between long public experience, socially acceptable and scientific evidence and theories.

The structure of human body, and how it is made, the way it works, the normal functions of a living body, the chemical process that changes the food and water we have take into energy, and materials for growth into new cells, and waste products by means of chemical process, steroid substances produced naturally in the body which can be used to treat various diseases, like anobolic steroids, secretion like urine containing multiples of medicinal chemicals are all the wonders of creation not made by the so called science.

The physical science is just knowing the secrets of the body functioning only. There is no evidence base for body creation by the Creator.

Professor B.M. Hegde says, the present Randomised Controlled Trials and Linear Relations helps generate billions of dollars in chemical therapeutics even if that results in thousands dying of our efforts directly or indirectly.

What is Evidence-Based Medicine Today

Hegde quotes, A study by researchers in a respectable US University of the placebo-based RCT s did show that the contents of the placebo capsule, which need not legally be made known to the regulating agencies like FDA [Federal Drug Administration] were very potent substances that would show the company drug as very effective in comparison.

To cite an example, anti-diabetic drugs are usually compared with sugar filled placebo capsules! Many such glaring criminal activities have come to light now in the filed of evidence based medicine today.

10. Thriving on Diseases

There is a hue and cry from different quarters of the society that modern medicine is no longer a safety and harm-free healthcare system. It has become almost an organised commercial professional and exploitation establishment rather than health caring field.

Malpractices, exaggerated expenses, unnecessary operations, wrong counselling, stealing organs from the patients for sale and transplantation, creating fear, lack of professional talent, long list of prescription drugs, unnecessary investigations, check-ups, even surgeory costly tests like an x-ray for cough of short duration, ECG for any chest pain, CT for headache, abuse and over prescription of powerful medicine like antibiotics, painkillers, opiates, costly treatment for minor ailments and many more have become a common news everywhere.

Today, healthcare industry is run by money. Everyone involved in the medical industry is running after money. The need and greed for money is ever increasing in competitive way. There is no sympathy for patients, and humanitarian considerations are conspicuous by their obsence, no concern for suffering.

Today, it is clearly visible in the industry that there is a decline in the expression a strong feeling of sympathy for patients who are suffering from ailments and lack desire to help them.

11. Prescription Drugs

The published research findings on just how bad modern medicine really is has become so overwhelming. The number of people who die every year due to "correctly prescribed" prescription drugs has been estimated between 1,20,000 to 1,60,000 and this has been published in "peer journal "Death by Medicine". Even though strict laws, regulations are there for medical doctors, it cannot prevent or even reduce the number of annual deaths by medicine.

Though the public is well aware of all these on medical intervention and prescription drugs, they are continued to rely, approach drug physicians whenever they have a health problem.

It shows how ignorant the public really is in this area?

Although a large percentage of people do in fact do not know the adverse effects they receive from drugs, they still ask their MSs and MDs, surgeons for health advice.

I, therefore, appeal the public to be better and more aware, cautious and more aware dangers of drugs, before opting for alternatives. Some, however, will still seek advice from MDs, MSs, for the natural living, diet, life styles, occupational styles. This is very sad and occasionally even fatal mistake for worry. They are asked about something commons of healthcare of which he/she knows very little and worse still, they will generally prescribe drug, vitamins, hormones supplements instead of saying, that they have no adequate expertise in that area.

Some are so scarced of visiting specialists.

12. Over-the-Counter Drugs

In India particularly, the over, the counter medicine is very common and popular. It means availability of drugs and medicine that can be purchased at any medical store, by any body without a prescription by a qualified medical practitioner.

A prescription is an official piece of paper on which a doctor writes the type of medicine the patient to buy, which alone enables him to get required drug from a chemist or pharmacist. It is writing a prescription for a particular medicine.

The presription of a drug is a doctor's responsibility, on its basis the patients have to buy and use for a particular treatment.

A chemist or pharmacist should not sell certain drugs like painkillers, antibiotics, opiates, analgisics, poisonous and other harmful to health medicine and they should be made available only on doctor's prescription.

But this practice has been violated by the chemist, and they are selling liberally whomsoever approach a pharmacist, ignoring side effects, and reactions.

People are liberally buying and using without consulting doctors, it would have dangerous consequencies.

Over the counter prescription medicine, they are only substitutes, give symptoms relief, masking cause of malady, temporary, neutralisers, quick relief, healers, repetitive nature, blockers and they do not get out the root of the problem. For instance, the fermentation, gas, bloating and the use of over the counter drugs antacids only offer symptomic relief, acts only as a blockers, cannot cure cause.

Every person must be aware of the most common over the counter and prescribed killer drugs and antibiotics. The pharmaceuticals rank among the five highest causes of deaths in the US and that the US medical system is responsible for more deaths in the USA than anything else.

In India there are no strict restriction on over the counter sale of antibiotics especially high end antibiotics and other dangerous drugs. The medical stores are dispersing without prescriptions. It has become a common practice for doctors to prescribe liberally antibiotics, painkillers for all common conditions. There is no stringent policy on the use of antibiotics, painkillers.

Time is now ripen to introduce the systems like medical rating and cancellation of doctors registration if they violate.

13. Real Drug – Placebo Drug Trials

A drug before legally to be prescribed, it is generally put to test to decide in advance what is going to happen. The information is processed in a random order as the drug is put to test among random respondents. The test medication also may hamper the body's performance and wellness. Nearly, all drug trials scientifically are invalid due to the influence of the mind.

Mind is the main factor of determiner of the effectiveness of many drugs.

Some drugs have failed to out-perform placebo, and some drugs appear to out-perform placebo, and some drugs appear to out-perform.

Placebo in Clinical Trials : Drugs are tested among randomised respondents, placebo controlled studies. Under placebo trials, they are usually hoping to get the real drugs, not the placebo drugs.

The real drugs have the impact of negative side effects like constipation, sexual disorder, nausea, headache etc. It means among the randomised those who have used real drugs face these problems. The real drug show toxic side effects because the drug excites them. Those who have received placebo drugs, and no side effects, it means they are not receiving real drug.

The question of scientific validity remains, because of every randomised, double blind placebo-controlled drug study that have ever been conducted. There is a possibility of the researchers set the expectation of drug's results in the minds of the patients. It is whose minds make the effect real, not necessarily the drug. We cannot ignore the psychological effects of the minds of the patient but not just the drug itself.

So, the trials are not designed based on truly scientific, clinical trial using drugs. Cancer drug trial, blood pressure drug trial, painkiller drug trial or many other drug trial are of the some type.

Placebo is a substance with no effects that a doctor gives to a patient instead of a real drug. Placebos are used when testing a new drug or sometimes when a patient has imagined his illness.

14. Not An Exact Science

Modern medicine is not exact science, means, it is not correct in every detail, in every way. For instance, inspite of all scientific tests, to which a patient is subjected to in these days, different doctors are giving different diagnoses, and medicine for the same ailment. It is the best illustration to say that modern medicine is an inexact science. But just average approximation, trial and error.

Medicine is not an exact science. A good deal of what they were being taught was not true when they came to deal with life, they knew so little about the living body that they could not be dogmatic. They could only lay down hypotheses which would hold for a day and then pass away, and just as the teaching of seventy years ago seemed to them very curious and not very sound, so it would be exactly the same forty years hence [Surgeon General Sir Watson Cheyne, *The Times*, Oct. 2nd 1918].

To illustrate, a patient was suffering from simple ailment as headache. He consulted no less than ten doctors, in succession, ten different doctors have given ten different opinions. Their opinions are as follows:

First doctor told him he had an obstruction in his nose and must see a nose specialist.

Second doctor told him that there was nothing with his nose, but he must see an oculist.

Third doctor told him he had low blood pressure, and must have injections.

Fourth doctor told him he had high blood pressure and must diet himself to lower it.

Fifth doctor told him his liver was enlarged and he must have electrical treatment.

Sixth doctor told him his liver was not enlarged but it secreted insufficient bile.

Seventh doctor told him that his pituitary gland was not functioning properly, and he must have glandular injections.

Eighth doctor told him he was suffering from intestinal poisoning and he must cut down his eating and smoking.

Ninth doctor told him that his was a case of nervous debility and he must take some pills for the trouble.

Tenth doctor told him there was nothing really with him, and that his headaches were just headaches! [American Journal, *Liberty*, January 22nd, 1938].

15. Doctors Ring and Drugs Ring

With all these before us, I still feel that nothing concrete to change this has happened. It is why then every allopathic doctor so certify that he is right or they are right. Today, it is the only mainstream medicine and no other therapy, or healthcare system should enter and complete.

They formed as a ring. Great power, in the name of science. It means they are a group of professional people with expertise who are working together especially in secret, illegally, technically, scientifically, in the name of scientific progress.

Today, it is a common sight to see to have a drugs rings, pharma ring, doctors ring. It is owned and managed by vested interest, people who work for them together, and help each other in order to achieve their aim. It has become a global phenomenon today, a medical syndicalism. They have complete freedom or authority to do whatever they like. They are a group of separate practitioners which agrees to earn more by fixing fees arbitrarity, not allowing other pathies and therapies to complete with them. It is high time to protect the public from this dangerous health ring.

16. Dangers are not Revealed

Every chemical substance is not a natural substance but synthetic and has side effects gives reaction and as such harmful to the body.

The label, slip or tag attached on the bottle, or pack, pills strip do not give the buyer the useful information about the side effects, after effects, or reactions that the medicine gives that the patients do not know before.

This amounts to non-disclosure of material facts amounts to misleading, the important facts are suppressed. So, the effects of drugs which should be made known to the regulatory authorities and to the public.

Neither the physicians nor the pharmaceutical companies are voluntarily revealing nor educating the patients about their reactions, side effects, no one is caring the natural vitality of the body to promote and maintain, it is strong flaw.

17. Not A Universal Medicine

Prime Minister Manmohan Singh himself described the rising cost of healthcare as a challenge. He remarked, "Impact of high medical costs places an unconscionable burdon on the poor". He also advocated the need to work towards hassle-free and cashless out patient care in public hospital. "We are, therefore, focussing our attention on social security of the poor with regard to their healthcare".

"Thanks to our sustained high growth rates in recent years, we have been able to provide the higher levels of public investments needed in the health sectors. Public expenditure on health has increased from less than one per cent of our GDP in 2006-07 to an estimated 1.4 per cant of GDP by the end of the Eleventh Five Year Plan. But we will need to work harder and do more if we have to reach our goal of increasing public expenditure on health to at least two and half per cent of the GDP. Education and health will be the key prorities of the Twelfth Five year Plan."

18. Cashless

Prime Minister said, on a broader level, we need to accelerate our efforts to achieve our goal of providing universal access to health care at affordable cost for all our citizens. We are moving towards the creation of public health cadres to work for the prevention and control of diseases.

Cashless out patient care and specialised cadre for public health are major recommendations of high level expert group of the Planning Commission on universal healthcare which had also proposed cashless health package for all.

19. Decentralised Health

Universal healthcare requires to unite all pathies and therapies in a concerned effort to preserve, protect and promote every one's helath.

Urinopathic medicine has greater capabilities for decentralisd, individualised, household healthcare management. This will require greater awareness and focus on this therapy and information system that can support such decentralisation of healthcare.

20. Long Run Impacts

It is a open secret and everybody's personal experience that there is nothing new about the fact of harmfulness of prescription drugs for all ills come loaded with variant possible side effects, reactions ranging from mild, severe, acute killing, suicidal, life threatening. The dangerous adverse effects are not always immediately clear, know, exhibit until widely taken medication have been used for long term.

Many of the drugs in the young throughout life, for mood disorders, many vaccines, immunization medicine, pain may cause in adult physical, mental, nervous, immunity, psychiatric disorders. Varient drugs are taken since pregnancy, during labour, after delivery, child, adult, adoloscncy, old age. Many research studies have been conducted to study the effects of prescription drugs and side effects. They bring no benefit in any way except temporary masking of cause of disease.

21. Relevance of Vaccines and Sera

There are many physicians who do not have much commonsense for common ailments and prefer prescriptive pharmaceutical drugs. One must see the cause or root of the illness rather just masking symptoms of the illness. Though there are efficacious simple treatment for the complex problem, but they do not follow.

Today, it has become a practice of giving people variety vaccines especially by injection or drops in order to protect them against diseases. For instance, vaccinations against polio, vaccination against hepatitis B, and measles, vaccine diphtheria, asthma and immunisation against this or that disease and veneral diseases. The vaccines or serums, etc. have adverse effects and after some time produce chronic affections. Nevertheless, these facts do not made known to the general public.

Remember that there are many roads to health and many methods and means of treating disease. If we think for a minute what is the state of human blood, but what will be the impact on the immunity system, when one has been inaculcated with a variety of poisonous doses against various conditions. Dr Benchetrit remarked that vaccines and sera are to be chiefly responsible for the increase of those two really dangerous disease like cancer and heart disease.

Other Vaccines :

1. Two Types – Inactivated polio vaccine (IPV) (Imovax polio) and Oral Polio Vaccine (OPV), Pentaxim, too, has IPV.
2. Diphtheria toxoid contained in DTwP, DTaP, (Tripacel), DT or Td vaccines and Pentaxim.
3. Pertussis Vaccine contained in DTwP, DTaP (Tripacel), DT or Td vaccines and Pentaxim.
4. Measles Vaccine (contained in MMR [Trimovax], MR and measles vaccines).
5. Mumps vaccine (contained in Mumps and MMR).
6. Rubella Vaccine (contained in Rubella and MMR Vaccine).
7. Tetanus toxoid contained in DTwP, DTap (Tripacel) DT, TT or Td vaccines and Pentaxim.
8. Hepatitis – B Vaccine.
9. Hib (Acthib), Hib/DTwp(Tetrac thib) Hib//DTap (Acthib// Tripacel) Pentaxim.
10. Hepatitis A Vaccine (Avaxim 80 UPaediatric).
11. Varicella Vaccine (O Kavax).
12. Influenza Vaccine (Vaxigrip).

22. Tokens

It is the primary duty of a physician to teach, educate the patients by counselling about nutrition, life styles, self responsibility, health and wellness management rather than just resorting to a long list of prescription drugs. If they really do this I would applaud them.

They devote a very little time to each patient to clear off lot of tokens and wait list of patients every day at the cost of quality of consultation. Thus, modern physicians have their own way of doing things, some are outlawed, irrelevant, randomised. There are a very fewer citizen's healthcare practitioners working in public interest.

Truly, holistic doctors would actually be taking a step forward.

23. Regular Health Check up

These are the days of fast emerging specialists, super specialists, and multi-specialists physicians and surgeons. They are a group of doctors who are experts in a particular area of medicine, having professional degree with a specialisation in particular organ, or part/or parts of the body.

To cite for instance, a cancer specialist, cardio specialist, urology specialist, nephrology specialist, generalist, a gynaecologist, arthritist, opthomologist, neuro-surgery, etc., they are the doctors, physicians, surgeons, consultants treat the medical conditions and diseases in which they are studied and not other conditions.

The trend to day is that the public prefer to consult specialists. Sometimes they formed as a ring.

A human body has many organs or parts all are subject to disorders or diseases. It means a patient necessarily has to go around all the specialists. Every expert advices, as it has become a common practice today to have a regular health-check up. Just imagine for a movement the hell the patient visiting all the days for regular diagnosis, consultation, as well as consuming pretty prescription drugs. Nothing could be more dangerous than this to the health.

When one is good at immunity system one should ever go for regular checkup. A change in mode of living leads to a healthier one rather controlling with drugs.

24. Cancer

For over nearly seven decades the allopathic cancer researchers were fully engaged in the cause and cure of this deadly human ailment. But still they could not succeed more than nothing better than surgical, radium and chemotherapy. They themselves proved highly unsatisfactory results from these curing modalities.

Urinopathic medicine has been instrumental in preventing and curing many ailments where the allopathic medicine has evidently failed with thousands of pretty drugs.

"What cannot be cured by the forces of the body cannot be cured by the forces outside the body" [Dr T.W. Deachman].

There is no effective preventing nor curing medicine in allopathy for cancer/AIDS/HIV Positive and found failed to discover a medicine. Besides, after allopathic treatment many patients have suffered lingering, long term pain, and painful death. Antibiotics, surgeries, radiation treatment, chemotherapy and other related modern therapies are the lastest therapies, patients who have undergone these treatments have experienced nausea, vomiting, depression, sweats, diarrhea, numb finger toes, dry, irritated skin, sleep distruptions, fatigue weight loss, etc.

A Danish study findings published reveal that women who have undergone allopathic breast cancer treatment experience pain long after completing treatment. [Journal of American Medical Association, 11 issue November, 2009].

25. Monopoly of Medicine

Qualified physicians have come plenty as just another sect interfered with natural and traditional household medical practices. They are attempting to monopolise the health care industry in the name of science, proof and evidence at the expense of many other. They began to popularise pharmaceutical drugs and conspired against with natural therapies.

The medical doctors have taken control over of the largest part of the health care industry, and it has become as a mainstream system, as a result other health care systems and professions are prevented from sharing.

There are many alternate and traditional healthcare systems by which many medical conditions can be prevented and cured like clinical nutrition, botanical medicine, naturopathic obstetrics, homeopathic medicine, physical medicine, oriental medicine and psychological medicine, etc.

26. Attitudinal Changes in Patients

There are many roads to health. There are many effective complementary, alternative, traditional and naturopathic ways for treatment. The drastic change in life style changed the way that people think and feel about their health and selection of a suitable pathy or therapy. Today, the expectations of patients are quite different. They are in their hurry, very quick or more quick than usual, do not have enough time to attend to their health problems, impatient towards medical care.

They are not willing to spend time on slow and effective cure, but want quick results, no time to wait, and pressurise doctors for quick relief even at the cost of their health and side effects. Some diseases take time to get cured.

It has become a common sight at dispensaries requesting doctors for powerful medicine like antibiotics, painkillers and other opiates, quicker investigations, even minor puncturing skin. If quick results are not there, patients attribute as inefficient doctor, or otherwise they would like to go to another doctor.

So, to get quick results to keep the patient with him only, they prescribe powerful synthetic pharmaceutical drugs harmful to the health. The patients want quick recovery, but he does not know the drugs affects the immunity system leads other complications of degenerative diseases.

27. Repetitive Clinical Visits

Bulk of Indians are poor, some belong to the poorest section of the poorer. Illiteracy is high. Many are living below the poverty line, on poverty line and many are at average income bracket. When we look of all these encompassing facts and the trend of the direction in which modern medical industry is moving affecting every one of us in mainstream medicine. The medicine is prohibitive, costly, beyond the earning capacity to afford these prescriptive drugs, surgery and radiational needs. Many drugs typically proved themselves ineffective in combating the menance of cancer, AIDS, arthritis, asthma and other degenerative and opportunistic infections.

Finally, the natural, traditional household medical practice eliminates your more common, frequent and repetitive visits to your healthcare allopathic physician's clinics because no or less manifestations are realised. Let your body enjoy health and protect it by nature to be natural.

28. Drugs Killings and Road Killings

Drugs kill more people than road and vehicular accidents, according to recent reports. For many years, the predominant cause of injury related deaths in the USA has been traffic accidents. The data released by the Centre for Disease Control and Prevention, and the National Centre for Health Statistics, USA, indicate that 16 states now see more drug related deaths.

"How do we address these drugs as social concern?"

Drug companies are inventing expensive synthetic killing drugs, instead of people can use inexpensive natural, traditional, alternative medicine plenty available.

29. Loss of Health Bacteria

Human race is subject to many of common ailments people experience in modern days due to pollution, adulterated food, contaiminated water, lack of hygienic environment and other factors. We often visit allopathic physicians who play with us with antibiotics, pain relivers, symptoms masking prescriptions. However, common medications using for long term destroy our health bacteria, which is our first line of immune defence.

This leaves us wide open for numerous health problems later in life throughout. The modern medical remedies are not effective, unsafe, temporary reliever, healer as experience proved. It has been well felt by allopathic healers themelves in treating pain, discomforts, disorders, from a variety of ailments including common stomach-aches, fever flu, headches, sinus, bronchitis, asthama, cancer, arthritis etc.

30. Drug Abuse

A patient who has been undergoing drug treatment long suffers from depression, thought process, rational thinking, confusion, psychic side effects, suicidal urges, unintended effects, decreases state of mind, reduces in pulse control, psychological risk.

There is no any doubt about legitimate medication may adversely effects patients' body performance. It is true that many people do infact abuse narcotic, painkillers and other prescription drugs.

"There is currently a nation-wide epidemic of prescription drug abuse in this country. In a report by the National Centre on Addiction and Substance Abuse, it was revealed that this type of drug abuse had nearly doubled from 7.8 million to 15.1 million from the year 1992 to 2003". [quoting Dr Julian Whitaker in their book "*Side Effects*", Kenneth W.Thomas, Ron Gilbert and Gerd Schaller].

Abuse of prescription of drugs raised 400 per cent in 10 years. This is according to the study conducted by the Substance Abuse and Mental Health Service Administration of US Department of Health and Human service.

31. Drugs leads to Infertility

Constant use of common Painkiller drugs lead to male infertility and adverse effects on pregnant women also. For instance, the effects of phthalates, bisphenol-A and other toxins are already widely known that disrupt proper hormonal functions in human body. Recent studies also have revealed that common painkillers like asprin and Ibuprofen are far worse. These are the findings according to scientists from Denmark, Finland and France.

32. Poor Diagnositc Ability

In case of cancer, that every growth, lump or nodules that form on the human body is not a cancer, but in the name of medical science, or specialist, it is labelled as malignant. Operation treatment is advised or dangerous treatments are administered, breast or other part of the body is removed.

Dr Rabagliati, well known in the medical profession performed no fewer than 500 major operations for growths, and it was the uniform lack of success with the knife [Dr J.W. Armstrong].

There is always a conflict between the allopathic theories and evidence base and popular public experience, which proved that nature is far more efficient healer than are so-termed scientific methods which result in harm to the body, cutting and removing organs, besides the diagnostic ability of the physicians of medicine is not correct in all cases.

33. Autocracy – No Democracy

The treatment of this topic shows how little the spirit and philosophy of democracy prevails in modern medical profession, and should give citizens of the nation a slight knowledge of healthcare that is happening or about to happen. The physicians have no inkling they have that something is wrong in the system and inkling as to why so many modern diseases are still said to be incurable and why drugs are causing side effects.

It is more true to say that patients do suffer from damage of one organ or other by use of prescribed drugs. This poses a serious threat to search for more effectively treating natural methods. In many cases which are alleged by the doctors to be a particular complaint had been wrongly diagnosed

34. No Health Management

The result of suppressive treatment of poisonous drugs will have horrible after effects and the poison is absorbed into the body. We are not thinking what will be the after-effects of these synthetic drugs put into the body. Most people are now inclined to and familiar with modern medicine of dealing with common, chronic and acute diseases. Sufferers are preferred to go to clinics to get treated with injections, drugs and knifes. The drugs ignore the patients' wellness, wholeness and health management for the cause of disease curing. Allopathic physicians serve to treat by their own drugs from what they have studied.

Many poisonous drugs literally damage the tissues, nerve ends, destroy healthy cells which ought to be providing new cells for the knitting together of the skin elements. Burning, allergy, skin patches, destroying vitamins and balance are some other adverse effects of medicine.

35. Healthy Becoming Ill-healthy

A study on mild to moderate hypertension treatment showed that to save possibly one stroke death in the next five years in society we will have to unnecessarily treat 850 healthy human beings with powerful anti-hypertensive drugs intense side effects could seriously damage the health of at least 75 healthy people with some of them meeting their market prematurely. The number needed to treat in heart ailment drugs and cancer treatment could be much more than hypertension [Professor B.M. Hedge].

36. Silent Killers

All risk factors always are silent killers. Using antibiotics, painkillers, opiates, analgisics and other drug based medicines are silent killers in the healthy segment of the population. The existence evidence base is not science base. Medical science is not an exact science.

Human urine is a new evidence base for health and illness, Human health is a condition where human body cell is moving or working at exactly the same time and speed. Ill health, disorder, disease is a situation when cells do not move or work at exactly the same time and speed called synchronisation, (sync and out of sync). It is a sort of communication between them which breaks down.

37. Death By Medicine

According to the Centre for Disease Control and Prevention (CDCP), prescription of drugs kills about 40,000 Americans every year. And through over the counter drugs from pain relievers, cough medicine cause thousands of additional deaths. Drugs can sicken, and sometimes kill through side effects.

38. Drugs Lead to Vitamin Deficiency

It is true that certain drugs cause vitamin deficiency in the body, gas formation, pain, skin disorders. For instance cholesterol-lowering statin drugs are not safe to take for long because it may lead to vitamin 'D' deficiency in the body. Many realist of the allopathic medical professional are increasingly beginning to recognise the drugs leading to deficiency of certain natural substances in the body.

39. Drugs Accelerate Diseases

Recent studies have revealed that use of common pain medication accelerates the growth of cancer tumors. The author of the study is Dr Patrick Singleton. He revealed the analysed side effects of morphine that the chronic pain drug and opiate based pain medication contribute to the growth and spread of cancer cells. Use of urinopathic medicine is advised to prevent people from cancer.

Severe pain is experienced by the cancer patients. For relief, painkillers known as opiates are popularly used to treat both acute and chronic pain. In particular it is 'morphine' that is popularly used. But it fuels the growth and spread of cancer. Other painkillers are darvon and dorvocet. Taking high dose is risky. In united Kingdom and USA, they have banned them for some time.

40. Drug Resistance

The body becomes resistant to irrational use of antibiotics, gradually becomes multi-drug resistant. It poses high risk to the body. The multi drug resistant bacteria are E.coli, pseudomonas, acineto bacter and klebsiella they resist to powerful drugs to respond. The next higher potency drugs are carbapenems which are broad spectrum antibiotics. The next higher potency drug belongs to polymyxins. Later there is no higher drug. What next to the body?

In western countries, there is another predominant measure prevalent known as methicillin resistant staphylococcus aureus.

In India, there are no strict restrictions on over the counter sale of antibiotics especially high end antibiotics and other dangours drugs. The medical stores are dispersing without prescriptions. It has become a common practice for the doctors to prescribe liberally for all even common conditions, there is no stringent policy and enforcements on these aspects.

41. Suicidal Drugs

The allopathic physicians are generally prescribing powerful painkillers, antibiotics and other pharmaceutical drugs even for common human ailments. They are very harmful and dangerous to the body. They may be provoking people to suicide according to a study conducted by researchers in Ruhr University in Bochum, Germany. The painkiller drug's name is ziconotide. Painkillers no doubt certainly give temporary relief. This relief does not necessarily mean a cure. There is a lot of difference between temporary relief and real healing.

The modern approach is based on identifying and masking the symptoms, and suppressing the cause. It does nothing to address the underlying root cause of the problem.

42. Not Wellness Enhancement

Patients often become dependent on allopathic medication. They suffer from numerous side effects and most importantly the drugs worsen the overall health by repetitive and constant use of them. Every one must understand the difference between wellness enhancement real healing, masking disease, suppression of disease. This is the difference between disease cure, and disease management which underlines urinopathic medicine.

43. Doctors Produce Disease

It is a common observation that doctors produce disease. Morever, the whole system and philosophy of our dealing with disease is mistaken [Dr. W.H.White].

The vested intrests, corporate health care system, commercial orientation, highly specialisation, mass advertisement, publicity, etc. fostering fear in the minds of the public.

This led to the doctrine that the patients exist for the doctors, instead of doctors exist for the patients. There have been many more developments in recent years which are much to be deplored.

44. Surgical Effects

Drug prescription and surgery are generally the two main approaches of allopathic system. Even in surgery also many people suffered worse during post operation period. A new study findings published in the British journal of surgery found that surgical operations are not even always beneficial to the patients. Many patients end up in worse shape even after surgery than they were before.

According to the study findings, nearly 14 per cent of patients end up with more physical and emotional pain after the surgeries than before, and 25 per cent experience other effects.

45. Ignoring Alternate Healthcare

Most allopathic physicians still prescribe pharmaceutical drugs instead of effective natural therapies like urinopathic for many disorders, knowing well they continue to prescribe drug treatments to their patients like asprin, painkiller, antibiotics, brufin, etc.

46. Ulcers

Stomach ulcers and other ulcers can also develop as a result of excessive use of asprin and or non-steroidal anti inflammatory medications such as ibuprofen.

47. Loss of Natural Vitality

Many prescription medications may hamper a person's vitality, strength, body's performance and even affects health safety.

I do not think it should be the way as we see today, the situation will become worse if we depend more on prescription medication.

Drugs containing opiates which include many popular prescriptions like painkillers, antiobiotics, asprin, ibuprofen, statin, cancer drugs, surgeries whose legitimate medication may adversely affect everyone, children, adult, old men and all suffering from one or more invisible side effects, or after effects,

48. Legal battle

But many physicians do in fact abuse over prescription of narcotic and other harmful medication.

There is currently, global wise, nation wide epidemic of prescription of drug abuse. In a report by the National Centre on Additcion and Substance Abuse, it was revealed that this type of drug abuse had nearly doubled from 7.8 millions to 15.1 million from the year 1992-2003, there are instances wherein the patients are now suing the physicians, and the companies.

49. Pretty Pills

Pills, liquid look pretty good to swallow, but just suppress symptoms, masking symptoms, gives immediate and short relief, over the counter availability, but do not address the root cause of the disease, opiates, norcotic, aspirin, ibuprofen, seditious, analgesic, antacids, pantacids, painkillers, antibiotics, addictive pills, morphine, fuels cancer growth, etc. are harmful to the body.

50. Drug Testing

Any drug designed, invented, before putting into market is put to test in a clinical trial. Clinical trial participants are recruited through a trial that is advertised as testing a drug. Most of the results of the trial are average, sample, randomised under controlled conditions. Medical science is not an exactness but nearness, based on average results.

51. Allopathic philosophy believes only in the biochemistry, scientific basis, physical evidences, systematic recording of knowledge. But according to scientific prescription, the body is not made it is quite opposite to the principles of nature. Urine medicine is based on a holistic approach that goes beyond the above factors by focussing physical, mental, emotional and spiritual well-being.
52. Besides, another noteworthy feature is that the number of deaths either in hospitals or home under allopathic treatment amounted for more than the number under natural medical care systems. Many urinopaths have treated patients with auto-urine and not a single death was recorded among them all.

53. To Sum Up

All these factors collectively show an impact on the healthcare system which in turn is largely a reflection of the society and education system. One should not overlook the fundamental problems that lie in the educational system, and outside concerning political aspects.

Granting permission to medical colleges without necessary infrastructure, resource persons, faculty, laboratory, basic library and research facilities. Poor quality of teaching, privately managed colleges run with profit motives, lack of standards, uniformity. Medical education has become costly, more so with capitation fee of both graduate and undergraduate seats at an exhorbitant capitation fees and host of other known reasons are impacting on health industry. The healthcare system as well as industry is run by money, and run after money has become evident.

I have no spirit of hostility towards doctors, physicians and modern medical healthcare system. I am confined to the facts and personalities. I do not have any ulterior motives. I have no medicine to sell, I am not earning by practice, nor I have any magic remedy.

I must admit that I never fought against modern medicine on matters of principles, but I fight because it is affecting natural and national health of co-citizens on humanitarian grounds I write. It seems unnecessary to increase the volume of this book identifying the drawbacks and limitations of the modern medicine experienced by the present generation citizens.

I can say that definitely certain drugs have side effects and certainly affecting some parts or organs of the human body.

The physicians, or surgeons know pretty well, hope agree on this point, but keep the patients un-informed, or half-informed which is not ethical and human.

Dr J W. Armstrong remarked, "Most people died of the doctors and not of the disease."

With these few observations of public pulse I will end this topic, without prejudice.

I am sure that readers by now would have realised the dangerous effects of drugs and the impact of modern medicine. Never before we have any of these powerful pharmaceutical drugs that we have today.

Every one should be cautious and should use medicines with extreme caution.

"Think what means to your body it is open to you".

Stay out of the physicians office consult your own body's medicine. Most pharmaceuticals are toxic to the body.

We have deprived the nature of her power to do her work of healing. The nature should be given a chance to do her work in her natural way if we have faith in the Creator. We may not understand the mysteries of His power. Verily the Creator's ways are not our ways. Drink and believe.

Today, all over the world, people have been increasingly realising to go for alternative, traditional methods of healthcare for healing human diseases and disorders for most of the incurable conditions.

Drugs have toxic side effects and most pharmaceuticals are toxic to the body.

63
Epilogue

The exciting and thrilling primary healthcare therapeutic system of your own urine you have just read is though complete as completed in this volume, but is still incomplete. The subject of healthcare as medical area is an ocean, it is not possible to cover entirely here.

Whatever I have presented in this book, is only a part of it, but if followed is enough for good health and normal living as health management of wellbeing. This volume is developed by gathering shells and pebbles at the seashore, where the knowledge of medical science is unfathomable. In fact, it is based on my personal experience.

Thank you for sparing your valuable time to read what I have said about this ancient culturally accepted traditional household healthcare practice.

It is you, I aimed to delight. Changes are fast coming as conspicuously visible in health conditions, and emerging variety of innumerable and incurable diseases and disorders. It is also equally true in planetary system and the rest of cosmic field, environment. We are at crossroads, under healing crisis, looking at for something new to help the present and future generations to live happily with physical immortality and merry life.

By knowing and understanding the newness of urinopathic way of medical care, we hope to help the ailing human race with a mark for the better tomorrows' mankind. Our approach to this therapeutic practice sets us apart from knowing the miracles and implications and natural methods of public healthcare system, which we believe will allow us to aware, but practice and continuous researches are necessary to meet the fuller benefits.

Here are some of the features we have studied that made this book a noval and special. Read and re-read with open mind, without bias you feel newer, and newer experiences. It is exciting, enjoy.

This is being a new, disliked and hence a unpopular subject so far, is difficult matter to digest and convince the public. This reading may give rise to many queries, requiring additional information, seeking clarifications on certain things and doubts to be clarifited in the name of science.

The only remedy in such a case is to think and rethink, fresh and refresh your thoughts from new dimensions, put into practice, feel experiences so that all the things will be self explanatory, cleared and clarified.

But still those who may have any query personally to be clarified or wish to see further explanation on this thought provoking therapy please do so.

To end this book, I wish to say, that the therapy is though nauseate, to support the scientific approach to the subject is also emphasised.

In these words, even though inadequacy in the capacity of the author to discuss in more medical technical way of complex knowledge of human body. But the Creator who has designed this urinary mystery, and medicinal properties of the urine has the innate capability of prevention, healing and wellness.

The Creator's role has been demonstrated as emphasised in many religious texts. By reading these ancient, historical holy scripts we definitely, suitably alter and change our prior beliefs and fixed notions on urine as to how it is a waste product?

Many people including scientists, researchers, monks, yogis, investigators, ethists, logists, critics and general public are indeed being surprised by what the people tell, recovery stories, experiences and scientific supports.

It is open to the readers, critics and the medical doctors who say this therapy as mockery. It is only on the basis of such long experience, that this book has seen its completion and seen in this form, and light of the day.

So, I appeal to you the reader to read with open mind, and put into practice you reap the benefits like *Alladhin and Wonderful Lamps*. There will be no question of failure to cure when applied as it is the desire of the Creative Origin, designed by Him and arranged by Him, direct by the Origin in the creation of human form physical body itself.

So, it works from basic metabolic system, there is no question of changing the fucntioning, so the work is going on smoothly and continues utill human-form exists. As it is planned to be practised by the entire humanity, there is no discrimination and exception as to caste, creed, colour, sex, religion and the country.

This therapy is a life force vehicle of new life principle for good health, prolongation of life, longevity, deageing, physical without disease, decay and death. The genuine truth seeker can experience personally by travelling in this vehicle.

As repugnancy, the authors' ideas of this book may or may not be liked by the majority of the readers but I cannot avoid it. It is the nature of the subject, the fact is that the very nature of the natural therapy is that it is unavoidable and becomes indispensable to practice when there is no alternate curable therapy. This is the reason why urinopathy is often termed as last resort, but first choice.

To sum up, the author would like to appeal you that, if the reader finds anything in utility, use value or worthy of appreciation in this volume, that is the only reward and satisfaction to the author for his efforts in this useful and subject piss related. No doubt, the author would feel satisfied even if a few common, chronic and acute diseases be cured by external application of urine if not by drinking, are found to be of use by a reader.

I am deeply grateful to you all, for all this trouble I have given to you. Your interest demonstrates the lead for the literature on this therapy. As healthcare practitioners, you are telling us that this book adds value to your life.

As a result, you add value to me. We enjoy maintaining our dialogue with our friends. It is an exciting to read and talk to others.

Reread and enjoy. Thank you.

I heartly invite any comments, criticism, suggestions concerning this book and your recommendations to improve the quality of the book in its next edition.

All great thoughts begin as blasphemies.

Dr C.S. Rayudu

Address :
D. No. 28-3-393
Sarada Nagar
Anantapur (PO) 515001
Andhra Pradesh (India)
Phone : Land : 08554-272182
Cell : 9848618095
E-mail ID : rayudu.choudem@gmail.com

Index

A

Abdominal 223
Abominable 105
Abstract 250
Abu Yusuf commented 32
Abu Yusuf commented 32
Abuse of drugs 302
Accumulated toxins 54
Acid 46
Acid base 85
Acidity 46
Acne 131
Acne 183
Acquired Immune Deficiency Syndrome 201
Acupressure 130
Acute 11
Acute 11, 153
Acute diseases 129
Addictive pills 318
Adenylate cyclase 47
Adhesion 38
Adolescent 271
Adolescent age 271
Adoloscncy 309
Adulterated food 313
Adulteration 250
After effects 54
Aftershave lotion 172
Age of materialism 302
Agni 288
Agonising journey 220
AIDS 9, 11
AIDS 9, 11
AIDS, arthritis, sinus 13
AIDS, arthritis, sinus 13
Ailing human 12, 28
Ailing human 12, 28
Ailing human race 130
Ailing human race 221
Ailing humanrace 216
Ailment 24
Ailment 24
Ailment of anaemia 166
Ailments 153
Ailments 98
Ailments of asthma 163
Ailments of human race 131
Ajna chakra 287, 288
Ajna chakras 288
Alimentary canal 22, 192
Alimentary canal 22, 43
Alkali 46
Alladhin and Wonderful Lamps 322
Allergic reactions 234
Allergy 181
Allopathic 13
Allopathic 13
Allopathic medicine 33
Allopathic medicine 33
Allopathic physicians 216
Allopathy 13, 17
Allopathy 13, 17
Alternative 99

Alternative healing agents 42
Alternative medicine 230
Alternative therapeutic modalities 95
Amar 27
Amar 27
Amar 27
Amar 27
Amaroli 29
Amaroli 29, 248
Amaroli 9, 27
Amaroli 9, 27
Amicable 54
Amino acids 135
Ammonia 191
Ammonia 46
Ammonia products 135
Amniocentesis 35
Amniotic fluid 191
Amniotic fluid 35, 37
Anaemia 48
Anahata 288
Analgesic effects 167
Analgisics 218
Analgisics 305
Anatomical 253, 272
Anatomy 19
Anatomy 19, 286
Ancient nature-based system 233
Ancient roots 14
Ancient roots 14
Ancient texts 215
Ancient therapy 301
Anecdotal 211
Anger 277
Angina 173
Animal's urine 149
Aniretrovial 207
Annihilater of senility 283
Annihilator of senility 247
Annihilator of senillty 141
Anobolic 304
Antaratma 294
Anti cancer agent 192
Anti-ageing 12
Anti-ageing 12
Antibiotic treatment 65
Antibiotics 117
Antibiotics 302
Anti-bodies 12, 13
Anti-bodies 12, 13
Antibodies 55
Antibody 192
Anti-body agent 65
Anti-carlivogenic 65
Anti-convulsive 65
Antidote 30
Antidote 30
Antidote 65
Anti-fungal medicine 210
Antigen 64
Antigen receptors 181
Antigens 13
Antigens 13, 192
Antineoplaston 12
Antineoplaston 12
Anti-neoplaston 65
Antineoplastons 48
Anti-obesity 12
Anti-obesity 12
Antiperspirants 171
Anti-poison 65
Antiseptic 184
Antiseptic 39
Anti-urinopathic movement 122

Anti-viral 65
Anti-viral and anti-bodies 209
Anu 291
Anu 293
Anus 22
Anus 22
Anxiety 266
Anxiety 271, 280
Armamentarium 228
Art of meditation 97
Arteries 23
Arteries 23, 172
Arteriosclerosis 176
Arthritis 180
Arthritis 97
Artificial heart 175
Artificial intelligence 255
Asanas 283
Assemblage of cells 20
Assemblage of cells 20
Asthma 22
Asthma 22, 64
Astral body 289
Astral centres 286
Atma sakthi 254
Atom 52
Atomised form of life 291
Atoms 86
Aura-powers 29
Aura-powers 29
Autogeneous 28
Autogeneous 28
Autogenous 40, 101
Autogenous urine 129
Auto-immunity system 64
Automatic muscular pump 23
Automatic muscular pump 23
Auto-urine 14, 23, 25
Auto-urine 14, 23, 25
Auto-urine 23
Auto-urine 23
Auto-urine therapy 13
Auto-urine therapy 13
Auto–urine therapy 14
Auto–urine therapy 14
Auto-urine therapy 14, 25
Auto-urine therapy 14, 25, 41
Aversion to drink urine 14
Aversion to drink urine 14
Ayurveda 13
Ayurveda 13, 95
Ayurveda 8, 30
Ayurveda 8, 30
Ayurvedic 13
Ayurvedic 13
Ayurvedic medicine 229

B

Bacteria 257
Bacteria 65, 72
Bacterial properties 131
Bad energy 283
Baldness 183
Bandage 60
Barbarous superstitions 14
Barbarous superstitions 14, 147
Barometers 293
Bathe 60
Bbloating 306
Bblood pressure 307
Bbroad minded physicians 303
Beauty parlors 172
Bedrock philosophy 98
Behavioural disorder 152
Beverages 78

Bhavprakasha 30
Bhavprakasha 30
Bible 220
Bible is the holy 31
Bible is the holy 31
Biochemical analysis 12
Biochemical analysis 12, 89
Bio-chemistry 28
Bio-chemistry 28, 42
Biological 11
Biological 11, 64
Biological characteristics 45
Biological indicators 235
Biological process 71
Biology 231
Bio-mechanism 57
Bio-medicine 91
Biopsy 196
Bisexuality 212
Bisphenol 314
Bitter sharp taste 46
Bitter taste 133
Black water fever 222
Bliss unhappiness 265
Blisters and herpes 187
Blisters fistules 183
Blocked sinuses 60
Blood and lymph 225
Blood capillaries 84
Blood circulation 86, 98
Blood clot 173
Blood Derivative 76
Blood filter 72
Blood filter process 72
Blood glucose 234
Blood moves 86
Blood pressure control 98
Blood product 78
Blood sugar 84
Blood vessels 22
Blood vessels 22
Bloodstream 74
Blossom of Bud 292
Blow drying 182
Bodily disorder 181
Bodily disorders 40
Bodily medicine 40
Bodily secretion 84
Body excrete 131
Body excrete 243
Body Mind Spirit 297
Body tissues 39
Bodycell 316
Body-heat 20
Body-heat 20
Body-made 19
Body-made 19
Body-made liquid 247
Body-made medicine 181
Body-mind-spirit medicine 249
Body-Mind-spirit-medicine 251
Boiled urine 164
Boiled urine 59
Bone cancer 180
Bone marrow 166
Bones 23
Bones 23
Boredom and fatigue 272
Botanical medicine 31
Botanical medicine 31
Bowel disorder 152
Brahma nadi 288, 289
Brahmadwara 289
Brahman 289

Brahmananda 282
Brahmanandam 249
Brain 254, 259
Brain and spinal cord 279
Brain cells 254
Brain damage 254
Brain tumour 185
Bramha Granthi 288
Breast 195
Briktha 291
Bronchi 22
Bronchi 22
Bronchial 216
Bronchiatic 60
Bronchitis 22
Bronchitis 22, 101
Bruises 215
Brushing 108
Bubbles 60
Budhic 295
Builds vitality 66
Burns 183
Butter 78
By-product 71
C
Calcium 182
Calcium 49
Camel's urine 32
Camel's urine 32, 149
Canalis centralis 289
Cancer 13
Cancer 13
Cancer cells 191
Capacity 271
Capillaries 21
Capillaries 21
Capping 217
Capricious practices 303
Carbamide 135
Carbohydrates 50
Carbon 50
Carbondioxide 22
Carbondioxide 22
Cardiac 21
Cardiac 21
Cardiac transplantation 175
Cardiovascular 12
Cardiovascular 12
Cardio-vascular 131
Care product 182
Cartilage 180
Cashless out patient 309
Catasteroids 47
Catechol amines 47
Causative factors 92
Causes of diseases 53
Cavity 37
Cell 19
Cell 19
Cell banks 38
Cell treatment 223
Cells 19
Cells 19
Cells 19
Cells 19, 47, 78
Cellular level 131
Cellular structure 225
Cementing 217
Centenarian 220, 222
Central Nervous System 21
Central Nervous System 21
Central nervous system 261, 279
Cervical 207
Cervix 38

Chakras 286
Changing cosmic material 249
Changing life styles 302
Chap 183
Chebula 31
Chebula 31
Cheese 78
Chemical element 30
Chemical element 30
Chemical fertilisers 228
Chemical imbalance 253, 256
Chemical imbalances 227
Chemistry of a drug 256
Chemotherapy 186
Chest discomforts 173
Chewing food 164
Chickenpox 43
Chief life 296
Chief wave 296
Chitra 288
Chlorine 51
Chocolates 78
Cholesterol 173
Cholesterol 316
Chronic 11
Chronic 11, 63
Chronic ailment 24
Chronic ailment 24
Chronic aliments 101
Chronic Diseases 153
Chronic internal ailments 149
Chronic pain drug 316
Chronic-acute disease 301
Circulatory System 23
Circulatory System 23
Circulatory systems 225
Cistern 31
Cistern 31, 220
Claustrophobic 269
Cleaning process 65
Cleans bowels 43
Cleansing agent 65
Cleansing bowl 192
Clinical investigations 231
Clinical Nutrition 231
Clinical nutrition 96
Clinical trial 234
Clot formation 173
Clotting dissolving agent 173
Coating 292
Code of conduct 258
Co-exist 13
Co-exist 13
Cold sweat 173
Colloids 51
Colon 195
Colonialism, 33
Colour baldness 183
Combating the menaces 12
Combating the menaces 12
Complementary medicines 41
Complex problems 133
Comprehensive treatment 42
Conceptual-cu 8
Conceptual-cu 8
Condensed energy 291
Condifolia 31
Condifolia 31
Conjunctivitis 164
Consciousness 258
Conspiracy 242
Constipation 187, 223
Constitutional change 67
Consumptive 221

Contaiminated water 313
Contamination–free 230
Contaminations constituents 230
Contraception 177
Contraceptive 48
Conventional medicine 94
Coping 271
Copious vomiting 187
Cornification 37
Coronary disease 172
Corporeal existence 247
Corpuscles 48
Cortico-steroids 39
Cosmetic cream 135
Cosmetic products 69
Cosmetic purposes 171
Cosmetic purposes 69
Cosmetic surgery 69
Cosmic influence 286
Cosmic Kundalini 292
Cosmic life 284
Cosmic troubles 248, 250
Co-terminus 13
Co-terminus 13
Counseling 97
Counselling 231
Counselling urinopaths 99
Counsellors 101
Cow's urine 149
Cranial nerves 21
Cranial nerves 21
Crbapenems 316
Creatinine 52
Creative Origin 296
Creator of the body 147
Crippling 180
Critics 322culturally accepted 321
Crollary 259
Crowning glory 182
Crusaders 9
Crusaders 9, 99
Crystalline 35
Cuboidal 20
Cuboidal 20
Cultural acceptability 25
Cultural acceptability 25, 101
Culturally acceptable 238
Culturally accepted medicinal 281
Cum-analytical 8
Cum-analytical 8
Curative 79
Curative efficacy 9
Curative efficacy 9, 101
Curative medicines 55
Curative modalities 111
Cure infections 65
Cure par excellence 210
Curing 110
Curing medicine 312
Customisation 42
Customotised 231
Cytoplasm 20
Cytoplasm 20
D
Daily treatment 208
Damara Tantra 26
Damara Tantra 26
Dandruffs 171
Danger of drugs 57
Dangerous limitations 302
Dangers of drugs 305
Dark colour 45
Ddrug abuse in 314
Dead cells 67

Deadly disease 201
Deafness 167
Deageing 295
Deageing 66, 92
Death bed patient 246
Death by Medicine 305
Debilitation of the body 302
Debility 250
Decentralisation 309
Decentralisation of healthcare 309
Defence mechanism 205, 225
Deficiency syndrome 65
Degenerative 11, 13
Degenerative 11, 13, 101
Degenerative diseases 223
Degenerative diseases 51
Dehydroepi 12
Dehydroepi 12
Dehydroepiandrosternoe 178
Delicious 78
Delusive 303
Demons 29
Demons 29
Denialists 122
Density 46
Deodorants 171
Deoxygenated 23
Deoxygenated 23
Depression 264
Depression 279
Dermis 21
Dermis 21
Destroying senility 247
Deter ageing 178
Deteriorating health condition 7
Deteriorating health condition 7
Detoxification 42, 57
Detoxifying agent 13
Detoxifying agent 13
Detrimental bacteria 211
Devoid 250
Diabetes 174
Diabetic 46
Diagnose 54, 68
Diarrhea 187, 210
Dictum 189
Diet 45
Dietary proteins 135
Dietary style 173
Dietary styles 162
Dietary styles 302
Dietetic 96
Digestive problems 223
Digestive System 22
Digestive System 22
Digestive system 22
Digestive system 22, 77
Dilute 108
Diphtheria 220
Diphtheria 310
Directin 194
Discomfort 91
Disease causing bacteria 131
Disease progression 206
Disease-free 147
Disease-free body 13
Disease-free body 13
Disease-resistant 68
Diseases 12, 28
Diseases 12, 28
Disguest beliefs 147
Disgust 77
Disgusting 78
Disorders 314

Disposable syringes 213
Dissolved substances 84
Dissolving cancer cells 192
Distal 84
Distils 48
Distressing features 302
Diuretic 136
Diuretic effect 167
Divine nectar 26
Divine nectar 26
Divine panacea 12
Divine panacea 12
Divine radiance 126
Divine radiance 247
Divine sight 92
Divine vision 247
Doctor of Divinity 161
Doctor to doctor 220
Documentary evidence 122
Documented sources 119
Dogmatic 307
Domicilliary care 175
Double blind placebo-controlled 306
Dramatic health 9
Dramatic health 9
Dramatised diagnosis 241
Dropsy 33
Drug 40
Drug abuse 318
Drug consumption 217
Drug industry 300
Drug physicians 305
Drug qualities 51
Drug resistance 166
Drug substances 111
Drug therapies 230
Drug trial 307dDrug trials 306
Druggist 137
Druggists 242
Drugless 40, 103
Drugless drug 12
Drugless drug 12, 218
Drugless natural drug 40
Drugless Therapy 8
Drugless Therapy 8
Drugs Killings 313
Drugs rings 308
Dry hair ends 182
Dsiscomforts 314
Ducts 23, 24
Ducts 23, 24
Duodenal ulcers 163
Dup dup 23
Dup dup 23
Dysfunction 227
E
Ear deficiencies 167
Ear drum 167
Earth kundalini 292
Ecstatic delight 249
Eczema 11
Eczema 11
Edema 43
Effectiveness 17
Effectiveness 17
Efficacy 17
Efficacy 17
Electric charge 19
Electric charge 19
Electro-cardiogram 234
Elixir of life 39
Embryo 37
Emotion 277
Emotional 53

Emotional disorder 152
Emotional Imbalances 155
Emotional outburst 277
Emotional problems 264
Emotionally 42
Emotions of a body 260
Empirical studies 110
Endocrinal glands 142
Endocrinal systems 259
Endocrine 297
Endocrine glands 24
Endocrine glands 24
Endocrine System 24
Endocrine System 24
Endodermis 21
Endodermis 21
Endometiosis 179
Endometriosis 223
Enema 24
Enema 24, 190
Energetic medicine 127
Energises the senses 125
Energy 283
Enzyme 175
Enzyme 50
Enzymes 226
Epidermis 21
Epidermis 21
Epilepsy 196
Epithelium 21
Epithelium 21
Equilibrium 302
Era of rejuvenations 117
Eruptions 171
Erythropoietine 166
Erythropoietine 47
Erythro-poietine 48
Eshical imperatives 300ethists 322
Eternity 248, 258
Etheric matrix 249, 282
Ethical base 258
Ethnical 101
Etio pathological entities 235
Euphoric 277
Evil eyes 29
Evil eyes 29
Exact science 307
Excited 277
Excitement 279
Excretory glands 85
Excretory system 22
Excretory system 22
Exhalation 22
Exhalation 22
Exigencies 101
Expert system 20
Expert system 20
Expulsion of carbon-dioxide 252
Extensive bibliography 9
Extensive bibliography 9
Exthusiasm 50
Extracellular fluid 37
Exuberance 67
Exuberant 66
Exuberant health 222
Eye opener 220
Eyelids 21
Eyelids 21
F
Fabulous efficacy 14
Fabulous medical 36
Fabulous medicinal 147
Fabulous quality 66
Fabulous unknown capability 12

Fabulous unknown capability 12
Face cream 172
Face-beauty 172
Facial expressions 277
Fallacious 303
Family practice 101
Fasting 98
Fatal 245
Fatal 91
Fatigue 173
Fatty food 174
Fbulous efficacy 14
Federal structure 120
Fermentation 306
Fertilisation 36
Fertility drugs 67
Fertility hormones 176
Fetas urine 35
Fibromyalgia 97
Fiction 250
Figure change 67
Filtration 83
Filtration process 105
First-aid 215
First-choice 237
Flawless complexion 171
Flow of urine 167
Fluid retention 223
Foetus babies 35
Food allergies 223
Force 92
Foul smells 217
Foul wound odour 184
Friendly-interaction 301
Frightened 166
Frustration 252
Fumigation agents 230
Function 64
Fundamentalists 122
Fungal 225
Fungus 183
Future agenda 17
Future agenda 17
Future anxiety 272
Future Medicine 13
Future Medicine 13
G
Gaduchi 31
Gaduchi 31
Gall bladder 87
Gangrene 221
Gargle 146, 147
Gargling 61
Gases 72
Gas-like pain 173
Gastric ulcer 43
Gastric ulcers 163
Gastrointestinal 297
Gauls 165
Gauls 32
Gauls 32
Gender 182
Generalisations 110
Genes 19
Genes 19
Genetic 53
Genetic inheritance 206
Genetic material 19
Genetic material 19
Genetics 265
Genital area 108
Genital organs 23
Genital organs 23, 178
Genital urinary track 139

Germs 53
Gestures 278
Giddiness 295
Gland 24
Gland 24
Glands 249
Glaucoma 222
Glaucoma 43
Global market 233
Global relevancy 119
Globular 20
Globular 20
Glucose 49, 83
Glutamine 136
Glutamine 191
Glutamine level 191
Goal of health 10
Goal of health 10
God Shiva 248
God's healing 208
Goddess Parvathi 249
Gonorrhea 43
Gonorrhoea 204
Good memory 29
Good memory 29
Gout 180
Gradhisthana 287
Grey hair 183
Gum problem 165
Gum problem 217
Gum problem 61
Guru 28
Guru 28
Gyanendrias 289
Gynochology 303

H

Hair follicles 21
Hair follicles 21, 216
Hair loss 182
Hair pulling 271
Hair-pulling 271
Hallucination 27
Hallucination 27
haos 303
Harm-free healthcare 304
Harmful substances 64, 71
Harmful treatments 187
Harmless drug 27
Harmless drug 27
Harmless urine therapy 12
Harmless urine therapy 12
Hashimoto's disease 223
Hassle-free 309
Hatha' yoga 252
Havoc 33
Healing crisis 118
Healinghuman diseases 320
Health 97
Health enhancement 7
Health enhancement 7
Health for all 234
Health management 187, 215
Health package 309
Health Philosophy 7
Health Philosophy 7
Health practice 233
Health promotion 101
Health service 8
Health service 8
Health service landscape 7
Health service landscape 7
Health strategy 8
Health strategy 8
Health treasure 11

Health treasure 11
Healthcare hierarchy 8
Healthcare hierarchy 8
Healthcare industry 7
Healthcare industry 7
Healthcare system 7
Healthcare system 7, 118
Heart attack 172
Heart attacks 175
Heart disease 97
Heart muscles 175
Heart pounding 172
Heart surgery 173
Heavenly nectar 129
Heaven–Urine 75
Heightens visualisation 141
Hemoglobin 133
Hepatitis 195
Herb 46
Herbal auto-urine 31
Herbal auto-urine 31
Herbal beauty parlour 172
Herbal medicine 223
Herbal medicine 95
Herbal mixture 29
Herbal mixture 29
Herbal plants 31
Herbal plants 31
Heredity 53
Heritage 234
Hermits and yogis 238
Hetrosexulality 212
Hhepatitis B 310
Hherbalism 303
Hidden medicine 218
High blood pressure 175
Himalayan yoga guru 215
Hindu God Lord Shiva 41
Hindu philosophy 27
Hindu philosophy 27
Hindu Scriptures 25
Hindu Scriptures 25
Hindu society 25
Hindu society 25
Hindu texts 26
Hindu texts 26
Hindus believe 237
Hippies 97
Hippocrates 300
HIV 11
HIV 11
Holism 81
Holistic 24
Holistic 24, 42, 117
Holistic 311
Holistic approach 54
Holistic combination 62
Holistic medicine 25
Holistic medicine 25, 53
Holistic Medicine 69
Hollow viscus 87
Holy Bible 31
Holy Bible 31
Holy spirit 257
Homeopathy 13
Homeopathy 13, 223
Homeostasis 92
Homosexual 207
Homosexuality 212
Hooping cough 60
Hormonal imbalance 176
Hormonal imbalance 47
Hormonal system 252
Hormone 47

Hormones 24
Hormones 24, 35
Household medical 94
Household medicinal practice 7
Household medicinal practice 7
Household practice 11
Household practice 11
Human ailments 79
Human anatomy 19
Human anatomy 19
Human excreta 71
Human Immunodeficiency Virus 201
Human kingdom 138
Human nectar 132
Human organism 48
Human physical figure 285
Human race 118
Human spirit 257
Human system 53
Humanitarian grounds 319
Humanitarian service 222
Humanrace 201
Humilitation 270
Hydration 46
Hydrogen 46, 84
Hydrotherapy 231
Hydrotherapy 96
Hydroxy-steroids 47
Hygienic 184
Hygienic 72
Hyperactivity 272
Hyperactivity 66
Hypertension 174
Hypertonic 142
Hypophysical hormones 48
Hypotheses 307

I

Ida 287
Idleness 166
Ill-effects 54
Illnesses 192
Ills 63
Illusion 250
Image devices 234
Immemorial 117
Immigration 33
Immortal physically 249
Immunisation 65
Immunity deficiency 226
Immunity system 12, 13
Immunity system 12, 13, 48
Immunization 209
Immunotherapy 192
Immutability 250
Imperishability 27
Imperishability 27
Impotency 176
Improve protective mechanism 209
Impurities 139
Impurities 192
Inactiveness 187
Incidence of deaths 210
Incredible cure 189
Incredible urine 243
Inculcating awareness 188
Incurability 218
Incurable ailments 281
Incurable diseases 12, 14
Incurable diseases 12, 14, 48, 109
Incurable human ailments 111
Incurable human ailments 152
India's cultural system 94
Indian culture 230

Indiscriminate doses of drugs 187
Individualised 215
Industrial medicine 117
Industrial Medicine 33
Industrialisation 7
Industrialisation 7, 33
Infallible 245
Infections 64
Infertility 176
Infertility 314
Infertility 67
Infertility problems 81
Inflammation 61, 97
Inflammatory 318
Ingestion 22
Ingestion 22
Ingredients 170
Ingredients 77
Inhalation 22
Inhalation 22
Inhaling and exhaling 163
Inherent Tendencies 155
Initial aversion 107
Injected 61
Innate capability 189
Innate natural power 92
Inner kingdom 282
Innocent unwary 130
Innovative studies 122
Innumerable 12
Innumerable 12
Inoculation 65
Inoculations 129
Insulin 47
Insulin secreted 84
Intangible power 127
Intelligence 254
Inter cellular substances 20
Inter cellular substances 20
Internal organs 64
Intervention 54, 80
Interventional material medicine 234
Interventional strategies 261
Intestines 24
Intestines 24, 86
Intoxicating 192
Intravenous drug 212, 213
Intravenously 141
Intrinsic 103, 132
Intrinsic Medicine 41
Intrinsic therapeutic properties 217
Intrinsic value 151
Introspection 254
Intuition power 247
Invading bacteria 226
Invading lassitude 187
Invasive 185
Investigations 109
Iodine 49
Ions 84
Iron 49
Irritability of temper 221
Irritable mood 277
Irritation 164
Islamic Scriptures 32
Islamic Scriptures 32
Isolating 111
Isopathy 151
Itching 98

J

Jaundice 195
Jaundice 220
Jeevanmukti 294
Jelly 20

Jelly 20
Joints 59
K
Kamam 287
Kanda 287
Kapalis 159
Karma 295
Karmendriyas 290
Karmic conditions 245
Ketones 46
Kidneys 23
Kidneys 23, 47
Kidneys 303
Kindling Kundalini Power 290
Knees 180
Koshtha 31
Koshtha 31
Kundalini 26
Kundalini 26, 282
L
Label 308
Larynx 22
Larynx 22
Lemon 46
Leprosy 125
Leprosy 167
Leprosy ailment 167
Leucocytes 195, 211
Leucocythaemia 222
Leucoderma 183
Leukaemia 222
Life 92
Life cycle 19
Life cycle 19
Life force 249
Life of changelessness 250
Life style 173
Life Style of Yogis 28
Life Style of Yogis 28
Ligaments 180
Light colour 45
Linga 'sarira' 289
Lingering 301, 312
Lingual gland 22
Lingual gland 22
Locomotion 20
Locomotion 20
Logists 322
Long teeth stay 217
Longevity 17
Longevity 17, 66, 92, 131
Longevity 27
Longevity 27
Lord Shiva 26, 28, 29
Lord Shiva 26, 28, 29, 249
Lose of sensation 166
Lub lub 23
Lub lub 23
Lumbago 43
Lumbar region 85
Lump 185
Lumps 173
Lung diseases 176
Lung fluid 37
Lungs 22
Lungs 22
Lungs bronchial 65
Lympatic system 253
Lymphatic membrane 21
Lymphatic membrane 21
Lymphatic system 94
M
Madina 149
Magic liquid 39, 40, 111

Magnetic therapy 130
Mahabharata 25
Mahabharata 25
Mainstream 25
Mainstream 25, 215
Mainstream allopathic 80
Mainstream therapy 237
Malady 25, 151
Malady 25, 69
Malaria 222
Male hormone 177
Male impotency 176
Malfunction 227
Malignancies 205
Malignancy 185
Malnutrition 209
Malnutrition 96
Malpractices 304
Mammary glands 24
Mammary glands 24
Manas 290
Mandibular gland 22
Mandibular gland 22
Mania 271
Manna 103
Manna from heaven 208
Mapping of the brain 258
Marital separations 272
Marriage maladjustments 272
Marvelous medicinal 67
Masking symptoms 91
Masking the symptoms 25
Masking the symptoms 25
Massaging 59
Massaging 97
Mastectomies 312
Material evidence 256
Maya 295
Mca and sulpher 126
Measles 310
Mechanism 225
Medical dogma 218
Medical purposes 32
Medical purposes 32
Medical science 9
Medical science 9
Medical secrets 11
Medical secrets 11
Medical therapy 11
Medical therapy 11
Medication 309
Medicinal 31
Medicinal 31
Medicinal constituents 33
Medicinal drug 11
Medicinal drug 11
Medicinal plants 95
Medicinal secrets 8, 11
Medicinal secrets 8, 11
Medicinal substances 39
Medicine 117
Medicine bag 40
Meditation 251
Meditation 29
Meditation 29
Meditation 96
Melanin pigments 21
Melanin pigments 21
Melantonin 28
Melantonin 28
Menstrual problems 179
Mental abennation 252
Mental abilities 97
Mental age 263

Mental illness 21
Mental illness 21
Mental practice 282
Mental predisposition 57
Mental pressure 271
Mental state 45
Mental system 260
Mentally depressed 188
Mentally ill 263
Mentarium 228
Mercury activity 293
Mercy of the Creator 208
Merry life 286
Mesmerising effect 158
Metabolic activities 191, 194
Metabolic functions 36
Metabolic processes 65
Metabolism 252
Metabolism 50, 85
Metabolites 22
Metabolites 22
Metaphysical 238
Metaphysics 258
Methicillin resistant 3
Methodologies 81
Microbial toxins 230
Microscope 155, 202
Microscopic 86
Mid-stream urine 139
Migraines 97
Migration 33
Millennium 7
Millennium 7, 281
Mimic physical illness 267
Mind 254
Mind concentration 29
Mind concentration 29
Mind-body-spirit 91
Mineral compounds 131
Mineral substances 47
Mineral supplementation 209
Mineral water 71
Minor ailments 215
Minor ailments 304
Miracle cure power 190
Miraculous 66
Miscarriages 223
Misleading 308
Mmagic remedy 319
Mminor puncturing skin 313
Mockery 122
Mockery 299
Modalities 91
Modality of treatment 217
Modern human race 218
Modern medicine 12
Modern medicine 12, 233
Modern scientific world 119
Mohammad 149
Moisturisers 143
Molecular 39
Molecular robotic 256
Molecular structure 35
Molecule 52
Molecules 86
Monks 322
Mononucleosis 223
Monopoly of Medicine 312
Mood flying 260
Moola prakriti 291
Mooladhara chakra 287
Morarji Cola 222
Morarjin 222
Morbidity 234

Morbility and mortality 210
Morphine 316
Mortal 247
Mortal physical 249
Mortality 175, 234
Mortem 247
Mother of all creations 290
Motor 21
Motor 21
Msssulti-specialists 302
Mucins 50
Mucous membrane 21
Mucous membrane 21
Mucucolitis 222
Mud therapy 130
Mudras 25
Mudras 25
Mukti 294
Multi coloured bottles 241
Multi-cellular organism 19
Multi-cellular organism 19
Multi-drug resistant 245
Multi-drug resistant 316
Multi-drugs resist 204
Multifarious conditions 94
Multifarious diseases 133
Multiple complaints 80
Multiple micronutrients 209
Multiple-scleroses 11
Multiple-scleroses 11
Multi-therapy 91
Multivitamin supplementation 209
Muscle discomforts 217
Muscle fibers 20, 21
Muscle fibers 20, 21
Muscles 20
Muscles 20
Muscular System 20
Muscular System 20
Muscular tension 280
Musculature 253
Musty pungent 46
Mutable 282
Mycobacterium tuberculosis 211
Myriad of generations 237
Myriad of pharmaceutical drugs 215
Mysteriously 63
Mythological subjects 147
Mythyle glyoxal 194

N

Nadi 286
Nail 21
Nail 21
Narcotic 314
Narcotics 218
Narcotics 54
Nasal congestion 60
Nasal passages 167
National heritage 25
National heritage 25, 119
Natural agent 118
Natural diet 26
Natural diet 26
Natural drug 67
Natural elixir 39
Natural healing power 103
Natural Immunity system 205
Natural immunity system 233
Natural methods 315
Natural self-system 14
Natural self-system 14
Natural substances 13
Natural substances 13
Natural tendencies 221

Natural therapy 7, 12
Natural therapy 7, 12
Natural tonic 228
Natural urea 135
Natural vaccine 159, 192
Natural vaccine 65
Nature Cure 8
Nature Cure 8
Nature's elixir 26
Nature's elixir 26, 216
Nature-cure-treatment 157
Nature-friendly 103
Naturopathic manipulation 231
Naturopathic medicine 42
Naturopathic modalities 91
Naturopathic Urine Therapy 41
Naturopathy 226
Naturopathy 8
Naturopathy 8
Nausea 173
Nauseating 78
Neem tree stick 217
Neo-classical people 259
Neomedical science 251
Nephritis 222
Nephrons 23
Nephrons 23, 71
Nephropathy 208
Nerve 286
Nerve cells 21
Nerve cells 21
Nerve endings 21
Nerve endings 21
Nerve fibers 21
Nerve fibers 21
Nervous break-down 196
Nervous System 21
Nervous System 21
Nervous system 248
Neuro endocrine 260
Neuro-cognitive disorders 208
Neuro-endocrine 261
Neuro-endocrine system 261
Neurological 297
Neurological condition 167
Neurological system 260
Neuron 21
Neuron 21, 279
Neuropsychiatric disorders 210
Neurosis 21
Neurosis 21
Neurosis 260, 279
Neurotransitters 271
Neutrons 19
Neutrons 19
New 7
New 7
New entrants 8
New entrants 8
New Testament 31
New Testament 31
Nitro Glycerin 176
Nitrogen 130
Nitroglycerine 175
Nocturna 222
Nodules 185
Nomeostasis 272
Non-absorbable food 22
Non-absorbable food 22
Non-allopathic 81
Non-disclosure of material facts 308
Non-drug urine medicine 120
Non-self recognition 194
Non-steroidal 318

Non-tonic 132
Non-toxic therapies 95
Non-violence 258
Normalisation 90
Nose 21
Nose 21
Notoriously difficult 216
Nourished 49
Nuclei 19
Nuclei 19
Nucleus 19
Nucleus 19
Numb finger 312
Numbness 166
Numbness 33
Nutrient glucose 84
Nutrients 46
Nutritionally rich urine 209
Nutritious deficiency 211

O

Oath 300
Obesit 180
Obesity 222
Obscurity 26
Obscurity 26
Obstetrics 101
Occupational diseases 33
Occupational hazards 217
Occupational styles 302
Oculist 307
Oddball 12
Oddball 12
Odour 14
Odour 14
Odour a fishy 46
Oestrogen 176
Oestrogen 47
Oily scalp 182
Ointments and lotions 135
Old Testamen 31
Old Testamen 31
Old therapy 43
Older brain 260
Omnel 29
Omnel 29
Omnipotent 292
Omniscient 247
Opiates 218
Opiates 302
Opportunistic infections 54
Opportunistic diseases 13
Opportunistic diseases 13
Opportunistic infections 11, 204
Opportunistic infections 11, 98
Opthomologist 311
Optimal balance 92
Optimal health 42, 91, 97
Optimise health 131
Oral consumption 59
Orange urine 46
Orchitis 222
Organic chemicals 228
Organic chemicals 52
Organic molecules 46
Organic Molecules 52
Organism 259
Organism of the cosmos 259
Organs 20
Organs 20
Organs of the human body 319
Oriental Medicine 8
Oriental Medicine 8
Orthodox 189
Orthodox 245

Orthodox beliefs 14
Orthodox beliefs 14
Orthodox medical system 303
Orthodox tenets 147
Orthodox treatment 195
Osteoarthritis 23
Osteoarthritis 23
Osteology 23
Osteology 23
Osteopathy 130
Osteopathy 303
Osteoporosis 180
Out-perform placebo 306
Ovaries 24
Ovaries 24
Over prescription 122
Over the counter drugs antacids 306
Over the counter shops 218
Overcome the barriers 107
Over-the-counter pharmacy 302
Oxygen 22
Oxygen 22, 50
Oxygenated 23
Oxygenated blood 23
Oxygenated blood 23
P
Pacemakers 175
Paid medication 98
Pain killers 301
Pain relivers 313
Pain-aching 59
Painful death 187
Painkillers 117
Painkillers 302
Palate 22
Palate 22
Panacea 28, 221, 245
Panacea 28, 57
Panam 26
Panam 26
Pancreas 84
Pandemic 201, 207
Panic disorder 267
Paradigm 81, 96
Paradoxical surprise 30
Paradoxical surprise 30
Paramatmic 294
Paranormal medicinal practices 299
Parasites 257
Parasitic 225
Parotid gland 22
Parotid gland 22
Part of science 110
Pathies 64
Pathogens 226
Pathological examination 89
Pathological situations 192
Peer journal 305
Pelvic pain 223
Pemphigus 183
Penacea 40
Pencillin 122
Pencilliosis 204
Penicillin injection 61
Peptic ulcer 163
Perenium 292
Pergonal 12
Pergonal 12
Peripheral nervous 301
Peripheral Nervous System 21
Peripheral Nervous System 21
Personal doctor 131
Pesticides 230
Petalled lotus 287

Pharma ring 308
Pharmaceutical company 40
Pharmaceutical drugs 259, 281
Pharmalogical treatment 229
Pharynx 22
Pharynx 22
Phobia 217, 268
Phthalates 314
Phylotherapy 31
Phylotherapy 31
Physical body 253
Physical harm 79
Physical immortality 247, 248
Physical Injuries 155
Physical Kundalini 292
Physical stimulation 67
Physicians 300
Physico-etheric body 294
Physiological 11
physiological 11, 130
Physiological characteristics 68
Physiological functions 256
Physiology 286
Phytotherapy 95
Pigment 22
Pigment 22
Pigments 50
Pills 241
Pills strip 308
Pimples 183
Pineal gland 28
Pineal gland 28, 141
Pineal gland 301
Pineal hormone 141
Pingala nadi 288
Piss 39
Placebo 109
Placebo 255
Placebo capsules 304
Placebo drugs 306
Planet 258
Plants 31
Plants 31
Plasma ultra filtrate 76
Plenty of Prana 284
Plexus 286
Poisonous 315
Poisonous preventives 129
Poisonous substances 24
Poisonous substances 24
Polio 149
Polio 310
Political transformation 33
Pollen 163
Pollution 182
Polymyxins 316
Possible affection 55
Post industrial era 219
Potassium 180
Potassium ammonia 84
Power of Creator 237
Power of spirit 254
Practice 8
Practice 8
Prana 283
Prana Treats 283
Pranic energies 249
Pranic energy 283, 289
Pregnancy 177
Pregnancy tests 89
Premature death 249
Premature death 67
Premature old age 222
Prescription drugs 304

Prescription drugs 92
Prescriptive drugs 218
Present mental 260
Pretty 210
Pretty drugs 312
Prevention 229
Prevention 54
Prevention and cure 42
Prevention and curing 111
Preventive maintenance 13
Preventive maintenance13, 101, 108
Preventive medicine 63
Previews 9
Previews 9
Priceless way 54
Primary atom 291
Primary healthcare 26
Primary healthcare 26
Primary healthcare system 231
Primary origin of Life 291
Proactive drug 42
Profasi 12
Profasi 12
Profassi Injections 177
Progesterone 177
Projestrogen 47
Prolongation of life 285
Promoting optimal health 237
Propagators 9
Propagators 9, 99
Properties 110, 111
Prophet Muhammad 32
Prophet Muhammad 32
Prophylactic 177, 194
Prostaglandin 47
Prostaglandin 48
Prostitution 212
Proteins 50
Protocol 42
Protons 19
Protons 19
Proved curable with 218
Psoriasis 183, 222
Psychiatric 301
Psychiatric disorder 152
Psychiatric disorders 263
Psychic centres 289
Psychic energy 289
Psychic side effects 314
Psycho Disorders 263
Psychodrama 264
Psychological weakness 76
Psychological disorders 152
Psychologically 108
Psychologically prepare 108
Psychomatic disorders 264
Psychometric 264
Psycho-neuro-immunology 260
Psychos 263
Public experience 111
Public opinions 122
Pulling 217
Pulmonary disease 204
Pulmonary embolism 176
Pure memory 247
Pure memory 254
Pure spirit 248
Purification 247
Purified blood 86
Purified derivative 76
Purified internally 125
Purunas 25
Purunas 25
Pyrrhoea 222

Q

Quackery 123

R

Radiance Gods 126
Radiation therapy 187
Radioactive substances 187
Radio-active wastes 76
Radioactivity 230
Radium 243
Rajasic 288
Rapid diseases progression 206
Rasa sadhana 25
Rasa sadhana 25
Ravages 126
Re-absorption 84
Reactivation of cells 208
Realm of philosophy 210
Recovery stories 109
Rectum 62
Recurring hospitalisation 175
Recycling 75
Red blood 19
Red blood 19, 48
Red blood corpuscles 133
Re-drink 77
Redundant 233
Refill the system 227
Refilling 91
Refilling deficiency 205
Refilling deficient immunity 208
Refilling immunity system 207
Refilling power 79
Refills immunity system 217
Reflex system 260
Regenerative effect 142
Regenerative power 21
Regenerative power 21
Regimentation 101
Regimentation 190
Regression of tumors 190
Rejuvenate 30
Rejuvenate 30
Rejuvenation 245
Rejuvenation 69
Relaxation 251, 261
Relieve muscle spasm 217
Remodelled healthcare 281
Renaissance 117
Renal artery 85
Renal tubules 84
Repetitive visits 216
Reproduction system 179
Reproductive System 23
Reproductive System 23
Repugnance 78
Repugnancy 77
Repugnant medicine 188
Research laboratories 111
Resistance deficiency disorders 227
Resistance power 57
Respiratory ailments 163
Respiratory Congestion 11
Respiratory Congestion 11
Respiratory route 204
Respiratory System 22
Respiratory System 22
Respiratory track 253
Respiratory tract 22
Respiratory tract 22
Restoration 245
Restorative 29
Restorative 29
Retinene 194
Retrovirus 202

Rheumatoid arthritis 180
Ribs 23
Ribs 23
Rich vitamins 216
Ripe old age 33
Rishi 220
Rishies 252, 254
Rishies 283
Rituals 141
Robust self-repair 228
Root canal treatment 217
Root cause 53
Root cause of the disease 189, 257
Root causes 69
Root of beejam 287
Roots of divination 161
Roster-one 12
Roster-one 12
Roughness itches 183
Rubbing 107
Rudra rupa 288
S
Sack 36
Sagacious 141
Sagacious practitioners 29
Sagacious practitioners 29, 142, 283
Sahasrara 26
Sahasrara 26
Sahasrara chakra 288
Sahih Bukhari 149
Saktirupa 287
Saline solution 62
Saliva 37
Salivary gland 22
Salivary gland 22
Samadhi 29
Samadhi 29, 284, 295
Samina 66, 131
Sanitary 32
Sanskrit text 26
Sanskrit text 26
Sarcoma 207
Satkriya 25
Satkriya 25
Scalp 183
Scanty literature 9
Scanty literature 9
Scarce substance 191
Scars 183
Sceptics of urinopathic medicine 121
Sciatica 221
Science 12
Science 12
Science of Yoga 29
Science of Yoga 29
Scientific laboratories 33
Scientific literatures 119
Scientific studies 118
Scorpion 165
Sebaceous glands 21
Sebaceous glands 21
Sebum 22
Sebum 22
Secret power of treating 158
Secrets of body's 12
Secrets of body's 12
Sediments 139
Self-achievement 282
Self-cure 33
Self-delusion 256
Self-healing 11
Self-healing 11, 53
Self-healing power 42
Self-preservation 67

Self-realisation 252
Self-refilling mechanism 228
Self-therapy 7
Self-therapy 7
Self-therapy 8, 10, 12, 14
Self-therapy 8, 10, 12, 14
Semen 178
Semipermeable membrane 37
Senile 247
Senile degeneration 126
Sense-organs 20
Sense-organs 20
Sensitiveness 53
Sensory organ 22
Sensory organ 22
Sensory experience 259
Sensory organs 21
Sensory organs 21
Serious ailments 216
Serious mental illness 264
Serum 25
Serum 25, 39
Setting fracture 94
Sex hormones 47
Sexual debility 176
Sexual glands 48
Sexual organ 243
Sexual organs 20
Sexual organs 20
Sexual power 178
Shampoo 183
Shivambu 26
Shivambu 26
Shivambu 26, 29, 31
Shivambu 26, 29, 31, 41
Shivambu Kalpa 26, 28
Shivambu Kalpa 26, 28, 39
Shivambu Kalpa Vidhi 26
Shivambu Kalpa Vidhi 26
Shivambu rishi 222
Shortness of breath 173
Shrugs off stress 97
Side-effects 54
Single celled parasites 210
Single organism whole 297
Sinus 22
Sinus 22
Sinus disease 60
Sinuses 60
Skeletal system 130
Skeleton System 23
Skeleton System 23
Skimmed milk 78
Skin blemishes 172
Skin disorders 59
Skin infections 183
Skin puncture 94
Skin System 21
Skin System 21
Smoking 192
Sneezing 60
Sniffing 59
Soaked stockings 164
Social anxiety disorder 269
Social groups 28
Social groups 28
Social ostracism 212
Social stigma 212
Social well-being 235
Sodium 51
Solar system 20
Solar system 20
Solid waste 62, 86
Solubles 51

Somatic 21
Somatic 21
Sorcerer 158
Sore throat 164
Soul 252, 257
Specialised organs 191
Specific disease cure 157
Specific gravity 46
Specific health disorder 89
Specific medicine 68
Specific opportunistic infections 204
Specific Phobia 269
Sperm 178
Spices 72
Spinal card 253
Spinal cord 287
Spindle-shaped 20
Spindle-shaped 20
Spirit 257
Spirit linking 259
Spirit of the universe 28
Spirit of the universe 28
Spirit spectrum 259
Spiritual 25
Spiritual 25
Spiritual aspirants 29
Spiritual aspirants 29
Spiritual energy 29
Spiritual energy 29
Spiritual power 147
Spiritual powers 36
Spirituality 251
Spiritually 42
Sprinkle 59
Sri Gurumurthy 288
Stem cells 38
Sterile 184
Sterile watery 86
Sternum 23
Sternum 23
Steroid hormonal metabolism 38
Stigmatisation of people 212
Stimulate cell growth 208
Stimuli 272
Stimulus agent 67
Stimulus to stress 271
Stomoach 195
Strain 280
Strep throat 32
Strep throat 32
Stress 271
Strong holistic 132
Structure of a cell 20
Structure of a cell 20
Stupid behaviour 271
Substances filled 83
Subtle energy 127
Subtle lifeforce 250
Subtle workings 254
Sukshma prana 287
Sulpher 126
Sunni Islam 149
Sun-protection 171
Super-medical panacea 147
Supernatural 29
Supernatural 29, 111
Supernatural healing qualities 26
Supernatural healing qualities 26
Supernatural life 28
Supernatural life 28
Supernatural vision 248
Superstitious 189
Support 111
Suppressing 25

Suppressing 25, 69
Suppressing the symptoms 13
Suppressing the symptoms 13
Suppressive drugs 117, 123
Supreme fountain source 282
Supreme Super Personality 296
Sure-cure 245
Sure-cure 64
Surgery 193
Surgical 91
Surgical cotton 60
Surgical Effects 317
Surpressing symptoms 53
Surveillance system 205
Surya 288
Suryanamaskar 25
Suryanamaskar 25
Susceptibility 53
Sushumna 284
Sushumna' nadi 284
Suspicious water 208
Sustainable health 234
Swallowing 22
Swallowing 22
Swamootra 26
Swamootra 26
Swellings 217
Symptoms treatment 117
Synchronisation 316
Syndicalism 308
Syndrome 202
Synthesises 258
Synthetic drug 259
Synthetic drugs 301, 315
Synthetic pharamaceuticals 31
Synthetic pharamaceuticals 31
Synthetic substances 302
Syphilis 204
Syphilis 222
System 20
System 20
System 301

T

Tantric religious traditions 27
Tantric religious traditions 27
Tantrik yoga culture 27
Tantrik yoga culture 27
Tasty 78
Techno-centric approach 233
Technological 7
Technological 7
Tech-pharmacology 118
Temporary relief 317
Tendons 180
Tension 280
Tension and depression 175
Terminal arthritis 196
Terrible ailments 215
Testosterone 12
Testosterone 12, 178
Testosterone 177
Textual evidence 109
Theory 8
Theory 8
Therapeutic properties 14
Therapeutic properties 14
Therapeutic purposes 11
Therapeutic purposes 11
Therapeutic value 12
Therapeutic value 12, 76
Therapies 99
Therapies and pathies 223
Therapy 8
Therapy 8

Thermometer 293
Threatening 309
Thrimoorthies 293
Thrombosis 173
Thromobosis 195
Tinospora 31
Tinospora 31
Tiny tubes 86
Tiredness 271
Tissue organisms 21
Tissue organisms 21
Tissues 20
Tissues 20
Tissues 47
Tobacco 185
Tobacco 46
Toes 180
Tolerance 258
Tongue disorders 165
Tonic 40, 66
Tonsillitis 168
Toothaches 165
Torn 67
Torn out tissues 67
Tornado 219
Toxic bacteria 184
Toxic substance 73
Toxicity 24
Toxicity 24, 62
Toxicity-free 230
Toxicological studies 230
Trachea 22
Trachea 22
Tradition of medicine 92
Tradition of yoga 27
Tradition of yoga 27
Traditional empirical evidence 109
Traditional healthcare methods 215
Traditional medicine 25
Traditional medicine 25
Traditional uropaths 99
Tranquiliser 28
Tranquiliser 28
Tranquility 28, 141, 258
Tranquility 28, 92
Transformation 261
Transformative 29
Transformative 29
Transmissible 204
Transmutation 77
Transpierced 192, 194
Transpierced 75
Transplantation 304
Transumulation 193
Trauma 274
Treasury of lustre 125
Treatable human disease 130
Treatment modality is 147
Trembling of legs 166
Tribes 229
Trichotillomania 271
Trick working 295
Trinity 103
Trinity 251
Trinity of Hindu Gods 293
Trinity of the life 257
Triple Coated Kundalini 292
Triple energies 291
Triple nerves 287
Tropical diseases 46
Trouble and discomfort 152
Tuberculosis 125
Tuberculosis 165, 220
Tubules 84

Tumour 185
Turmoil 219
U
Ulcer 189
Ulcer complaints 163
Ulcerative colitis 223
Umani Avastha 288
Unblocking coronary arteries 175
Unclothed examination 103
Unconscionable 308
Under nutrition poor immunity 209
Unfathomable 321
Unit of life 291
Universal healthcare 309
Universal medicine 110, 131
Universally accepted 151
Unknown medicine 219
Unorthodox 245
Unparalleled mystic powers 248
Unpleasant 105
Unpleasant feeling 164
Unpleasant drinking 242
Unrelenting pain 215
Unsoluble substance 192
Uraina tribe 149
Urbanisation 7
Urbanisation 7, 33
Urea 52
Urea substance 73
Ureters 23
Ureters 23
Urethra 23
Urethra 23
Urethra 23
Urethra 23
Uric acid 180
Uric acid 52
Urinals 23
Urinals 23
Urinalysis 75, 89
Urinary bladder 23
Urinary bladder 23
Urinary ketone 89
Urinary ketone bodies 90
Urination 23
Urination 23
Urination 39
Urine 52
Urine bladder 87
Urine bladder. 31
Urine bladder. 31
Urine density 46
Urine ingredients 170
Urine pack 60
Urine therapy 11, 17
Urine therapy 11, 17
Urine Therapy 24
Urine Therapy 24
Urine therapy 8, 13
Urine therapy 8, 13
Urine track infections 301
Urine urea 191
Urine-herb 31
Urine-herb 31
Urinetherapy 10
Urinetherapy 10
Urine-therapy 9
Urine-therapy 9
Urinopathic application 9
Urinopathic application 9
Urinopathic medicine 8, 9, 11, 25
Urinopathic medicine 8, 9, 11, 25
Urinopathy 8, 14
Urinopathy 8, 14

Urinotherapy 11, 14
Urinotherapy 11, 14, 41
Urogastrone 163
Urokinase 12
Urokinase 12
Urokinase 48
Urology 41
Uropathy 41
Urotherapists 13
Urotherapists 13
Urotherapy 12
Urotherapy 12
Urotherapy 41
Uterine cavity 38
Uterus 195
Uterus 48
V
Vaccine 64, 65, 130
Vajra nadi 288
Valuable drug 11
Valuable drug 11
Valuable hormones 77
Valuable moisturiser 171
Vaporated milk 78
Vasodilatation 175
VDS 11
VDS 11
Vedas 25
Vedas 25
Veins 23
Veins 23, 173
Venereal 204
Venereal diseases 155
Venous blood 213
Verifying its propensity 121
Vertebral column 85
Vigour 248
Vigour 50, 65
Violent reactions 187
Viral infections 225
Virucidal effects 193
Virus 202
Visceral 21
Visceral 21
Visualisation 28, 29
Visualisation 28, 29
Vital energy 127
Vital energy 287
Vital force 54, 92
Vital matrix 258
Vital power 25
Vital power 25
Vital substances 74
Vital tissue 221
Vitality 12, 248
Vitality 12, 50
Vitality 318
Vitamins 182
Vitamins 49
Vortex 289
W
Water of Life 208
Water of Life 219
Water of Life Foundation 238
Water of Lord Shiv 26
Water of Lord Shiv 26
Watery solution 71
Web 259
Wellness enhancement 210
Whirlpool 289
White blood 19
White blood 19
Whooping cough 163
Wide array of ailments 159

Will of action 292
Will power 247, 292
Womb 35
Womb 35
Wonder 67
World wide epidemic 96
Worry 271
Worry 280
Wrapped 164
Wrinkled 105
Wrinkles 126
Wrinkles 183
Wrong counselling 304
Y
Yellow amber 45
Yellow Fountain 15
Yellow Fountain 15
Yoga 25, 28
Yoga 25, 28, 281, 283
Yoga texts 25
Yoga texts 25
Yoganadis 287
Yogic life 29
Yogic life 29
Yogic practice. 29
Yogic practice. 29
Yogic religion 28
Yogic religion 28, 141
Yogic tradition 27
Yogic tradition 27
Yogis 12, 14, 26, 28
Yogis 12, 14, 26, 28
Yogis 28
Yogis 28
Yuga 13
Yuga 13
Yugas 29
Yugas 29, 281
Z
ZSSiconotide 317